Work

and the

Health of Women

Author

Vilma R. Hunt
College of Human Development
The Pennsylvania State University
University Park, Pennsylvania

With Special Assistance From:

Kathleen Lucas-Wallace, J.D.
Labor Lawyer
San Francisco, California

Jeanne M. Manson, Ph.D.
Kettering Laboratory
University of Cincinnati
Cincinnati, Ohio

CRC Press, Inc.
Boca Raton, Florida

Library of Congress Cataloging in Publication Data

Main entry under title:

Work and the health of women

Bibliography: p.
Includes index.
1. Women—Diseases. 2. Work—Physiological aspects.
3. Women—Health and hygiene. 4. Occupational
diseases. 5. Women—Employment. I. Title.
RC963.6.W65H86   613.6'2   78-26039
ISBN 0-8493-5301-7

© 1979 by CRC Press, Inc.
Second Printing, 1982

International Standard Book Number 0-8493-5301-7

Library of Congress Card Number 78-26039
Printed in the United States

PREFACE

The impetus for writing *Work and the Health of Women* resulted from a concentrated interest which developed among women themselves. At the 1974 annual meeting of the Women's Equity Action League (WEAL) a resolution was passed calling for more attention to the occupational health of women workers and was directed to the secretaries of the U.S. Department of Health, Education, and Welfare and Labor. The American Association for the Advancement of Science annual meeting in 1975 included a panel on the subject, sponsored by its affiliate group, Graduate Women in Science. The Coalition of Labor Union Women at its formation in 1975 included the occupational health of women as an important part of its purpose. Since then, workers both men and women (most particularly those in unions), have asked questions of the medical and legal professions, industrial hygienists, the academic community and management. And they have questioned many of the answers.

We hope this book will be a resource for those who are responsible for providing answers and influencing the quality of our work environment.

We would like to acknowledge the contribution of Margaret M. Quinn to the section on the jewelery industry in the chapter on The Chemical Environment. The information is derived from an undergraduate investigative project by Brown University students. Richard M. Gioscia prepared the information for the effects of sound on the reproductive system in the chapter on The Physical Environment, when he was a graduate student at the Pennsylvania State University. Ruth Simon, research assistant at the Kettering Laboratory, Cincinnati, Ohio, assisted Jeanne M. Manson in the preparation of the Chapter, Influence of Environmental Agents on Male Reproductive Failure.

Particular appreciation goes to the many students, who over the years, shared and encouraged our concern for occupational health. They can scarcely realize the importance of their interest and support.

Vilma R. Hunt
Jeanne M. Manson
Kathleen Lucas-Wallace

THE AUTHORS

Vilma R. Hunt is Associate Professor of Environmental Health, College of Human Development at the Pennsylvania State University, University Park.

Ms. Hunt received her B.D.S. degree in dental surgery in 1950 from the University of Sydney, Australia, and her A.M. in physical anthropology from Radcliffe College, Harvard University. She was among the first group of scholars at the Radcliffe Institute for Independent Study when it was established in 1961 and became a Research Associate in Physiology at the Harvard School of Public Health. She was Assistant Professor of Environmental Health at Yale University School of Medicine and Research Associate at the John B. Pierce Foundation.

Ms. Hunt is a member of the Health Physics Society, the Radiation Research Society and the American Public Health Association.

Her research has resulted in publications on naturally occurring alpha emitting isotopes, lung function, infant mortality, occupational hazards for pregnant women and risk assessment in occupational and environmental health.

Kathleen Lucas-Wallace is a practicing Labor Lawyer in San Francisco, California. She earned her Juris Doctor from George Washington University, Washington, D.C. in 1974.

Ms. Lucas-Wallace also earned her M.A.T. in 1968 at Oklahoma City University and her B.A. from Manhattanville College, Purchase, New York in 1967.

Jeanne M. Manson is Assistant Professor of Environmental Health at the University of Cincinnati School of Medicine. She received her Ph.D. from Ohio State University, Columbus, and her B.A. degree from Emmanuel College, Boston.

To all the young women and men who will follow in
Alice Hamilton's footsteps.

TABLE OF CONTENTS

Chapter 1

THE DEMOGRAPHY OF WOMEN WORKERS

I. INTRODUCTION

Between March 1971 and March 1975 the number of women working or looking for work in the U.S. increased by about 4.8 million. The comment has been made that such rapid growth "has taken most analysts and policymakers by surprise".[1] The surprise may have been due in part to the general view that women were part of a shadow work force. The actual increase in labor force participation of women was 2.75 million, of which 800,000 or 29% could be accounted for by more young women entering the work force than in previous years. Most of the increase occurred among women under 35, particularly married women with children under 6 years of age. There is no simple explanation for these marked changes in work participation patterns over a period of less than 10 years. The social impact however has had the effect of identifying the woman worker as an integral part of the labor force, despite the fact that she has always been there.

An extensive literature in the 19th and early 20th century describes the conditions of work for women in Europe and the U.S.[2] It is not so long ago that women and children were the beasts of burden, harnessed to the coal carts they dragged through the underground mines of Europe and Britain (illustrated in the First Report of the Children's Employment Commission, London, 1842). Charles Dickens described graphically the work of women in the lead mills of East London in 1869 and noted that "they bear the work much better than men: some few of them have been at it for years. . . Even so, he was compelled to quote his Irish informant twice in *The Uncommercial Traveller*. She was a captive of London's slums and described a "poor craythur" in her care.

The lead, sur. Sure 'tis the lead-mills, where the women gets took on at eighteen pence a day, sur, when they makes application early enough, and is lucky and wanted: and 'tis lead-pisoned she is, sur, and some of them gets lead-pisoned soon, and some of them gets lead-pisoned later, and some but not many, niver; and 'tis all according to the constitooshun, sur, and some constitooshuns is strong, and some is week; and her constitooshun is lead-pisoned, bad as can be, sur; and her brain is coming out at her ear, and it hurts her dreadful; and that's what it is and niver no more, and niver no less, sur.[3]

The inevitability of sooner or later and for "some but not many, niver" was vividly impressed on Dicken's perception of the lead mills before and after he visited them, but there is little to indicate that he saw much difference between the men and women in their mutual struggle to survive at whatever job they could get in mid-19th century London.

Fifty years later in the U.S. Elizabeth B. Butler's *Women and the Trades, Pittsburgh, 1903—1908,* also left little to the imagination. Stogy and garment factories, foundries, textile mills, and laundries produced anger and energy enough in women to try to improve their sweat shop conditions.

Butler described the work conditions and the women who were forced to tolerate them as the industrial revolution gained momentum. They were immigrant women, working in sweat shops worse than those they had left behind in Tsarist Russia and Victorian Ireland, and the native-born who were moving from an agrarian society into a fast-growing industrial holocaust of exhaustion, disease, and filth. The class differences between the women who worked and the women who spent were most blatant early in the century, yet strength and leadership came from both classes of women —

the working class and the privileged. Social legislation resulted in maternal and child health programs, the trade union movement became more responsive to the needs of women members (though more so in some unions than in others), and the worst excesses of exploitation of workers were moderated.

II. WORKING WOMEN IN THE 20TH CENTURY

The number of women in gainful employment in the U.S. increased from 4,005,532 in 1890 to 10,752,116 in 1930. The increase was from 17.4 to 22% of all women 10 years of age and over. Of all women wage earners in 1890, 13.9% were married, but in 1930, 28.9% were married. The Women's Bureau in reporting these statistics in 1934 noted:[5] "With the data available it is impossible to estimate the number of women who are exposed to occupational conditions in various ways detrimental to health. The inadequacy of data on which to base programs of control is significant."

The Women's Bureau together with the Children's Bureau of the Department of Labor had been the voice of conscience during the first quarter of the century. Maternal and infant mortality rates were excessive and extensive epidemiologic studies were published by both bureaus. The eight studies of U.S. cities published from 1915 into the 1920s by the Children's Bureau were in large measure designed to examine the effect of mothers' employment on infant mortality. Two communities, New Bedford, Mass.[6] and Manchester, N.H., were textile mill towns with a high proportion of mothers working before and after their confinement. The infant mortality rate in New Bedford in 1913 for women "gainfully employed" prior to birth was 154.5 as contrasted with a rate of 108.8 for infants of mothers not employed. The frequent association of poverty of the family and return to work soon after giving birth contributed to the high rate for the working group. In Manchester, N.H. in 1914[7] the infant mortality rate for babies whose mothers had been gainfully employed was 199.2 and 133.9 for those whose mothers were not. When the "gainfully employed" were broken down to those who worked away from home the infant mortality rate was 227.5, and for those who worked at home it was 149.8. These two communities showed the most extreme conditions of harsh employment for women combined with poverty. Education and welfare programs of the state and federal government in the following years reflected the national concern.

Alice Hamilton advised the Women's Bureau on the industrial substances known to endanger pregnancy: lead, carbon monoxide, tobacco, benzene, carbon disulfide, and nitrobenzene (the latter a popular abortifacient in Europe!). In the textile industry the general health of women operatives was reported to be far below that of men. Warnings came from the New York Department of Labor[8] that there could be increased susceptibility to poisoning during pregnancy, for example from benzol.

"The unassailable point on which special protection for women rests is that fact of maternity. Not only is the health of future citizens endangered by exposure to industrial hazards, but the combined action of occupational influences and the strain of pregnancy constitute considerable danger for women. Pregnant women are more easily fatigued by the monotony of unskilled machine operations, and fatigue lowers their resistance to intoxications."

"In connection with the effect on children of poisoning of mothers, lead has been proven to be a specific cause of stillbirths, abortions and sterility. It has been found that poisons are eliminated from the body to some extent and that one path for the elimination of poisons including lead, arsenic and mercury is the lacteal secretion. This should be remembered when women who are breast feeding are employed on work which involves risk of such poisoning."

Despite these obvious adversities for the working woman, the economic necessity of continued employment maintained the high proportion of women, both immigrant and native born, in the work force. The Women's Bureau continued to point out through the decades that women worked because they *had* to work and that their health and safety had to be protected.

The Public Health Service also included the woman worker in industry-wide studies. Menstrual and reproductive histories were included in these analyses. A detailed reference manual was prepared for conducting industrial hygiene surveys and pregnancy was included as a diagnosis appropriate for statistical analysis.[9] The objective was to analyze the health of the worker in terms of pregnancy rate, disability rate, severity rate, fatality rate, and mortality rate specific for age, sex, color, department, and occupation. Presumably the wartime conditions of the 1940s precluded full development of these survey plans which were not implemented.

When World War II increased the number of women in the work force the Women's Bureau continued to publish pamphlets to inform women of safety precautions, etc. One example is a special bulletin published in 1944, "The Industrial Nurse and the Woman Worker"[10] which with modifications could be useful today. A Maternal Policy in Industry is reviewed

The problem appears to be of some moment to employers at this time for several reasons. The majority of working women are in the child-bearing years, and the inexperience of some employers with women workers causes them a bit of panic in the face of possibilities that they scarcely know how to handle. It is the usual practice in plants not to hire women who are known to be pregnant; and it is almost equally common to discharge them as soon as pregnancy is discovered. Such a policy, however, encourages women to conceal their pregnancy as long as possible. Under such circumstances a woman may continue to work at a job or in a place that offers considerable hazard to her health and safety. Moreover, the first three months of pregnancy, which are the most easily concealed, are also more precarious than the next three months. At this early date, then, women particularly need protection; but unless there is a policy in the plant that will encourage them to report their condition, they cannot avail themselves of protection. The plant also will profit from knowledge of the women's condition by assuring itself that women will be kept on suitable jobs and thus experienced workers will not be lost, and by being protected against the risk of accident among women doing heavy or hazardous work at a time when they are not fitted to do it.

The points to be considered for such a maternity policy are: the importance of judging each case individually; the time at which a woman should stop work before the birth of her child, and how soon afterward she may return to work; the types of jobs that should be avoided because of danger of physical strain or injury from toxic substances; the preservation of seniority rights, the opportunity to return to her job, the length of hours and rest periods, and other conditions of work.

There has been little added in the 30 years since those words were written. The Women's Bureau turned away from its concern for health conditions in the years following the war, when presumably most women returned to the kitchen — or so it was believed. Their emphasis was directed to economic and legal issues, and for the most part the woman worker has not had a health advocate for over a quarter of a century.

III. SOME DEMOGRAPHIC CHARACTERISTICS OF THE FEMALE WORK FORCE

The total number of women in the work force increased 18% during the decade 1960 to 1970 to a total of 33.3 million.[11] The 20 occupations employing the largest number of women in the U.S. comprised 53% of the total female work force in 1970, an increase from 47% in 1960.[12] Occupations which could be considered the most hazardous in this group are shown in Table 1.

Generally, it appears that there has been an increase in the number of women entering the more dangerous of the 20 largest occupations, the comparison being with teaching, secretarial, and telephone operators.

Projections for the rest of the century show that the number of women in the labor force will continue to increase. Table 2 provides a detailed breakdown of the number

TABLE 1[11,12]

Leading Female Occupations with Known Hazards

	Number of Women in the U.S.		
	1970	1960	Increase (%)
Sewers and stitchers	812,716	534,258	34
Registered nurses	807,359	567,884	30
Nursing aides, orderlies, etc.	609,022	485,383	20
Assemblers	454,611	270,769	40
Hairdressers and cosmetologists	424,873	267,050	37
Checkers, examiners, inspectors (manufacturing)	327,530	215,066	34
Packers and wrappers	314,067	262,935	16

of women in particular industries in 1970, Table 3 shows the age of employed women by detailed occupation in 1970, and Table 4 shows the percentage distribution of women 16 years and over for the major occupational groups in 1974.[13-16]

Department of Labor statistics on occupational mobility have been developed primarily for purposes of identifying common skills and other shared characteristics within groups of occupations.[17] An important finding has been the extremely large volume of occupational movement among workers. The likelihood of consistent exposure to the same occupational conditions therefore varies, with some occupations maintaining a higher proportion of single occupation workers than others. Men generally have higher proportions of transfers than do women of the same age. Opportunities are far less for women in terms of earning power (a transfer incentive for men) and alternative occupations. When major occupation groups were compared for the changes occurring from 1965 to 1970 the transfer rate for men ranged from 43.6% for nonfarm laborers to 17.7% for farmers and farm managers. The range for women was much smaller, from 36.0% for nonfarm laborers to 17.2% for professionals. Greater variations can be seen in the detailed occupations shown in Table 5. Lowest transfer rates were for professionals, private household workers, service workers, and operatives. The highest were for nonfarm laborers, farmers, transport operatives, and managers. However, men have considerably lower separation rates than women in all categories and at all ages. The high proportion of women who experience job separation during their work lives provides a discontinuity which may be of some advantage for their future health status, in contrast to the economic disadvantages which also have long-term impact on seniority and retirement income. The particular characteristics of each occupation shown in Table 5, nonemployment, death, and transfer are affected differentially by factors within each category of occupation — education level, technical skill, and the age distribution in the occupation. Fluctuations in the economy had a differential impact on women and men in the same occupations and there are only rare examples where a higher proportion of women has remained in the same occupations when compared with men, examples being bus driving and some of the female intensive occupations such as sewing and cleaning service workers.

IV. OCCUPATIONAL SAFETY AND HEALTH

In the Occupational Safety and Health Act of 1970 (PL 91-596) Section 2(b) the Congress "declared it is to be its purpose and policy to assure so far as possible every

TABLE 2[12]

Occupations by Industry: Number of Women — 1970

	No. of women
Health Industry	
Registered nurses	807,359
Nursing aides, attendants, orderlies	609,022
Clinical laboratory technicians	84,641
Radiologic technicians	35,463
Health technicians (NEC)[a]	33,525
Physicians	25,824
Dental hygienists	14,863
Dentists	3,110
Chiropractors	1,127
Engineering and science technology	
Agriculture and biological — technicians (excluding health)	10,060
Chemical — technicians	9,034
Electrical, industrial, mechanical	11,515
Draftsmen	22,257
Surveyors	1,690
NEC[a]	33,189
Agricultural scientists	1,011
Biological scientists	10,254
Chemists	12,887
Physicists and astronomers	866
Manufacturing	
Durable goods	
Electrical machinery, equipment, supplies	107,332
Radio, TV and communication equipment	29,907
Electrical machinery, equipment	71,903
Nondurable goods	
Paper allied products	40,092
Chemicals and allied industries	23,800
Rubber and miscellaneous plastic products	53,875
Rubber products	17,853
Miscellaneous plastic products	36,022
Footwear, except rubber	13,434
Operatives, except transport	
Assemblers	459,134
Checkers, examiners, inspectors	332,668
Clothing, ironers, and pressers	136,772
Cutting operatives	44,079
Laundry and dry cleaning	105,146
Meat cutters and butchers	28,724
Meat wrappers — retail	42,340
Metalworking	152,407
Packers and wrappers (not meat or produce)	313,356
Sewers and stitchers	816,441
Shoemaking machine operatives	37,228
Textile operatives	232,985
Miscellaneous	
School teachers	1,934,798
Secretarial	5,396,061
Sales — retail and cashiers	2,160,168
Waitresses, cleaners, cooks	2,075,129
Telephone operators	384,543

[a] Not elsewhere classified.

TABLE 3

Age of Employed Persons by Detailed Occupation: 1970[13]

Females	16 and 17 years	18 and 19 years	20 to 24 years	25 to 29 years	30 to 34 years
Printing craftsmen	689	2,671	7,799	6,411	5,651
Upholsterers	70	208	943	901	1,041
Assemblers	2,909	18,673	65,421	50,854	45,942
Checkers, examiners, and inspectors manufacturing	1,560	8,956	32,760	29,820	30,281
Clothing ironers and pressers	1,286	3,475	10,286	10,516	12,453
Cutting operatives, NEC[a]	502	1,394	5,082	3,938	4,628
Laundry and drycleaning operatives, NEC[a]	2,698	3,832	7,682	6,545	7,761
Meat cutters and butchers, except manufacturing	187	649	878	906	1,294
Meat cutters and butchers, manufacturing	200	646	2,088	2,133	1,580
Meat wrappers retail trade	918	1,513	3,295	3,637	4,679
Metalworking operatives, except precision machine	827	4,926	17,698	17,410	16,187
Packers and wrappers, except meat and produce	6,657	13,931	34,051	29,134	29,192
Sewers and stitchers	6,466	28,213	88,188	80,992	74,050
Shoemaking machine operatives	597	1,760	4,675	3,674	2,846
Textile operatives	1,921	8,228	28,411	23,905	23,913
Miscellaneous and not specified operatives — occupation	7,941	28,680	88,777	73,976	70,265
Miscellaneous and not specified operatives — industry					
Manufacturing	5,686	23,464	77,550	66,537	62,535
Durable goods	2,031	11,091	39,773	34,449	31,952
Machinery, except electrical	43	652	2,602	2,491	2,575
Electrical machinery equipment and supplies	668	4,431	15,491	13,348	11,314
Radio, TV, and communication equipment	193	1,492	4,652	4,217	3,415
Electrical machinery, equipment and supplies, NEC[a]	312	2,444	8,598	7,724	6,546
Nondurable goods	3,632	12,080	36,734	31,531	29,918
Apparel and other fabricated textile products	1,044	2,899	7,345	6,376	6,096
Paper and allied products	184	1,052	4,918	3,555	3,948
Chemicals and allied products	172	662	2,906	2,545	2,264
Rubber products	69	584	2,053	1,958	1,628
Miscellaneous plastic products	270	1,798	4,934	4,230	4,195

TABLE 3 (continued)

Age of Employed Persons by Detailed Occupation: 1970[13]

Females	16 and 17 years	18 and 19 years	20 to 24 years	25 to 29 years	30 to 34 years
Footwear, except rubber	160	666	1,826	1,521	1,043
Secretaries	22,657	157,033	611,920	339,358	240,712
Typists	26,383	113,863	235,898	92,029	69,071
Miscellaneous clerical workers	22,704	70,046	170,443	83,624	69,906
Office machine operators	3,623	35,850	113,964	61,128	43,428
Waiters	106,439	92,483	127,071	91,024	83,505
Airline stewardesses	26	332	19,640	8,735	1,925
Hairdressers and Cosmetologists	3,822	22,957	108,644	57,069	34,488
Health service workers	31,542	72,320	178,810	101,552	89,796
Dental assistants	4,615	11,540	24,826	9,697	6,378
Health aides, except nursing	5,274	7,007	19,211	10,053	8,063
Health trainees	276	5,110	9,412	718	473
Nursing aides, orderlies	20,884	43,641	88,786	55,736	54,567
Practical nurses	472	5,022	36,535	25,220	20,243
Registered nurses	792	5,263	116,283	107,825	89,766
Health technologists and technicians	873	6,975	52,452	33,651	19,173
Clinical laboratory	380	2,420	23,629	16,830	16,830
Dental hygienists	44	62	5,085	3,636	1,568
Radiologic technologists and technicians	99	2,397	13,402	6,427	3,530
Health technologists and technicians	292	1,751	8,565	5,554	3,303
Agriculture and biological technicians	82	349	2,104	1,122	1,084
Chemical technicians	58	330	2,302	987	749

Note: U.S. Census of Population 1970. Occupational Characteristics - PC(2) - 7A Dept. of Commerce. (1973)

a Not elsewhere classified.

TABLE 4

Major Occupation Group of All Women 16 Years Old and Over[14-16] March 1974 (in thousands)

		16—19	20—24	25—34	35—44	45—54
Total women 16 years and over	78,108					
Employed	33,200	3,329	5,281	7,331	6,057	6,438
Percent	100.0	100.0	100.0	100.0	100.0	100.0
White collar workers	62.0	52.0	68.4	67.1	61.5	60.2
Professional, technical, and kindred workers	15.5	2.4	15.4	22.7	16.1	13.2
Managers, administrators, except farm	4.9	.6	2.6	4.3	5.7	6.9
Sales workers	6.7	11.4	5.6	4.6	6.1	6.9
Clerical and kindred workers	34.9	37.6	44.8	35.5	33.6	33.2
Blue collar workers	15.5	11.7	13.1	15.2	17.8	17.6
Craft and kindred workers	1.7	.9	1.2	1.6	1.8	1.7
Operatives, including transport	12.9	8.8	10.8	12.7	14.9	15.0
Laborers, excluding farm	0.9	2.0	1.1	.9	1.0	.9
Farm workers	1.3	1.7	.7	1.0	1.6	1.8
Laborers and farm managers	0.3	—	.1			
Farm laborers and supervisors	1.0	1.7	.6			
Service workers	21.2	34.6	17.8	16.8	19.2	20.4

working man and woman in the nation safe and healthful working conditions and to preserve our human resources."[18]

Thirteen statements outline how Congress intended the purpose to be achieved. Four of these are particularly pertinent to our concern for the health and safety of women workers:

·   By encouraging employers and employees in their efforts to reduce the number of occupational safety and health hazards at their places of employment, and to stimulate employers and employees to institute new and to perfect existing programs for providing safe and healthful working conditions;
·   By providing that employers and employees have separate but dependent responsibilities and rights with respect to achieving safe and healthful working conditions. . .
·   By providing for research in the field of occupational safety and health, including the psychological factors involved, and by developing innovative methods, techniques, and approaches for dealing with occupational safety and health problems;
·   By exploring ways to discover latent diseases, establishing causal connections between diseases and work in environmental conditions, and conducting other research relating to health problems, in recognition of the fact that occupational health standards present problems often different from those involved in occupational safety.

An important link in the successful implementation of the Occupational Safety and Health Act (OSHA) is the involvement of workers who are aware of and informed about hazards in the work place.[19] The right to know includes an understanding of the hazard potential of dangerous substances and working conditions in addition to being informed about and trained in safe work practices.

Unfortunately, the progress to a uniformly high quality of enforcement of OSHA has been slow indeed. For some time to come, we can expect that workers and their representatives will have to demand labeling of dangerous substances and posting of appropriate information to ensure safe working conditions. Men and women must be able to make an evaluation of the work environment in terms of any potential hazard should they plan to procreate. OSHA defines the right to safe and healthful work conditions. The Undersecretary of Labor, Eula Bingham, has stated that workers also have a right to procreate healthy children.[20]

TABLE 5

Percent Distribution by 1970 Status of Women Employed in 1965 by Occupation in 1965[17]

	Occupation in 1965			
		Status in 1970		
	Not in the labor force	Dead	Transferred to different occupation	Employed in same occupation
All occupations	26.04	3.95	25.56	42.12
Professional, technical and kindred workers	22.87	3.87	8.16	63.97
Librarians	20.50	5.15	16.38	57.01
Physicians	—	4.76	—	66.63
Registered nurses	22.15	3.82	11.15	61.82
Dieticians	20.43	4.80	17.39	56.17
Therapists	26.37	2.72	—	56.65
Clinical laboratory	24.70	1.94	13.92	58.65
Dental hygienists	—	1.89	—	63.43
Radiologic Technologists	29.20	1.61	—	56.70
Other health technologists	—	2.11	22.85	50.66
Teachers	23.67	4.16	9.04	62.33
Managers and administrators	21.70	5.83	22.41	48.57
Salesworkers	28.49	4.86	23.08	41.49
Clerical and kindred workers	26.63	3.06	8.36	60.21
Craft and kindred workers	20.92	4.52	20.95	50.85
Printing craft workers	23.18	3.53	21.40	48.85
Operatives, except transport	24.45	3.84	10.46	56.71
Assemblers	23.99	2.76	21.84	46.38
Bottling and canning	35.48	—	—	28.87
Semiskilled packing and inspecting workers[a]	25.88	3.45	16.60	49.63
Clothing ironers and pressers	24.48	4.41	18.40	48.97
Laundry and dry cleaning	26.66	5.37	26.04	39.22
Punch and stamping press	22.89	3.22	20.16	48.54
Solderers	24.46	2.78	24.31	41.95
Sewers and stitchers	23.86	4.22	13.27	53.98
Shoemaking machine	23.81	3.83	27.13	40.27
Textile operatives	19.92	3.51	19.38	53.05
Transport equipment operatives	16.49	3.23	24.47	53.69
Laborers, except farm	25.49	3.74	33.91	33.12
Farmers and farm managers	30.37	7.71	28.89	31.81
Farm laborers and supervisors	45.58	4.03	22.05	23.77
Service workers, except private household	28.52	4.15	15.01	49.84
Cleaning service workers	25.63	6.36	18.34	47.03
Food service workers	30.84	3.82	20.92	41.10
Health service workers	26.22	3.58	17.55	50.61
Flight attendants	—	0.63	—	38.41
Hairdressers and cosmetologists	26.11	2.89	10.40	59.21
Private household workers	27.49	8.04	13.61	48.54

Note: Absence of data denotes standard error greater than 10%.

[a] Includes checkers, examiners, inspectors, graders, and sorters in manufacturing, meat wrappers in retail trade, other packers and wrappers.

V. OCCUPATIONAL HEALTH AND PROTECTION

The concept of protection of women workers began to appear at the end of the 19th century in industrialized countries with the extenson of laws and orders concerning the employment of women and children. In 1919, the International Labour Conference compiled international comparisons of protective legislation which were intended to prevent excessive toxic exposure of women and children to lead, mercury, phosphorus, and arsenic.[21] In the U.S., Connecticut, Massachusetts, New York, and Vermont had mandatory pregnancy leave ranging from 4 to 8 weeks before and after delivery. In contrast to some other countries, there was no right to reinstatement after absence and no requirement to provide facilities for nursing mothers.

Even prior to the enforcement of Title VII of the Civil Rights Act (1972) the concept of "protection" in relation to pregnancy was not commonly accepted or practiced throughout the jurisdictions of the U.S. Under the legislation designated "protective" only two states and Puerto Rico provided maternity benefits and only Puerto Rico had some provision for job security during absence for childbirth. Six states and Puerto Rico prohibited employment for periods before and after childbirth. (See Chapter 8 for further discussion of legal aspects).

Consideration of paternal protection has been rare. Some countries, e.g., New Zealand and Japan, have calculated the procreation profile of their radiation work force, but there is no evidence that protection of a particular group of men has been seriously recommended.[22]

Overall, we do not know the full range of possible effects of hazardous agents on reproduction, whether it is the male worker being exposed or the female worker.

The long-term neglect of women workers in research studies of occupational health has been examined in relation to the difficulty which now confronts us in obtaining good epidemiologic information. It is not presently possible to identify an adequate data base to establish whether women are more or less vulnerable than men to work hazards. It seems unlikely that there would be biological equality, but from a practical point of view it may be that the concept of differential vulnerability is specious for optimal formulation of social policy.

The crude death rate for the total U.S. population in 1975 was 8.9 deaths per thousand population, which was the lowest ever recorded.[23] There has been a relatively stable rate of about 9.4 for the past 25 years, and before the introduction of antibiotics the overall death rate had been about 11. The lower rate for 1975, a 3.3% decline since 1974, may be a short-term fluctuation, though the reduction appeared in all age groups. However, the ratio of the age-adjusted death rate for males to females has remained constant from 1973 to 1975 at 1.8. This high ratio is eventually seen as a 7.8-year differential in life expectancy, 68.7 years for men and 76.5 for women. Throughout the entire human life span for the period up to 1 year, from 1 to 4 years, 5 to 9 years, or any 5-year increment to 85 years and over, the male death rate exceeds that for females. A generalization believed by many is that the life expectancy differential between men and women is largely attributable to the stress of the work experience on men, one rationale for the protective legislation in force before the Civil Rights Act. The age-adjusted female death rate and sex mortality ratio for the leading causes of death are shown in Table 6. Except for diabetes mellitus, the only condition with a female to male rate ratio more than one, all the other conditions listed could be associated directly or indirectly with conditions of work. There is little possibility that the effects of occupational hazards alone could be sufficient to explain the very low sex ratios which have declined even further since 1952. A more systematic evaluation of work experience could conceivably show that men are more vulnerable to work stresses, as they appear to be for many other physiological and psychological stresses,

TABLE 6

Age-adjusted Female Death Rate and Sex Mortality Ratio
for Leading Causes of Death, U.S. 1952 and 1973[23]

Cause of death	1973	1952
All causes		
Female age-adjusted rate	513.1	658.9
Age-adjusted sex ratio[a]	0.56	0.67
Diseases of the heart	167.4	225.6
Sex ratio	0.49	0.60
Malignant neoplasms	108.7	118.8
Sex ratio	0.68	0.89
Cerebrovascular diseases	58.4	84.6
Sex ratio	0.83	0.93
Accidents	27.4	32.0
Sex ratio	0.35	0.37
Influenza and pneumonia	15.2	19.7
Sex ratio	0.57	0.69
Certain causes of mortality in early infancy	11.8	33.5
Sex ratio	0.68	0.69
Diabetes mellitus	13.3	16.4
Sex ratio	1.03	1.43
Arteriosclerosis	7.3	13.9
Sex ratio	0.82	0.82
Bronchitis, emphysems, and asthma	4.5	3.2
Sex ratio	0.25	0.48
Cirrhosis of the liver	9.9	6.2
Sex ratio	0.17	0.48
Suicide	6.6	4.3
Sex ratio	0.37	0.28
Congenital anomalies	6.0	11.4
Sex ratio	0.81	0.81
Homicide	4.5	2.4
Sex ratio	0.27	0.28
Nephritis and nephrosis	2.5	11.8
Sex ratio	0.68	0.77
Peptic ulcer	1.6	1.8
Sex ratio	0.39	0.22

Note: Leading causes of death are as of 1969. Based on
age-specific death rates per 100,000 population in
specified group. Computed by the direct method,
using as the standard population the age distribution
of the total population of the United States as enum-
erated in 1940.

[a] Ratio of female rate to male rate.

a question that has apparently not been seriously raised, particularly in relation to
setting of standards for conditions of work and exposure to hazardous substances.
Psychological stresses on men appear to have a more adverse impact particularly in
the 15- to 24-year age group, where for accidents the death rate in the male is 2½
times to 3 times that for females and for suicide and homicide 3 to 3½ times. Such an
excess vulnerability certainly must be considered as a serious indictment of the social
and work environment which young people pass through. Yet there seems to be reti-
cence in acknowledging the sociological and physiological factors which make men so
vulnerable at a time when young women are also likely to be experiencing the most

physically and psychologiclly stressful period of their lives, childbearing, child rearing, and working. It is necessary to note also the adverse experience of those designated "all other", that is blacks and other racial minorities. Although the male to female ratio is comparable, the female mortality rate is lower than for the white male but considerably higher than for white females.

Goldsmith analyzed Social Security data from the Longitudinal Employer-Employee Data file (LEED) and the file of Social Security covered decedents.[24] Table 7 shows the mortality rates for persons having earnings in 1960 covering a 13-year period (1960 to 1972 inclusive) and confirms the marked sex and race difference for a working cohort. On the basis of his identification of some high-risk industries for young workers, Goldsmith has suggested that more extensive use of these data files be made. There were significantly high standardized mortality ratios for white males in agricultural production, metal mining, real estate, military, and reserves and for white females in miscellaneous business services and eating and drinking establishments (Table 8). More detailed analyses of this nature would go far in establishing the relative importance of factors which contribute to complex occupational and social interactions.

VI. THE YOUNG WORK FORCE

In the 1980s the youth labor force size will begin to decline as the smaller number of babies born in the 1960s attain working age. In 1980 there will be about 18.25 million women aged 16 to 24 years and it is likely that an increasing proportion of them will be employed, a trend seen from 1966 when 47% of this age group was employed compared with 58% in 1976. In part, the trend is reflected in the decline in the proportion of young women not working because they are "keeping house", from 27 to 18% over the same period, though some of these women make up the 19% in the age group (16 to 24) attending school.[25] The occupations of employed young women somewhat differ in pattern from those of men of the same age (Table 9). The conditions of health and safety vary markedly from one occupational group to another and men are underrepresented in the less hazardous white collar jobs. Over 80% of the young men are in service and farm work where there is likely to be risk of exposure to toxic agents and dangerous work practices. In contrast, only about 40% of young women are operatives and service workers, the latter including the health professions where hazardous work conditions are poorly controlled.[26]

VII. FERTILITY AND EMPLOYMENT

Demographers warn us of the pitfalls of prophecy when reviewing fertility patterns in particular populations, for example, placing reliance on specific variables such as urbanization, education, social mobility, etc. However, Blake proposes that the employment of women outside the home may be one of the most likely sources of a desire for small families.[27] "Such employment will often entail satisfactions, alternatives to children (companionship, recreation, stimulation and creative activity) or the means to such satisfactions in the form of financial remuneration." Labor force participation bears one of the strongest relationships to family size of any variable. An inverse relationship between labor force participation of married women and their family size has been observed in Europe and the U.S. for many years. Collver examined the hypothesis that a high rate of participation of women in the labor force tended to reduce birth rates in a community, following on his earlier observations that working women have fewer children than nonworking women.[28] Measures were obtained from the 1960 U.S. Census of women's work participation, fertility, the percentage married, and the percentage who completed high school for four age groups and for whites and nonwhites

TABLE 7

Mortality Rates for Leed Cohort Covering 1960—1972[24]

		White		Black	
Year of birth	Age in 1960	Males	Females	Males	Females
1940—44	16—20	0.017	0.005	0.038	0.015
1935—39	21—25	0.020	0.009	0.044	0.017
1930—34	26—30	0.025	0.014	0.057	0.028
1925—29	31—35	0.037	0.020	0.077	0.042

From Longitudinal Employer-Employee Data File (Leed File).

TABLE 8

Standardized Mortality Ratios of Industries Among Employees Age 11 to 30 in 1960[24]

	White males[a]	White females
Agriculture production	136.3	
Metal mining	216.6	
Real Estate	158.2	
Military and reserves	119.9	
Eating and drinking places		133.2
Miscellaneous business services	71.9	171.7

[a] Significantly different from 100 $p \leq 0.05$.

TABLE 9

Employed Persons 16 to 24 Years Old, by Occupation Group, Age, and Sex: 1976[25]

	Male		Female	
Occupation group	16 to 19 years	20 to 24 years	16 to 19 years	20 to 24 years
Total employed (thousands)	3904	6742	3365	5534
Percent Distribution				
Total employed	100.0	100.0	100.0	100.0
White-collar workers	16.2	30.2	49.1	67.4
Professional, technical, and kindred workers	2.0	10.1	2.8	15.2
Managers and administrators, except farm	1.5	6.0	0.7	3.1
Sales workers	6.3	5.9	11.6	6.1
Clerical and kindred workers	6.4	8.2	34.1	43.0
Blue-collar workers	53.0	55.6	11.4	12.8
Craft and kindred workers	9.6	19.6	1.1	1.3
Operatives, including transport	19.5	23.8	7.8	10.2
Laborers, except farm	23.9	12.3	2.5	1.3
Service workers	23.0	10.6	37.9	19.1
Private household workers	0.3	—	7.6	1.3
Service workers, except private household	22.7	10.6	30.2	17.7
Farm workers	7.8	3.6	1.6	0.7
Farmers and farm managers	0.4	1.1	0.1	—
Farm laborers and supervisors	7.4	2.5	1.5	0.7

Note: Civilian noninstitutional population. Annual average data.

separately. The negative association of women's work participation and fertility was again observed, though it was accounted for primarily by whites. Both delayed marriage and low marital fertility were typical of communities with high women's work participation rates. In contrast, work participation of nonwhites had only a slight negative association with fertility indicators. Education was a better predictor of fertility than work participation, whereas for whites work participation was independent of education.

It is important to note that the statistical evidence shows only that work participation and fertility are associated, not that high work participation causes fertility to fall. The mobility of married women and many female heads of families is more limited than that for single women, so their chances for employment have been more dependent on the demands of employers in the locality and economic conditions. Depressed family incomes may result from layoffs and also be associated with a reduction in the birth rate. The multitude of factors form extremely complex and open systems which can change drastically over an extended interval of time.

The nature of a causal relationship has been difficult to examine because the relationship between work participation and reduced fertility is observed to be almost independent of the level of fecundity. It is not yet clear whether the small-family ideal is solely a result of labor force participation by women or whether the intention of working precedes the desire for small families and is established before the onset of a woman's family experience or intensive work experience.

Sklar and Berkov have made the most detailed and recent analysis of the American birth rate based on data from California,[29] which was one of the first states to liberalize abortion laws and to show high rates of legal abortion. They conjecture that the reduction in the general fertility rate for the U.S., which reached the lowest point ever recorded in 1973 (69.2 live births per 1000 women aged 15 to 44), must be coming to a halt and that we should soon see an upturn. The proportion of childless young women is now very high and if they are to reach their reproductive goals they will have to begin their families soon. The latest data show a rise in birth rates in California in 1974. Although Sklars prediction is far from universally accepted, support comes from the Current Population Survey (1975) which showed that among all married women under age 30 in 1974, only 16% expected to have no children or only one child.[30] Yet almost one third of all women under age 30 who have ever been married have not yet borne any children.

Table 10 shows the trends in legitimate and illegitimate birth rates in California, New York, Hawaii, Washington, and Oregon where legal abortion has been in effect longest.[29] The downward trends have been relatively consistent over a period of time and approximate short-term predictions for the purposes of estimating the need for maternity disability insurance and health benefits would appear to be possible for working women. Whether increased insurance and health coverage for working women who have postponed childbearing would affect the conjectured delay remains to be seen. There is the likelihood that the total expected births per woman will remain close to two for some time and the number of women of childbearing age will continue to increase (Table 11). It is worth noting that a completed family of two children in the 1970's does not pose the same logistical problems experienced by parents in the 1960s. The time absent from work is likely to be very short relative to a woman's total work experience. The likelihood is that many more women will choose to remain childless and in the work place, many more will bear children and work most of the time, and proportionately fewer will bear children and leave the work place permanently.

The relative contribution of each of these groups to the total number of childbearing women in the future is unpredictable although estimates based on different patterns of childbearing have been made.[31] The number of women under 30 years, that is the

TABLE 10

Estimated Birth Rates — Ages 15 to 44[29]

	1966		1973	
	Legitimate[a]	Illegitimate[b]	Legitimate	Illegitimate
New York	135.8	22.6	92.1	21.4
Hawaii	136.9	22.1	122.2	22.8
Washington	115.1	16.5	91.8	13.9
Oregon	118.8	16.1	98.4	14.2
California	122.4	22.5	94.3	22.2

Note: Rates computed by relating total births, regardless of age of mother, to estimated number of women aged 15 to 44.

[a] Legitimate rates are births for 1000 married women.
[b] Illegitimate rates are births per 1000 unmarried women (single, widowed, divorced, and separated).

TABLE 11

Lifetime Births Expected per 1000 Wives: 1971, 1976, and 1977[30]

		Age at date of survey			
Year, race, and origin	Total, 18 to 39 years	18 to 24 years	25 to 29 years	30 to 34 years	35 to 39 years
All Races					
1977	2.4	2.1	2.2	2.5	2.9
1976	2.4	2.1	2.2	2.5	3.0
1971	2.8	2.4	2.6	3.0	3.3
White					
1977	2.4	2.1	2.2	2.4	2.9
1976	2.4	2.1	2.2	2.5	2.9
1971	2.7	2.4	2.6	2.9	3.2
Black					
1977	2.8	2.1	2.3	3.0	3.9
1976	2.8	2.3	2.5	2.9	3.6
1971	3.3	2.6	3.1	3.7	4.2
Spanish origin[a]					
1977	2.8	2.3	2.5	3.1	3.5
1976	2.8	2.4	2.4	3.3	3.5

[a] Persons of Spanish origin may be of any race.

age group experiencing the most childbearing, will be decreasing in number from 1980 to the year 2000 (Table 12).

Earlier quantitative information on employment during pregnancy in the U.S. came from the National Health Survey of 1963.[32] The survey included only women who had legitimate live births in 1963 and therefore had a number of associated limitations. For our purposes, it is useful in that it gives the estimate that approximately 31% of these women were employed outside the home at some time during pregnancy. Almost 60% of those women having their first legitimate child were employed compared with 22% of women who already had other children. Of those women who worked, 47%

TABLE 12

Projection of Number of Women of Childbearing Age (in Thousands) by Age.[31] 1980 to 2000[a]

	1980	1990	2000	Percent change 1980—2000
Total	50,722	55,581	56,021	+ 10.4
15—19	9,984	9,006	9,737	− 2.5
20—24	10,298	10,011	8,734	− 1.8
25—29	9,641	10,321	8,406	− 1.5
30—24	8,295	9,660	9,059	− 10.0
35—39	6,770	8,281	9,929	+ 46.7
40—44	5,734	6,715	10,156	+ 77.1

Note: The peak number of 25 to 34 year olds is reached in 1990, a 14.9% increase over 1980.

Assumptions: Fertility — Both white and nonwhite populations decline linearly from their age-specific fertility rates in 1972 to replacement level by 1990, and remain constant thereafter. Mortality — Levels of white mortality as of 1969 are extended to 2000 for white population. Nonwhite mortality is expected to trend linearly to equal white mortality by 1990, and thereafter the two are expected to be identical. Migration — From an annual net immigration of 4 million per year a linear decline to zero net migration by the year 2000 is projected.

were still employed during the third trimester of pregnancy, 32% reported that they did not work after the second trimester, and 14% did not work after the first trimester (Table 13). Part-time and full-time employment patterns are also shown in Table 13. Educational attainment affected employment rates, particularly among those having their first child, to the extent that 28% of those with an elementary school education , 66% of high school graduates, and 82% of the college graduates were employed.

A more recent survey of the National Center for Health Statistics on family growth found that in a 12-month period 1972 to 1973 pregnant workers made up about 8.8% of the estimated 14,357,000 ever-married women of reproductive age in the labor force.[33] The number of women 15 to 44 years of age who worked during pregnancy ending in a live birth divided by the number of ever-married women 16 to 44 years of age who were in the labor force in March 1972 provides a crude index of the probability that women will be working while pregnant during a year period in the labor force. The index was 88 per 1000 women 15 to 44 years of age in the work force. For the ages 15 to 24 years of age, 206 per 1000 women worked during their pregnancy, but only 53 per 1000 of those 25 to 44 years. The number of women 15 to 44 years of age who worked during pregnancy per 1000 women who had a live birth in the same period was 415, i.e., 41.5% of all pregnancies in 1972 to 1973. For the age group 15 to 24 years, 46.9% of all women who had a live birth worked during pregnancy and for those 25 to 44 years, 36.6% worked during pregnancy. These percentages represent 1,260,000 live born children who were in the work place in utero at some time during their mother's pregnancy in a 12-month period from 1972 to 1973.

Table 14 shows the educational attainment of employed women in 1976, an indirect guide to the pattern of employment during pregnancy for a variety of occupations.[34]

TABLE 13

Number of Mothers and Percent Distribution of Mothers, by Last Trimester of Pregnancy During Which They Were Employed According to Color of Mother and Employment Status: U.S., 1963 Legitimate Live Births[32]

Color and employment status	No. of mothers in 1000s	Total	Not employed	Trimester (% distribution)				Unknown
				1st	2nd	3rd	Unknown	
All mothers (total)	3797	100.0	67.5	4.3	9.9	14.6	2.2	1.4
Not employed	2564	100.0	100.0	...	...	...	...	—
Employed	1179	100.0	—	14.0	31.7	47.1	7.2	—
Full time only	855	100.0	—	15.3	32.8	45.9	5.9	—
Both full and part time	91	100.0	—	0.8	22.0	69.2	8.0	—
Part time only	232	100.0	—	14.1	31.6	42.5	11.7	—
Unknown	55	100.0	—	—	—	—	—	100.0
White (total)	3315	100.0	67.8	4.4	10.0	14.1	2.1	1.5
Not employed	2248	100.0	100.0	—	—	—	—	—
Employed	1016	100.0	—	14.5	32.7	46.1	6.7	—
Full time only	755	100.0	—	16.2	33.5	44.5	5.8	—
Both full and part time	83	100.0	—	—	24.1	69.6	6.2	—
Part time only	178	100.0	—	14.0	33.1	42.2	10.8	—
Unknown	51	100.0	—	—	—	—	—	100.0
Nonwhite (total)	482	100.0	65.5	3.6	8.8	17.8	3.5	0.8
Not employed	316	100.0	100.0	—	—	—	—	—
Employed	163	100.0	—	10.8	26.1	52.7	10.4	—
Full time only	100	100.0	—	8.8	27.8	56.7	6.8	—
Both full and part time	8	100.0	—	*	*	*	*	—
Part time only	55	100.0	—	14.7	26.8	43.8	14.8	—
Unknown	4	100.0	—	—	—	—	—	100.0

Note: * indicates that figure did not meet standards of reliability or precision as calculated by Division of Vital Statistics, National Center for Health Statistics.

TABLE 14

Occupation of Employed Women by Educational Attainment March 1976 (Percent Distribution)[34]

Occupation	Total employed 16 years and over	Elementary 8 years or less	High School		College	
			1—3 years	4 years	1—3 years	4 years +
All occupational groups						
Number (in thousands)	34,609	2,837	5,580	15,432	5,637	5,123
Percent	100.00	100.00	100.00	100.00	100.00	100.00
Professional, technical, and kindred workers	16.2	0.8	2.3	6.0	18.7	67.8
Managers and administrators	5.7	2.8	3.4	5.9	7.0	7.9
Sales workers	6.6	4.6	8.2	7.2	7.6	2.8
Clerical and kindred workers	35.1	8.0	19.1	47.9	46.7	16.0
Craft and kindred workers	1.4	1.6	2.2	1.6	1.1	.4
Operatives except transport	11.4	33.8	21.1	10.2	2.9	1.2
Transport equipment operatives	0.6	0.5	1.2	0.7	0.4	0.1
Laborers, except farm	1.1	2.2	2.3	0.9	0.6	0.2
Private household workers	3.2	12.5	7.8	1.6	1.0	0.2
Service workers, except private household	17.8	30.4	31.1	17.2	13.4	3.3
Farm workers	0.9	2.6	1.3	0.8	0.5	0.3

The Center for Disease Control (CDC) of the U.S. Department of Health, Education and Welfare reports the rate of legal abortions by state for women aged 15 to 44.[35] In 1975 the rate for the U.S. was 18 per 1000 women age 15 to 44 and ranged from none reported in West Virginia to 124 for the District of Columbia, neither of which are representative of the national experience although they reflect the widely varying rates throughout the country. California and New York report 33% of the abortions but only 17% of the live births, and their abortion rates are 30 and 37 abortions per 1000 women age 15 to 44, respectively. However, geographic mobility affects these rates markedly as the denominator (female population age 15 to 44 in the state) does not include all the out of state women who entered the state solely to obtain an abortion. The ratio of the number of abortions per 1000 live births has the same overestimate. For example, the District of Columbia had 22,721 abortions and 9759 live births in 1975. Those states with ratios of over 300 abortions per 1000 live births were California, Connecticut, Illinois, Maryland, Massachusetts, New York, Oregon, Rhode Island, Vermont, and Washington (ranging from 301 to 624). In most of these states women make up a high proportion of the work force. The total number of legal abortions and live births for the U.S. in 1975 was 854,853 and 3,119,648, respectively, giving a ratio of 274 abortions per 1000 live births. For 1977 CDC has estimated the number of abortions to be very close to one million. It is likely that working women with their relative economic independence make up a considerable proportion of those women who choose to abort, particularly when 60% of the total abortions reported in 34 states are in women 20 to 35 years of age (Table 15).

Birth registration data on illegitimate births show that there has been a marked increase since 1950, particularly among teenage women. By 1975, 38% of all births to women aged 15 to 19 and 12% of all births to women aged 20 to 24 were classified as illegitimate, an overall increase from 1950 when the comparable births were 13.3% (15 to 19 years) and 3.8% (20 to 24 years).[25] The decline in the legitimate birth rate has been the major factor in the overall reduced birth rate in recent years.

In 1972, the estimates of the percent of mothers sterilized following delivery of legitimate live hospital births was 7.8%.[36] However, regional differences are marked with the North Central region of the U.S. showing a much higher likelihood of sterilization for all other races, 16.6% compared with 6.9% for whites. There was a marked increase in postpartum sterilization after the delivery of the third child (15.8%) and the fourth child (19.9%). Sterilization increased markedly with age from 8.2% at 25 to 29 years to 22.4% at 35 years and over (Table 16).

For the purposes of this discussion a simple model can be used to extrapolate from reports of the Bureau of the Census, the National Center for Health Statistics, and

TABLE 15

Reported Legal Abortions by Age in 34 States[35]

	Total number	Mean % for 34 states
<15	9,454	1.5
15—19	199,000	31.2
20—24	201,081	31.6
25—29	114,854	18.0
30—34	61,151	9.6
35—39	31,895	5.0
40 Unknown	7,425	1.2
Total	637,195	100.0

TABLE 16

Estimated Percentage of Mothers Sterilized following Delivery of Legitimate Live Hospital Birth by Live Birth Order and Age of Mother U.S., 1972.[36]

| | Total | Live birth order | | | | |
		1st	2nd	3rd	4th	5th or higher
Total	7.8	1.9	5.3	15.8	19.9	18.7
Under 20 years	2.7	2.2	3.7	—	—	—
20—24 years	4.7	1.3	5.1	12.5	12.6	22.5
25—29 years	8.2	0.7	4.6	14.5	18.6	19.9
30—34 years	15.2	4.6	7.2	21.0	22.5	16.9
35 years and over	22.4	28.2	20.5	27.1	26.6	19.2

the Department of Labor to make rough estimates of the minimum number of women who know they are not fertile among the age group 30 to 55 years in the work force in the decade of the 1980s. For example, if we can assume a steady rate of sterilization during the decade of the 1970s comparable to 1972, an estimated total of 2,100,000 sterilizations will have been experienced by those aged 20 to 44 years. During the period 1980 to 1990 approximately 22 million women aged 30 to 55 years will be in the work force, about 61% of the total number of women of those ages from 1980 to 1990.[37] The minimum number who would know they were not fertile would be 1,281,000, in that the National Center for Health Statistics estimates stem from postpartum sterilizations and do not include sterilizations not directly associated with childbirth. That is, more than 6% of the cohort could specify that they were not fertile, or more than one working woman in every 16 aged 30 to 55 in the 1980s. This estimate is most certainly very conservative but allows us to consider the usefulness of vital statistics sources for evaluating reproductive risks to the working population.

In her study of sterilization and fertility decline in Puerto Rico, Presser calculated the percentage of mothers aged 20 to 49 in 1965 who were sterilized in terms of their usual activity and total number of births.[38] Table 17 shows the consistently higher percentage of sterilization for those employed. Although not directly applicable to the total population of the U.S., it provides some indication that a difference exists between the two portions of the female population, those who are employed outside the home and those who are not, in terms of sterilization.

The prevalence of abortion in women and sterilization in both men and women are two important characteristics of a working population. Epidemiologic studies of reproductive effects of hazardous agents must take them into account. It is aso likely that knowledge of adverse relationships may affect the decisions of workers of procreative capacity and management in terms of job choices and placement.

The number of women who remain childless by choice or circumstances makes up a considerable proportion of the work force.[39] In 1974 the percentage of employed women still childless at 35 to 44 years of age was 9.6%, a marked drop from 24.6% for those 25 to 34 years of age (Table 18).

Decisions concerning an individual worker and his or her reproductive experience cannot be based on limited criteria with general applicability. It is evident that the age profile of procreation, the abortion and sterilization rate, the number of men and women who choose to continue working during their childbearing years, and the proportion of childlessness of unknown cause are important factors.

Changing fertility patterns are of some significance in terms of the possible impact of hazardous work conditions on both parents. A body burden of toxic substances or their metabolites can develop over a period of time in men and women, for example

TABLE 17

Percent Sterilized of Mothers Aged 20 to 49 in 1965[38] by Usual
Activity and Total Number of Birth

Total number of births	Usual activity		
	Unemployed (at home)	Employed	Difference
1—2	27.9%	35.6%	+ 7.7
3—4	44.3%	51.8%	+ 7.5
5 or more	25.9%	33.3%	+ 7.4
Total percent	32.0%	40.1%	+ 8.1
Total number of mothers in study	778	277	

lead or organochlorinated compounds, so that the effect on germ cells of both parents can originate long before the pregnancy of concern. Adverse impact on the embryo and fetus may be attributable to the mother's immediate or past work experience. The relative contribution of each parent to the biological consequences of work-related influences on each fertilized ovum and its development is not known. Subsequent chapters will describe occupational hazards which may affect human reproduction. For most agents the effects may be better known for one sex than for the other because of different exposure patterns or inappropriate research emphases in the past.

The relationship of years of work experience to procreation can be quantified in the form of person years of occupational experience for men and women, assuming that everyone begins to work at 16 (Table 19). The vital statistics reported by the National Center for Health Statistics include birth rates by parental age.[40] For these estimates the assumption is made that the working population procreates at the same rate as the nonworking population, an assumption that is far more true for men than for women. That is, when relating birth rate for male parents (the number of live births for 1000 resident males) in each age group to the appropriate age group in the work force the estimate is more reliable than the same calculation for female parents, many of whom are not in the work force and are bearing a far higher proportion of babies than women in the work force. Therefore, the person years of occupational experience for women is very much more of an overestimate. With such limitations in mind it is evident from the results in Table 19 that the work experience in terms of person years for fathers of children born in 1976 was more than twice that of the mothers. The younger age of procreation for women and the smaller number in the work force in their prime child-bearing years account for the marked discrepancy between the work experience contribution of mothers and fathers over 25 years of age to their procreation.

VIII. HEALTH INSURANCE COVERAGE FOR MATERNITY CARE

Health insurance for maternity care may cover all or part of three components of pregnancy: (1) physician bills for office visits or home calls during pregnancy, (2) physician bills for delivery of the baby, and (3) hospital care at the time of delivery.

The National Natality Survey reported health insurance coverage only for legitimate live births during 1964 to 1966, so that there are severe limitations in extrapolating to current conditions.[40] For example, the father's employment would be the prime source of insurance coverage.

Of the married mothers who were employed during pregnancy, 63% had partial or complete coverage for maternity care as compared with 58% of the married mothers

TABLE 18

Percent Childless to Date Among Women Ever Married: June 1974 (Civilian Noninstitutional Population)[39]

	15—24 years		25—34 years		35—44 years	
	No. of women	% childless	No. of women	% childless	No. of women	% childless
Total	7,027	43.3	13,425	15.1	11,041	7.9
In labor force	3,747	57.7	6,291	24.6	5,856	9.6
Full-time	2,408	62.5	5,958	25.0	5,591	9.8
Part-time	940	50.9	4,051	29.4	3,765	11.1
Unemployed	399	44.9	333	17.1	265	6.0
Not in labor force	3,280	26.8	7,134	6.7	5,184	5.9

Note: Numbers in thousands.

TABLE 19

Person Years of Occupational Experience Preceding
Pregnancies Terminating in 1976[26,40]

	Male	Female	M/F Ratio
16—19	255,017	556,132	0.46
20—24	4,744,392	4,263,612	1.11
25—29	12,207,696	6,846,564	1.78
30—34	11,503,628	3,650,410	3.15
35—39	4,866,400	1,453,386	3.35
40—44	2,357,713	386,154	6.11
45—49	1,006,848	227,152	4.43
50—54	107,342	—	—
55 +	53,384	—	—
Total	37,102,420	17,383,410	2.13

Note: Calculated from published statistics.

From Employment and Earnings, Labor Force by
Age, 1976, Bureau of Labor Statistics, U.S. Department of Labor, Washington, D.C., 1977. Vital Statistics of the U.S., Vol. 1, Natality, National Center for
Health Statistics, U.S. Department of Health, Education and Welfare, 1976.

who were not employed during pregnancy (Table 20). Several factors are associated
with the higher rate of coverage for employed mothers — their higher median family
income and the possibility that their group health insurance plan at work provided
maternity benefits. The rate of coverage for employed mothers might have been higher
were it not for the fact that they had a higher percentage of first births (51%) than
did mothers not employed (20%). There has been a practice of no coverage for the
first-born conceived before marriage in many insurance plans.

It appears that employed women have some advantages in relation to maternity coverage compared with women not employed during pregnancy. The statistics of the mid-
1960s only provide indirect information concerning married mothers 15 years later,
and it is more difficult to obtain reliable information on maternity coverage for the
unmarried mother, whatever her pregnancy outcome. The availability of prenatal care
is generally accepted as a necessity for ensuring satisfactory pregnancy outcome, and
it seems reasonable to expect that maternity coverage would place a family in a lower
risk category by reducing economic barriers.

Information on corporation plans paying temporary benefits for disabilities arising
out of pregnancy is reported by the U.S. Department of Labor, Bureau of Labor Statistics, Digest of Health and Insurance Plans. In the 1971 edition, 69 corporations and
associations reported maternity coverage, 66 for 6 weeks, 2 for 13 weeks, and 1 for 20
weeks. In the 1974 edition, of the 154 plans covered, 96 mentioned maternity coverage;
30 of the 96 excluded maternity coverage, 54 provided 6 weeks, 5 reported 8 weeks, 1
reported 13 weeks, 4 reported 26 weeks, and 2 reported 52 weeks. In that the Digest
provides only summary information, these figures have been derived from interpreted
data. However, it would appear that there was a modest improvement over the 3 years
1971 to 1974.

The Sex Discrimination Guidelines issued by the Equal Employment Opportunity
Commission relating to pregnancy and childbirth and the Supreme Court decision concerning pregnancy coverage are discussed in Chapter 7.

TABLE 20

Number and Percent Distribution of Mothers by Insurance Coverage for Maternity Care, According to Employment of Mother During Pregnancy and Family Income: U.S., 1964—66 Legitimate Live Births[40]

Employment of mother during pregnancy and family income	All mothers		Percent with coverage						Percent without coverage
					Partial coverage				
	Number in thousands	Percent	Total	Complete coverage	Total	Hospital care and physician visits	Hospital care and delivery	Hospital care alone	
All mothers	3480	100.0	59.4	34.0	25.4	1.8	16.5	7.1	40.6
Less than $3,000	691	100.0	21.2	10.2	11.0	1.4	6.4	3.2	78.8
$3,000—$4,999	779	100.0	44.8	22.6	22.2	2.0	13.2	7.0	55.2
$5,000—$6,999	889	100.0	73.1	42.5	30.6	2.0	20.2	8.4	26.9
$7,000—$9,999	716	100.0	82.4	50.1	32.4	1.4	22.4	8.5	17.6
$10,000 or more	406	100.0	81.7	49.5	32.1	2.1	21.1	8.8	18.3
Employed during pregnancy	1045	100.0	62.7	36.8	26.0	1.9	16.7	7.3	37.3
Less than $3,000	165	100.0	25.9	13.1	12.9	1.0	8.9	2.9	74.1
$3,000—$4,999	214	100.0	49.9	26.9	23.0	1.7	14.2	7.1	50.1
$5,000—$6,999	265	100.0	68.8	38.4	30.4	3.1	17.2	10.1	31.2
$7,000—$9,999	250	100.0	78.8	48.3	30.4	1.3	21.1	8.0	21.2
$10,000 or more	150	100.0	84.1	54.8	29.3	2.2	20.9	6.2	15.9
Not employed during pregnancy	2436	100.0	57.9	32.8	25.1	1.7	16.3	7.0	42.1
Less than $3,000	525	100.0	19.7	9.3	10.4	5.6	3.2	1.5	80.3
$3,000—$4,999	564	100.0	42.9	21.0	21.9	2.1	12.9	6.9	57.1
$5,000—$6,999	624	100.0	74.9	44.2	30.7	1.5	21.5	7.7	25.1
$7,000—$9,999	467	100.0	84.4	51.0	33.4	1.5	23.1	8.8	15.6
$10,000 or more	255	100.0	80.2	46.5	33.8	2.1	21.3	10.4	19.8

IX. FAMILY HEALTH

A recent World Health Organization (WHO) study has examined some current family health statistics and noted that family patterns and changes are important in relation to the health of the individual members and affect their use of health services.[41] The WHO assumption is that the interrelation between health and the family is not a static phenomenon, but a dynamic process. The mother's employment becomes an important variable in the demographic analysis of family characteristics. For example, certain aspects of reproduction (in particularly rates of pregnancy wastage, childlessness, and infant mortality rates) can be analyzed according to this framework. Absenteeism and premature retirement from work are other important issues. When the demographic and social data can be linked with epidemiologic data, the impact of their interactions on the health situation of the family can be better examined. A change in the family conditions such as high employment rates for mothers is relevant to the planning of health services.

In the exploratory development of this approach the WHO report considers labor force status of women as a critical contributory social characteristic in the pattern of utilization of health services and health behavior. The claim is made that although family data are often included in the economics of health, there have been very few investigations of the economics of the family unit in this context such as the relationship between health (which in this context may mean illness) and productivity or on the use of health care resources.

In economic terms, households and families can be regarded as both production and consumption units and decisions on health care and practices are affected by the curative and supportive services available within the family, the perception of need, the relative cost of internal and external care, and the household's purchasing power. Each of these factors is in turn affected by the employment status of the mother. Additionally, it is evident that various combinations of these factors could result in a low demand for organized health services, but could reflect either effective functioning of the family or deprivation.

Studies of family usage of external health services have not been particularly successful though qualitatively it appears that purely economic factors are less important than social and cultural elements. In large measure, the problem of analysis results from the difficulty of assigning direct measures to health and illness. Demands for care may be the first and only evidence of illness.

Andersen provides a behavioral model of family use of health services diagrammed as follows:[42]

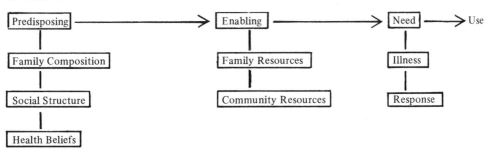

The mother's role in the predisposing, enabling, and need component is tacitly assumed, usually in terms of her availability for nursing care, her evaluation of the condition, and her decisions, i.e., the mother's expected role. How do mothers currently in the work force deal with the crises of family illness and ongoing dental and medical care? Medical services from private sources seldom respond to anybody's work schedule. The emergency service of hospitals, now perceived as a source of regular outpatient medical care, is likely to become more important as more mothers work at 9:00 to 5:00 jobs. Dental services are time consuming and seldom convenient in time or place. Large corporations place dental visits high on the list as a cause of absenteeism.

Preventive pediatric programs throughout the U.S. depend on the mother. She must perceive the need and take the child to a hospital, clinic, or private office. A major deterrent to work outside the home for many mothers is the need, as they see it, to be visibly present at all such encounters. The working mother of necessity usually finds she is dispensible but still suffers the mental stress when her presence is expected and she cannot be there. We have no information which would indicate whether or not the children of working mothers have more or less of their immunization series completed, more or less physical examinations, more or less dental care, etc.

In the context of the Andersen model the possibility that the mother's income enables the family to obtain these services may be just as important as the roadblocks to obtaining services for adults and children outside regular working hours. In contrast, there is the high likelihood that the woman who enters paid employment will find it economically feasible and esthetically necessary to invest in extensive dental treatment for herself, usually the last in a family to be treated.

In the U.S. there has been a marked increase in the number of women with children under 18 years of age in the work force. In March 1976, 49% of all mothers were employed (14.6 million) in contrast to 27% in 1955. About 5.4 million had children under age six, almost two fifths of all working mothers (Table 21). The Women's Bureau considers that the fivefold increase in labor force participation of mothers since 1940 is the most significant change ever seen in the U.S. labor market. In 1960 the labor participation rate for mothers was 30.4% and for all women 36.7%. In 1970 these rates were 48.8 and 46.8% respectively, i.e., 2 percentage points higher for mothers than for all women.[14]

Working mothers with husbands present worked in occupations comparable to all women, 34% clerical workers, 18% service workers (except private household), 17% professional and technical jobs, 13% operatives, and 5% managers and administrators.

Mothers who are heads of household are far more likely to be in the labor force. For those with children under 6 years of age, the participation rate is 56% compared with 37% for those who have husbands present (Table 22).[14]

X. OUR WORKING LIVES

A woman's perceptions of her work experience affect her entry and exit from the work force throughout her life. Most discussions emphasize her domestic commitments and educational background in relation to job opportunities. Very little information can be found on any relationship with her state of health.

TABLE 21

Percentage Labor Force Participation of Mothers by Age of Children:[14] March 1976

Age of children (years)	1971 (%)	1976 (%)	Increase (%)
3	27	34	7
3—5	38	44	9
6—17	52	56	4

TABLE 22

Mothers in the Labor Force, by Marital Status of Mother and Age of Children: March 1976[14]

Marital status of mother and age of children	Number (in thousands)	Percent distribution	As percent of all ever-married women in the population
Mothers with children under 18 years	14,598	100.0	48.8
Married, husband present	11,693	80.1	46.1
Widowed, divorced, or separated	2,904	19.9	63.8
Mothers with children 6 to 17 years only	9,239	63.3	56.2
Married, husband present	7,270	49.8	53.7
Widowed, divorced, or separated	1,970	13.5	68.1
Mothers with children under 6 years[a]	5,358	36.7	39.7
Married, husband present	4,424	30.3	37.4
Widowed, divorced, or separated	935	6.4	56.2
Mothers with children 3 to 5 years (none under 3)[a]	2,827	19.4	47.2
Married, husband present	2,227	15.3	44.1
Widowed, divorced, or separated	600	4.1	63.4
Mothers with children under 3 years[a]	2,531	17.3	33.8
Married, husband present	2,197	15.1	32.4
Widowed, divorced, or separated	335	2.3	46.7

Note: Mothers 16 years of age and over.

[a] May also have older children.

For the U.S. we know little about the rate of withdrawal from employment, least of all by category of occupation and industry, for reasons of health. For example, the manufacturing jobs in which women are heavily represented demand to varying degrees manipulative speed, manual dexterity, and powers of visual discrimination.[43] There may be considerable standing and/or movement demanded. There is some difficulty in extrapolating observations on men in manufacturing occupations to the many women in repetitive, boring jobs which have fallen to their lot as technological complexity and female employment have increased.[44] There are no data readily at hand which allow an evaluation of the relative tolerance of men and women in any work conditions as they age. Work in hot conditions is an exception. Several important factors which probably affect the choice to withdraw from the work force are retirement and pension privileges, industrial strain, or ill health. The need for maintaining workers in productive employment until retirement should be an encouragement to a more detailed evaluation of these relationships for women as well as men in all job categories.

Clark, in the monograph "Woman, Work and Age," expands on this rarely discussed topic — withdrawal of the older woman from the work force.[43] Although he examined British data there are enough similarities to U.S. conditions to consider his conclusions seriously, and in the U.S. we have little useful information on the ages at which older women leave paid employment and for what causes. His conclusion concerning the postchildbearing female work population was that "a woman's term of service and her self-determined age for withdrawal from wo. k can never be administratively assessed in the ways in which one would assess those of a man." This unequivocal statement stems from his empiric observation that he could not trace statistically the course of individual movements of women in and out of the labor market. Writing on female employment in the early sixties in England, his view was that "for most

mature women it is still somewhat incidental to their role as housewives and mothers.''
A full reading of his monograph, however, shows sensitivity and understanding of the
many necessary reasons for women's employment. For example, a discussion of impaired health and the rates of withdrawal from work is a rare published account of
the older woman worker based on national insurance statistics. He states that there is
only one question that is strictly relevant. ''Are mature women in any degree more
susceptible than men to such chronic or degenerative conditions as are likely to render
them more or less unemployable?'' Mortality rates are not applicable in the circumstances under discussion here because there are many chronic diseases which can reduce
working ability and efficiency without necessarily shortening the life span. Data from
the United Kingdom Ministry of Pensions and National Insurance for 1956 showed
insured persons certified sick for 6 months or more expressed as percentages of the
average populations of people similarly insured at that time (Table 23).

It is worth noting that the incapacity perceived by the medical practitioner (for purposes of certification in the study cited) was not necessarily related to medical conditions alone. The author's view was that ''women continue to cope with their domestic
tasks long after their physical condition has removed them from employment,'' so that
it is important to examine the forms of ill health that directly influence the working
woman if we are to explain the reasons for withdrawal from work. The older woman
has more experience to bring to her decisions on how well she can fulfill the total daily
commitment of employment plus domestic responsibilities, both in terms of her own
health status and the family expectations for her continuing care for them. The sex
differences in cases of long-term invalidity (i.e., inability to continue in paid employment) seen in England in 1956 are interesting in relation to the U.S. National Health
Survey Data (Table 24). The listed causes accounted for more than half of the long-
term invalidity at the time they were collected and it seems likely that women were
over three times more susceptible than men to nervous conditions, high blood pressure,
rheumatism, and arthritis. The high withdrawal rate from employment for older
women can well be understood in terms of the discomfort and physical debility which
to a large extent is not life shortening but must be tolerated in the adverse work settings
experienced by many older unskilled, service, or blue-collar workers. Similar sex differences in morbidity for these diverse categories were reported for the population at
large, derived from ''patient consulting rates'' of medical practitioners in England.

The National Center for Health Statistics of the U.S. Department of Health, Education and Welfare has published morbidity data on selected diseases over the past 10
years. Tables 25, 26, and 27 provide prevalence rates for three debilitating conditions
to which women appear to be more prone than men. More detailed information was
collected on hypertension in the U.S. for 1974 through the Division of Health Interview
Statistics. Demographic factors associated with a higher percentage of persons with

TABLE 23

**United Kingdom Ministry of Pensions and Na-
tional Insurance 1956**[43]

Insured persons	Percentages incapacitated for 6 months or more at ages		
	45—49	50—54	55—59
Men	1.2	2.0	4.1
Married women	4.2	5.7	8.9
Other women	4.1	5.6	7.9

TABLE 24

England — Approximate Percentage of Insured Persons Incapacitated, 1956: Expressed as Proportions of the Average Insured Populations in Each Age Group[43]

	Ages	45—54	55—59
All causes	Male	4.0	7.8
	Female	8.2	11.8
Psychoneurosis and psychosis	Male	0.3	0.5
	Female	1.1	1.2
Hypertensive disease	Male	0.07	0.2
	Female	0.4	1.1
Bronchitis	Male	0.3	1.7
	Female	0.4	0.7
Arthritis	Male	0.1	0.3
	Female	0.7	1.4
Rheumatism	Male	0.1	0.2
	Female	0.3	0.5

TABLE 25

Rheumatoid Arthritis — Prevalence Rates in Adults: U.S. (1960—1962)[45]

	Rate per 100 adults	
	Women	Men
Industry		
Agriculture, forestries, and fisheries	3.0	2.0
Manufacturing	3.7	1.2
Wholesale and retail trade	2.9	1.0
Finance, insurance, and real estate	2.1	0.0
Service and miscellaneous	3.3	1.2
Occupation		
Professional, technical, and managerial	2.5	0.5
Clerical and sales workers	2.0	1.4
Operatives and kindred workers	3.1	0.6
Private household and service workers	5.1	2.8
Usual Activity Status		
Usually working	2.8	1.0
Keeping house (women), retired (men)	5.5	6.8
Other	3.1	2.9

TABLE 26

Prevalence of Arthritis: U.S. 1969[46]

Number per 1000 persons	< 4 5 yr	4 5 — 6 0 yr
Usually working (17 years and over, men and women)	36.8	160.7
Usually keeping house (females 17 years and over)	65.5	288.6
Retired (45 years and over, Men and Women)	—	315.0

TABLE 27

Prevalence of Chronic Circulatory Conditions: U.S. 1972[47]

	Number per 1000 persons					
	Varicose veins		Hemorrhoids		Hypertensive disease	
	<45 yr	45—60 yr	<45 yr	45—60 yr	<45 yr	45—60 yr
Usually working (17 years and over, men and women)	23.6	53.5	60.8	73.1	39.5	108.9
Usually keeping house (females 17 years and over)	75.2	118.4	102.5	89.9	48.8	164.4
Retired (45 years and over, men and women)	—	72.5	—	106.1	—	133.4

TABLE 28

Percent Distribution of Persons with Limitation of Activity by Selected Chronic Conditions According to Sex and Age: U.S. 1974[48]

	Male		Female	
	45—64 yrs	65 yrs +	45—64 yrs	65 yrs +
Malignant neoplasms	2.5	2.8	3.9	1.8
Diabetes	5.4	5.7	6.2	7.7
Mental and nervous conditions	5.2	3.0	6.3	3.8
Heart conditions	24.2	25.2	15.6	22.2
Cardiovascular disease	3.2	5.8	2.4	4.3
Hypertension without heart involvement	5.9	6.0	11.8	10.9
Varicose veins	—	—	2.0	1.3
Other conditions of circulatory system	3.7	5.5	4.4	6.3
Chronic bronchitis	1.1	1.2	0.9	—
Emphysema	5.1	7.9	1.8	1.6
Asthma	3.0	2.8	3.0	1.6
Other conditions of respiratory system	3.4	3.3	1.2	1.1
Peptic ulcer	2.6	1.9	2.1	1.4
Hernia	3.2	3.2	2.6	2.4
Other conditions of digestive system	3.2	2.7	4.2	4.3
Genitourinary system	2.2	3.1	3.7	2.4
Arthritis and rheumatism	12.5	15.6	22.4	29.4
Paralysis, complete or partial	4.1	4.2	2.6	3.2
Impairment (except paralysis) of back and spine	7.5	3.1	7.1	3.3
Impairments of upper extremities and shoulders[a]	2.7	1.0	1.5	1.0
Impairment of lower extremities and hips[a]	7.0	5.0	4.4	6.9
Other musculo-skeletal disorders	7.8	3.0	7.9	3.4

[a] Except paralysis and absence.

From: Limitation of Activity due to Chronic Conditions U.S. 1974, Health Resources Administration, U.S. Department of Health, Education and Welfare, Washington, D.C., 1977.

hypertension were income less than $5000, 25.7% compared with 11.8% for those with incomes $10,000 or more. The older black population, particularly of low income, had the highest percentage of hypertension. For all women 45 to 64 years, 31.2% reported they had ever had hypertension whereas 24.3% of men reported ever having hypertension. For the age group of men and women 65 years and over the percentages were 47.2 and 32.5%, respectively. The self-reported experience of hypertension when viewed in relation to the limitation of activity of 11.8% for women and 5.9% for men indicates a high prevalence among both men and women over 45 who continue to work.[45-47]

These data provide only an indication of the health disadvantage experienced by women who continue to work in outside employment and/or at home. The essential difference between men and women in the older age group until retirement is that men are at higher risk from life-threatening diseases, but women experience debilitating chronic disease.

Women, from the foregoing data, appear to suffer more from chronic diseases likely to impair bodily activity or the will to work than they experience serious breakdown. More appropriate preventive and treatment programs need to be initiated in occupational health services to take this morbidity experience into account. Men at the same ages appear to suffer more life-threatening illnesses, an unknown proportion directly work related. Occupational health services, though inadequate, have been in recent years more intensively directed to their prevention.

Morbidity studies which provide information on sex differences are particularly necessary in a continued evaluation of the older work force. Table 28 provides more recent data on limitation of activity by selected chronic conditions. Overall the percentage of the population with limitation of activity was 25.3 for men and 23.0 for women age 45 to 65 years and 49.7 for men and 43.1 for women age 65 and over. Heart conditions, emphysema, and impairments of the upper and lower extremities were markedly more important causes for limitation of activity in men. In contrast, hypertension, arthritis, and rheumatism affected women very much more than men.[48]

We presume that we have the right to enjoy retirement, yet physical impairment is difficult to measure and predict. The female work force will continue to show an increase in the number of women with long years of work experience so that debilitating, non life-threatening chronic diseases can be expected to become more important factors in job placement and age of retirement.

XI. WORKER DISABILITY

Worker's Compensation provides cash benefits, medical care and rehabilitation services for workers who suffer work-related injuries and diseases. To be eligible for benefits, normally an employee must experience a personal injury by accident arising out of and in the course of employment. All 50 state laws plus five other jurisdictions and two Federal programs provide benefits for workers with occupational diseases although not all cover every form of occupational disease. The percentage of employees covered by State or Federal worker's compensation programs in 1972 was about 85% of all employees.

The National Commission on State Worker's Compensation Laws prepared a report in 1972 as specified under the Occupational Safety and Health Act of 1970.[49] The conclusion was that state workmen's compensation laws do not provide an adequate, prompt, and equitable system of compensation for workers who suffer disabling injury or death in the course of their employment. Another criticism was that the information base was "dismally sparse."

"The inequities of wide variations among the States in the proportion of labor force covered are compounded by the nature of the exclusions. The occupations typically excluded from coverage, such as household workers and farm help, are disproportionately low-income, less-education, non-white and female — those least able financially to carry the burden of disability by themselves."

Recommendations by the National Commission on State Worker's Compensation Laws in 1972 included the following:

1. Compulsory coverage of all employees by worker's compensation laws with no waivers permitted
2. No exemption of employers from worker's compensation coverage because of the number of their employees
3. Extension of worker's compensation coverage to all occupations and industries, without regard to the degree of hazard of the occupation or industry
4. Coverage of farm workers and all government employees on the same basis as all other employees
5. Coverage of household workers and all casual workers at least to the extent they are covered by Social Security

It is interesting to note that a Supplemental Study for the National Commission on States Workmen's Compensation Laws "Too Little and Too Late... The Economic Plight of Very Seriously and Permanently Disabled Men and Their Households in the New York City Metropolitan Area" (Volume II, 1973) concerned 121 men drawn from a survey universe of 319 men.[50]

This example is one of many for which the exclusion of women is tacitly accepted as appropriate. The authors in selecting their respondents state, "We further refined the sample, eliminating women, those known to be deceased, those with very early injuries, and those with addresses outside the survey area."

The next supplemental study, "Serious Industrial Injuries and Worker Earnings in Florida," for the Commission describes the population under study as workers, but a description of the final sample states that "All women were excluded so that we could focus on male earnings... with women one might expect more voluntary withdrawal from the labor force after the injury."[51]

"Sources of Information about Workmen's Compensation Recipients", another supplemental study for the Commission, in a review of previous surveys could not differentiate female workmen's compensation recipients into those receiving compensation due to their own work-connected disability or that of their husband.[52] In 1967, "Approximately 88% of those assumed to be recipients are male. The degree of error in terms of sex is probably small, but the inability to identify survivor's benefits separately precludes any determination of its real magnitude." Despite this conclusion the authors proceeded to study 919 males.

Makarushka in a study of worker's compensation benefits in New York State, Florida, Wisconsin, and Washington concluded that those women who qualify for worker's compensation are as seriously injured as men, both in terms of total permanent impairment and number of work weeks lost.[53] However, 5 years after the injury, women are far less likely to be working than the men and their absence from the labor force is related to marital status, household size, and age.

The National Longitudinal Survey of the Bureau of the Census included cohorts of women 30 to 44 and 18 to 24 as two of the four subsets and should provide some worker's compensation information over a long period, but data are not yet available.

Since 1935, Social Security programs in the U.S. have been extended to workers in nearly all kinds of employment including self-employment and work on farms, in private households, in state and local government, and in private nonprofit organizations. The majority of workers excluded from this coverage fall into three major caegories:

1. Those covered under Federal civilian staff retirement systems.
2. Household workers and farm workers who do not earn enough or work long enough to meet certain minimum requirements (workers in industry and commerce are covered regardless of regularity of employment or amount of earnings).
3. Persons with very low net earnings from self-employment.

Although coverage by Social Security appears broader than in Worker's Compensation, those covered must work a certain number of quarters in order to qualify for disability benefits. In contrast, under Worker's Compensation, a covered worker is eligible for benefits, if injured, from the moment employment begins. About 80% of persons of working age have worked long and recently enough to be eligible for Social Security benefits.

It seems likely that women make up a large proportion of the 20% of working persons ineligible for social security benefits. One of the natural improvements resulting from higher employment of women would be their improved disability coverage by Social Security.

Haber examined the relationship of functional capacities to the severity of disability using a national survey of the U.S. conducted by the Social Security Administration in 1966. The consequences of capacity limitations were examined in relation to employment and household participation. Disability was defined as limitations in work capacity of longer than 6 months duration resulting from chronic health conditions or impairments.[54]

The conclusion was that women, older people, the undereducated, and the unskilled appear to have less adaptive capacity to face more demanding requirements in that their ability to work was more affected by activity limitations. At work men appeared to be more able than women to cope with impairment by accommodation on the job.

Haber discusses the consequences of functional limitations, i.e., limitations in activity and physical performance which affect the ability to engage in expected role performance. Performance limitations may lead to loss of employment as a reflection of inability to meet requirements. The individual's perception of disability may change as a result, particularly among those with restricted labor market opportunities. Women have many reasons beyond disability to stay at home, although their work experience and labor force participation in this study were directly affected by the extent of functional limitations.

Their family demands may well explain much of the difference between men and women in the extent of severe disability. For example, the proportion of severely disabled men not employed ranged from just over two thirds for those with no loss in functional capacities to 80% of those with extensive limitations. For women the range was only from 31% to 62%.

It seems reasonable to conclude that the discrepancy in employment experience between disabled men and women who were severely impaired functionally also reflects differences in job opportunities and acceptance of physical impairment for men and women. The evidence presented here indicates that causes of disability and the subsequent employment experience may be quite different for men and women, though the data have been taken from studies not necessarily designed to show these differences.

The work force participation of women varies markedly with marital status and in March 1975 approximately 12.3% of the female labor force was either divorced or separated, an increase of 10.7% since 1970. The U.S. has the highest divorce rate in the world, 4.8 per thousand popuation. Divorced women had a higher work force participation, 72% of the 4 million divorced women, compared to 55% of the 3 million separated women, and 44% of the 47.5 million married women living with their husbands. For divorced women with children aged 6 to 17, 80% were in the work force, compared with 66% for those with children under 6 years of age.[55]

With the overall increase in life expectancy of women, there has been a marked addition to the number of years of working life. The additional life expectancy since 1900 has been 24 years and the work life expectancy of women at birth has increased from 6.3 years to 22.9 years. Since 1950 women have reduced the time spent out of the labor force so that work life expectancy has risen at a faster rate than overall life expectancy. Although the work life expectancy for men has been declining since 1960, it is still almost twice that for women. Women still tend to retire at an earlier age than men and the interruption for childbearing is not considered to be the equivalent of time spent by men in the armed services.[56]

Table 30 shows the entry rate of men and women into the work force in 1970 in relation to age. For women, the additional factors which influence their entry are the children reaching school age and becoming a widow. Separation rates for women are also affected by the presence of children, but more dramatically by early retirement (Table 31).[56]

XII. CONCLUSION

The age distribution of the work force will change by the year 2000 probably with fewer men aged 16 to 24 and 55 years and over. The proportion of women will increase from 20 years of age to 55 years and over (Table 29).[37] Their experience in the work place may affect their health and their reproduction. We should be able to apply the demographic information we have now to ensure that adverse effects will be minimized and positive effects will be optimized.

TABLE 29

Civilian Labor Force by Age and Sex[37]

| | Number in labor force (in thousands) | | | |
Sex and age	1975	1980	1985	1990
Total, 16 years and over				
Women	36,998	41,673	45,699	48,619
Men	55,615	60,000	62,903	65,220
16 to 19 years				
Women	4,038	4,226	3,762	3,649
Men	4,760	4,905	4,181	3,976
20 to 24 years				
Women	6,069	7,066	7,329	6,656
Men	7,398	8,069	7,795	6,671
25 to 54 years				
Women	21,614	24,636	28,694	32,550
Men	34,568	37,861	41,922	46,017
55 years and over				
Women	5,277	5,745	5,914	5,764
Men	8,888	9,165	9,005	8,556

Note: Actual 1975 and projected 1980, 1985, 1990

TABLE 30

Estimated Rates of Men and Women Entering the Labor Force, 1970[55]

	Total entry rate[a]		Entry rate relating to		
	Men	Women	Children reaching school age	Loss of husband	Aging
16—19	476.0	66.2	0	0	66.2
20—24	84.2	22.7	1.0	0	21.7
25—29	12.1	6.0	5.6	0.2	0.3
30—34	—	10.0	8.4	0.2	1.4
35—39	—	12.2	7.3	0.3	4.5
40—44	—	7.2	3.4	0.3	3.5
45—49	—	1.6	0.9	0.7	0
50—54	—	1.8	0	1.8	0
55—59	—	2.3	0	2.3	0
60—64	—	2.4	0	2.4	0
65—69	—	2.3	0	2.3	0
70—74	—	0.6	0	0.6	0
75—79	—	0.6	0	0	0
80—84	—	0	0	0	0
85 +	—	0	0	0	0

[a] Entries per 1000 persons in the stationary population.

TABLE 31

Estimated Rates of Men and Women Separating from the Labor Force, 1970[55]

Separation rate[a]

	Men			Women			
	Total	Due to death	Due to withdrawal	Total	Related to birth of children	Related to death	Related to aging
16—19	1.7	1.7	—	24.5	23.8	0.7	0.0
20—24	2.3	2.3	—	42.5	41.7	0.8	0.0
25—29	2.0	2.0	—	13.4	15.3	0.9	2.2
30—34	2.5	2.3	0.2	11.0	7.1	1.2	2.8
35—39	4.4	3.1	1.3	4.8	2.9	1.8	0.0
40—44	6.7	4.9	1.8	3.7	.9	2.8	0.1
45—49	11.0	7.6	3.4	15.0	.1	4.2	10.7
50—54	17.2	11.8	5.4	33.1	0	6.2	27.0
55—59	32.9	18.6	14.3	61.3	0	9.0	52.3
60—64	103.3	28.4	74.9	165.9	0	12.8	153.1
65—69	170.7	43.6	127.1	193.2	0	19.8	173.3
70—74	166.4	61.8	104.6	234.8	0	31.1	203.7
75—79	169.3	89.6	79.7	235.1	0	51.6	183.4
80—84	284.6	130.6	154.0	244.6	0	84.0	160.6
85 +				1000.0	0	354.0	646.0

[a] Separation per 1000 persons in the stationary labor force.

REFERENCES

1. **Smith, R. E.**, Sources of growth of the female labor force 1971—1975, *Mon. Labor Rev.*, 100, 27, 1977.
2. **Hunt, V. R.**, The Health of Women at Work, A Bibliography, Occasional Papers No. 2, Program on Women, Northwestern University, Evanston, Ill., 1977.
3. **Dickens, C.,** *The Uncommercial Traveller — All Year 'Round,* New Series 1(13) and (25), Chapman & Hall, London, 1861.
4. **Butler, E. B.**, *Women and the Trades Pittsburgh 1907—1908,* Russell Sage Foundation, 1909.
5. State Reporting of Occupational Disease Including a Survey of Legislation Applied to Women, Bulletin No. 114, Women's Bureau, U.S. Department of Labor, Washington, D.C., 1934.
6. Infant Mortality in New Bedford, Mass., Infant Mortality Series 10, Children's Bureau Publication 63, Children's Bureau, U.S. Department of Labor, Washington, D.C., 1920.
7. Infant Mortality in Manchester, N.H., Infant Mortality Series 6, Children's Bureau Publication 20, Children's Bureau, U.S. Department of Labor, Washington, D.C., 1917.
8. **Ross-Smith, A.,** Chronic Benzol Poisoning among Women Industrial Workers, Special Bulletin No. 150, New York, N.Y. Department of Labor, Albany, 1927.
9. A Preliminary Survey of the Industrial Hygiene Problem in the United States, Public Health Bulletin No. 259, U.S. Department of Health, Education and Welfare, Washington, D.C., 1940.
10. The Industrial Nurse and the Woman Worker, Women's Bureau, U.S. Department of Labor, Washington, D.C., 1944.
11. Handbook of Women Workers, 1962, Bulletin 285, Women's Bureau, U.S. Department of Labor, Washington, D.C., 1963.
12. Census of Population 1970, Detailed Characteristics, U.S. Summary PC (1) D 1, Bureau of the Census, U.S. Department of Commerce, Washington, D.C., 1973.
13. Census of Population 1970, Occupational Characteristics PC (2)-7A, Bureau of the Census, U.S. Department of Commerce, Washington, D.C., 1973.
14. A Statistical Report of Women in the U.S., No. 58, Bureau of the Census, U.S. Department of Commerce, Washington, D.C., 1976, 23.
15. **Grossman, A. S.**, Women in the labor force: the early years, *Mon. Labor Rev.*, 98, 3, 1975.
16. **Klein, D. P.**, Women in the labor force: the middle years, *Mon. Labor Rev.*, 98, 10, 1975.
17. **Sommers, D. and Eck, A.**, Occupational mobility in the American labor force, *Mon. Labor Rev.*, 100, 3, 1977.
18. The Occupational Safety and Health Act of 1970, 29 U.S.C. 651-678, 1970.
19. **Hunt, V. R.**, Effects of an informed work force, in Symp. Public Information on the Prevention of Occupational Cancer, December 1976, National Research Council, Washington, D.C., 1977.
20. **Bingham, E.**, Keynote Speech, in Workshop on Methodology for Assessing Reproductive Hazards in the Workplace, April 1978, Society for Occupational and Environmental Health, Washington, D.C., in press.
21. Report of the Employment of Women and Children and the Berne Conventions of 1906, *League of Nations, International Labour Conference,* Harrison & Sons, London, 1919.
22. Report of the U.N. Scientific Committee on the Effects of Atomic Radiation, Ionizing Radiation Levels and Effects, Vol. 1, United Nations, New York, 1972.
23. U.S. Department of Health, Education, and Welfare, National Center for Health Statistics, Advance Report, Final Mortality Statistis, 1975, Monthly Vital Statistics Report, (HRA) 77-1120, 25, 11 (Suppl). Washington, 1977.
24. **Goldsmith, J. R.**, Mortality and industrial employment, *J. Occup. Med.,* 19, 249, 1977.
25. Characteristics of American Children and Youth, Current Population Reports, Special Studies Series P-23, No. 66, Bureau of the Census, U.S. Department of Commerce, Washington, D.C., 1976.
26. Employment and Earnings, Labor Force by Age, 1976, Bureau of Labor Statistics, U.S. Department of Labor, Washington, D.C., 1977.
27. **Blake, J.**, Demographic science and the redirection of population policy, *J. Chron. Dis.*, 18, 1181, 1965.
28. **Collver, O. A.**, Women's work participation and fertility in metropolitan areas, *Demography,* 5, 55, 1968.
29. **Sklar, J. and Berkov, B.**, The American birth-rate: evidences of a coming rise, *Science*, 189, 693, 1975.
30. Current Population Reports, Fertility of American Women: June 1977, Series P-20, No. 316, U.S. Department of Commerce, Washington, D.C., 1977.

31. **Undry, J. R. and Huyck, E. E., Eds.** *Workshop on the Demographic Evaluation of Domestic Family Planning Programs,* Ballinger, Cambridge, Mass., 1975.

32. Employment During Pregnancy, Legitimate Live Births U.S. 1963, PHS Publ. No. 1000, Series 22, No. 7, National Center for Health Statistics, U.S. Department of Health, Education and Welfare, Washington, D.C., 1968.

33. Pregnant Workers in the United States, Advance Data No. 11, National Center for Health Statistics, U.S. Department of Health, Education and Welfare, Washington, D.C., 1977.

34. **Michelotti, K.,** Educational attainment of workers. March, 1976, *Mon. Labor Rev.,* 100, 62, 1977.

35. Center for Disease Control. Reported Number of Legal Abortions by State of Occurrence, 1975, Morbidity and Mortality Weekly Rep. No. 25, U.S. Department of Health, Education and Welfare, Atlanta, 1977, 39.

36. The Incidence of Sterilization following Delivery of Legitimate Live Births in Hospitals in the United States, Monthly Vital Statistics Report 26, No. 6 Suppl., U.S. Department of Health, Education and Welfare, Washington, D.C., 1977.

37. New Labor Force Projections for 1990, Special Labor Force Report 197, Bureau of Labor Statistics, U.S. Department of Labor, Washington, D.C., 1976.

38. **Presser, H. B.,** *Sterilization and Fertility Decline in Puerto Rico,* University of California Press, Berkeley, 1973.

39. Current Population Reports, Population Characteristics Series, P-20, No. 277, U.S. Department of Commerce.

40. Vital Statistics of the United States, Vol. 1, Natality, National Center for Health Statistics, U.S. Department of Health, Education and Welfare, Washington, D.C., 1976.

41. Statistical Indices of Family Health, Tech. Rep. Ser. No. 587, World Health Organization, Geneva, 1976.

42. **Andersen, R.,** A Behavior Model of Families Use of Health Activities Center of Health Administration Studies, Research Series No. 25, Graduate School of Business University of Chicago, 1968.

43. **Clark, F. L.,** *Women, Work and Age,* The Nuffield Foundation, London, 1962.

44. **Raphael, E. and Gillaspy, T.,** Population Redistribution and Industrial Change in a Non-Metropolitan Labor Force, Pennsylvania, 1940-1970, NIH-NICHD-72-2743, U.S. Department of Health, Education and Welfare, Washington, D.C., 1974.

45. Hypertension, United States, 1974, Advanced Data, Vol. 2, National Center for Health Statistics, U.S. Department of Health, Education and Welfare, Washington, D.C., 1976.

46. Prevalence of Chronic Skin and Musculoskeletal Conditions — U.S. 1969, PHS Publ. No. 1000, Ser., 10, No. 92, National Center for Health Statistics, U.S. Department of Health, Education and Welfare, Washington, D.C., 1974.

47. Prevalence of Chronic Circulatory Conditions, U.S. 1972, PHS Publ. No. 1000, Series 10, No. 94, National Center for Health Statistics, U.S. Department of Health, Education and Welfare, Washington, D.C., 1974.

48. Limitation of Activity due to Chronic Conditions, U.S. 1974, (HRA) 77-1537, Health Resources Administration, U.S. Department of Health, Education and Welfare, Washington, D.C., 1977.

49. United States National Commission on State Workmen's Compensation Laws, Report, Washington, D.C., July 1972.

50. Too Little, Too Late. The Economic Plight of Very Seriously and Permanently Disabled Men and their Households in the New York City Metropolitan Area, Vol. 2, U.S. National Commission on State Workmen's Compensation Laws, Washington, D.C., 1973.

51. Serious Industrial Injuries and Worker Earnings in Florida, U.S. National Commission on State Workmen's Compensation Laws, Washington, D.C., 1973.

52. Sources of Information about Workmen's Compensation Recipients, U.S. National Commission on State Workmens Compensation Laws, Washington, D.C., 1973.

53. Makarushka, J. L., Workers' compensation: The long-term consequences of work-related injury for women, in Proc. Conf. Women and the Workplace, Society for Occupational and Environmental Health, Washington, D.C., 1977.

54. **Haber, L. D.,** Disabling effects of chronic disease, Impairment II, *J. Chron. Dis.,* 26, 127, 1973.

55. **Grossman, A. S.,** The labor force patterns of divorced and separated women, *Mon. Labor Rev.,* 100, 48, 1977.

56. Length of Working Life for Men and Women, 1970, Special Labor Force Report, Bureau of Labor Statistics, U.S. Department of Labor, Washington, D.C. , 1976, 187.

Chapter 2

ERGONOMICS

I. INTRODUCTION

Just as the biochemistry of the human body limits our tolerance to toxic substances, physiological characteristics govern the range of human interaction with the physical conditions of the workplace. Temperature, noise, vibration, illumination, machine design, and materials handling must be within the range of human tolerance and the ergonomics literature deals extensively with the work conditions which can be considered optimal. In some areas of ergonomics there has been — in contrast to other occupational health areas — a consideration of women workers, particularly in regard to body mechanics, maximum work capacity, and temperature tolerance.

The current status of ergonomics research has been well summarized by Dukes-Dubos.[1] A diversity of disciplines has contributed to the evaluation of human anatomical, physiological, and psychological characteristics and their interaction with the work environment. Human factors engineering, biomedical engineering, and biomechanics have been research areas for physiologists, physicists, engineers, and social and behavioral scientists.

In 1971 Henschel presented to the annual meeting of the American Conference of Governmental Industrial Hygienists a summary overview of the role of women in industry.[2] His balanced evaluation of sex differences from the applied physiology perspective was the first following the passage of the Occupational Safety and Health Act but unfortunately received little notice because of his limited audience. The related implication of Title VII of the Civil Rights Act of 1964 was the impetus for his consideration of maximum work capacity, heat tolerance, response to toxic substances, and the physiologic changes of pregnancy. He concluded his comments with: "In spite of the evidence on differences in responses to stress, history has proved women capable of successfully meeting the challenges of the environment and of competing with men in most real life situations. The fact that they have a longer life expectancy attests to their adaptive capacities. In our world of constant change, adaptability is the key to survival. And it is beyond doubt and question that the changes today in law and custom will only contribute to womens continued progress in the industrial world."

The full range of human adaptability may well be the key concept in the critical area of ergonomics, particularly when women workers are being evaluated in relation to their work environment and where we can usually only rely on empirical studies of experienced workers. Currently, possible changes in women's work capacity can only be indirectly examined in light of studies in exercise physiology.

II. FUNCTIONAL STRENGTH

Chaffin's[4] extensive research on human strength capability, particularly in relation to low back pain has included women. Low back pain usually stems from discogenic disorders and is one of the leading causes of hospitalization and work incapacitation. It ranks with upper respiratory problems as a major cause of lost work days and for those whose work involves heavy labor the duration of disability is longest. The majority of people, as high as 70% (presumably reported for industrialized societies),

TABLE 1

Predicted Standard Strengths for Various Cases of Stature, Body Weight, Gender, and Age[4]

Age (years)	Height (ft)	Male Body Weight (lb)		Female Torso Strength	
		100	200	100	200
20	5	75.3	128.8	50.3	78.8
	6	88.5	155.2[a]	63.5	105.3
50	5	56.4	91.0	31.4[b]	41.1
	6	69.6	117.5	44.6	67.5
			Arm Strength		
20	5	72.5	88.3	41.2	55.9
	6	76.8	96.7[a]	44.4	64.3
50	5	64.6	72.4	32.3[b]	40.0
	6	68.8	80.8	36.5	48.4
			Leg Strength		
20	5	117.5	226.9	82.4	131.8
	6	187.4	246.7[a]	92.2	151.5
50	5	151.7	175.4	56.6[b]	80.2
	6	156.5	184.8	61.3	89.7

[a] Maximum.
[b] Minimum.

suffer low back pain at some time in their lives. The symptoms may be episodic, recurring every 3 months to 3 years, and are only rarely associated with an identifiable activity which precipitated the episode. Because identification of cause is so difficult, low back pain cannot be usually labeled as an "injury", but reflects the physical activity of the high-risk population. Chaffin et al. followed the weekly medical status of 551 new workers who were strength tested in an isometric simulation of individual jobs.[4,5] Physical stress evaluations were made for 103 different jobs. Standardized Position Strength Tests were used without any emotional appeals being directed to the subjects and were carried out in an industrial setting. Gender, age, weight, and stature were found to be very poor predictors of those at risk to back pain and injury, though these characteristics are important in determining population average strengths. When the Standard Position Strength Test was used, the mean strength of these working women was about 58% of the men, and the skewed distribution showed a modal value of 26 pounds for women which was 65% of the 40-pound modal value for men. Scandinavian and English studies have reported similar comparisons of the isometric muscle strength of women and men,[7,8] though Nordgren observed more pronounced sex differences in muscle strength in the upper extremities than in the lower extremities.[10] Table 1 shows the observed distribution of arm, leg, and torso lifting strength for 105 women and 446 men from Chaffin's study. The results are standardized for age, height, and body weight and, therefore, indicate lower average strengths and variability of strengths (between individuals) for the female population in relation to the male population. The jobs having increased incident rates of low back pain were those with the heaviest loads to be lifted, even occasionally. Those jobs with more frequent lifting of maximum loads on the job were associated with higher frequency and severity rates of musculoskeletal problems, other than back incidents and more severe contact injuries. More frequent and severe musculoskeletal problems resulted when the load center of gravity was remote from the body. The need for individual strength testing was confirmed by the observation that when the job was more physically demanding than the worker's relative strength, the extent of tissue damage in the back was more severe or the worker could not quickly return to the job. Although more epidemiologic investigation was suggested, it is apparent from the data presented that occasional heavy physical exertions can be as damaging as more frequent exertions when a person is lifting and moving loads close to her maximum strength. Chaffin et al.[4] emphasize that appropriate job placement based on well-controlled strength testing of all individuals and evaluation of the strength requirements of the jobs they are to perform is the best protection for all workers, given the high risk experienced by workers in materials handling jobs. Objective testing of a person's strength in relation to the job avoids indiscriminate placement of workers ill-suited to the task to be performed. There are few occupational conditions where individual characteristics can be so well defined in relation to risk, and further accumulation of epidemiologic data and refinement of testing techniques appear to be the best approaches for the protection of women and men, who are comparably vulnerable to adverse effect when mismatching of their strength to task load occurs.[4,5]

High compression forces impact on the lower lumbar discs when a load is manually lifted, and a weight of 100 lb held at forearm length in front of the body acts as a compressive force of 1400 to 1500 lb on the lower lumbar spine. For those with less massive skeletal mass than the average male, the spine compression capability and force-bearing area may be smaller by 15 to 20% so that the anatomical realities are an integral part of "occupational biomechanics."[11]

Unfortunately, very few efforts have been directed to the needs of women in jobs where lifting involves human loads, that is, in nursing and child care. Matching of the individual to the job is based on criteria other than strength and different means must therefore be used to reduce the risk of harm. Far more innovative approaches need to be introduced into the hospital setting particularly and the human services area generally, in that new design and refitting of hospitals is not going to be done in the immediate or even near future. Improved individual concern for health workers, better supervision, and team work are necessary to prevent individuals reaching beyond their strength limit in the many critical situations that arise in a day's work. The routine availability of physical therapy, physical training, and relaxation programs to hospital staff, for example, could go a long way in lessening the effects of unavoidable physical stress.

Snook and Ciriello[9] have examined the maximum weights and work loads acceptable to female workers. Thirty-one women, including 16 "housewives" and 15 who were second shift workers from a local industry (not identified in terms of chemical exposure conditions), were tested for six basic manual handling tasks — lifting, lowering, pushing, pulling, carrying, and walking. The authors again point out that the manual handling of materials is the principal source (23% in 1973) of compensable work injuries. The associated accidents also contribute to aggravation of existing disorders and are an indicator of the mismatch between the strength and endurance the worker brings to the job and the demands of manual handling tasks.

Statistically significant performance differences were observed for nonemployed and industrial women, and the authors speculate on "whether industrial women handle more weight than housewives because they can handle more weight." The maximum weight (force) acceptable to the nonemployed women was 25% less than for industrial women and we can at least infer that in one parameter, acceptable work load, the female industrial work force differs from nonemployed women, a difference that may well be associated with other physiologic parameters not examined in these studies. The average maximum weight acceptable to industrial women for lifting, lowering, and carrying tasks was 65% that for industrial men, which is the same result obtained by Chaffin and other investigators.[4] However, for pushing and pulling tasks it was 85% of that for industrial men, which confirms Nordgren's[8] observations of the sex differences in muscle strength for upper and lower extremities. For walking and 7-ft sustained pulling tasks the industrial women performed at 100% of the male work load. The American Industrial Hygiene Association's Guide to Manual Lifting[10] suggests for extrapolation that strength of the female worker be considered 70% of the male worker, based on European studies, primarily Scandinavian and performed in a laboratory setting. It will be particularly important that a continuing evaluation of women's strength be maintained as the female work force becomes more heterogeneous in terms of physical conditioning. If the recent increase in physical activity of American women continues with the encouragement of the enforcement of Title IX of the Civil Rights Act, it is unlikely that the relationship of 70% for female to male strength measures will remain constant. However, it is also apparent that the reality of individual anatomical and physiological characteristics must be taken into account for men and women carrying out manual materials handling.

Brown's epidemiologic approach involved a questionnaire survey in Canada which elicited information on factors related to causes of low back pain.[11] A large proportion of the women in the study were hospital workers so that the reported higher prevalence of back injuries when compared with men is not surprising. However, the study does not provide sufficient demographic data to allow a detailed critique of the results. Although there were 509 responses from 1000 workers, there is no tabulation of the number of women in the final sample. The results are presented as percentages with no statistical analysis so that it is not possible to draw firm conclusions based on the author's evaluation of his data. One could conclude that the worker's compensation system in Canada may have similar characteristics to that in the United States when 25% of the males and 6% of the females with back injuries received worker's compensation, although back injuries were more frequently reported by women.

Kelsey et al. in a preliminary study have examined the syndrome of herniated lumbar intervertebral disc in relation to pregnancy and have found that the more live births a woman has, the more likely she is to have a subsequent disc herniation.[12] No difference was observed in relation to the total number of pregnancies (including miscarriages). Women with herniated discs at the lumbar 5 level averaged 3.09 live births compared to 1.91 among their controls. For the lumbar 4 level, the number of live births was more comparable, 2.58 vs. 2.33 in their matched controls. Although dealing with a small population, the case control study has been done with statistical care and identifies the epidemiological limitations. The mechanical stress from carrying the fetus and the extent of the ligamentous laxity which develops as a result of relaxin derived from the corpus luteum toward the end of pregnancy are both important areas for further examination. In addition, behavioral and sociologic factors are involved in parental care of children in terms of the amount and kind of child lifting by father and mother. Men with and without the syndrome appear to have the same number of children. From Kelsey's study, it seems more likely that pregnancy itself is the important risk factor rather than the stress of child care alone, though the fact that the two factors are frequently combined during a woman's reproductive life must be remembered. In an earlier report, Kelsey had concluded that there was little evidence in the population under study that lifting on their jobs increased the risk of herniated lumbar discs in women.[13] People in sedentary occupations with prolonged sitting were at highest risk of acute herniated lumbar intervertebral discs, which did not exclude the contribution of lifting on the job as a precipitating event. However, the past work history was not included in the data analysis so that it is likely, in view of the high proportion of workers with episodic low back pain, that earlier experience and medical advice had led to a change to sedentary work some time before the eventual development of the herniated lumbar intervertebral disc.[4]

Diddle has commented on changes in posture during pregnancy and noted that the center of gravity for the average nonpregnant woman, when standing, falls through the instep of the foot.[14] Near the end of pregnancy, it falls through the base of the big toe. In the last trimester, the pregnant woman tends to throw her shoulders back and arch her spinal column forward in the lumbosacral region in order to maintain an upright posture. Presumably, a similar but more gradual adaptation occurs in men with the continuing deposition of excess abdominal adipose tissue through middle age and later.

One of the few studies directed to a particular female intensive occupation has been done through the Federal Aviation Administration on the functional strength of commercial airline stewardesses (now called flight attendants).[15] The authors note that pilots and flight engineers "have been studied in great detail from abdominal girth to zygotic selection."[15,16] However, the engineering design data for cabin and galley design have come from anthropometric studies of World War II Wafs, who were shorter, heavier, and possibly stronger than present-day airline attendants. Strength tests were designed for the study to be appropriate for comparison with flight activities and involved maximal static forces that flight attendants generally employ at various work levels. Isometric strength measurements were a leg lift (25 cm from floor), a back lift (50 cm from floor), an arm lift (100 cm from floor), and a push (110 cm from floor). Anthropometrically, these airline attendants were taller and lighter than the U.S. female population and the WAF population, not a surprising observation given their age and selection criteria.

Tables 2 through 5 provide the summary of values. It is noteworthy that 9.2% (14 women) did not participate in the back lift because of recent back injuries or other back problems. These data provide a good basis for evaluation of other occupational categories where the workers are experienced in the maneuvers under study. The emphasis was on maximum voluntary strength of the flight attendant, not maximum force which could be exerted under stress, as in the event of flight emergencies.

The occupations of flight attendant and nurse share the problem of a double standard in the job specification. A high level of constant physical activity must be maintained as part of the normal work flow but, additionally, there is the expectation that under emergency conditions the nurse and flight attendant can perform to maximum physical effort. Legal decisions have now been made concerning pregnant airline attendants' capacity for maximum physical effort though comparable considerations have not yet been directed to nurses, although it is a frequent practice for them to work during pregnancy.

The research on work and exercise physiology provides the basis for our understanding of the few data which have been systematically accumulated on women in the industrial sector. One of the most critical needs is an evaluation of the effects of physical conditioning and experience. It is not surprising that the nonemployed women in Snook's study showed considerably less strength for the same tasks performed by industrial women. There is a far larger body of data on physical conditioning available on female athletes than can be found for workers. Hanson and Nedde[17] in a study of the long-term physical training effect on sedentary women, reviewed earlier studies

TABLE 2

Summary Statistics for the Leg Lift for Flight Attendants[12]

Strength measures	Number of subjects	Mean	Standard deviation	Minimum	Maximum
Average plateau (1b)	149	111.4	33.85	47.3	213.1
Maximum force (1b)	150	130.9	35.44	55.0	253.0
Pulse (lb/sec)	149	103.7	30.38	46.2	200.2

TABLE 3

Summary Statistics for the Back Lift for Flight Attendants[12]

Strength measures	Number	Mean	Standard deviation	Minimum	Maximum
Average plateau (lb)	138	144.7	43.85	62.7	257.3
Maximum force (lb)	138	163.3	47.89	63.8	285.3
Pulse (lb/sec)	138	129.1	39.19	64.2	219.2

TABLE 4

Summary Statistics for the Arm Lift for Flight Attendants[12]

Strength measures	Number	Mean	Standard deviation	Minimum	Maximum
Average plateau (lb)	152	78.8	21.95	31.4	165.7
Maximum force (lb)	152	90.3	24.13	24.7	172.2
Pulse (lb/sec)	152	74.6	21.07	28.7	154.9

TABLE 5

Summary Statistics for the Push for Flight Attendants[12]

Strength measures	Number	Mean	Standard deviation	Minimum	Maximum
Average plateau (lb)	152	66.7	17.82	30.0	128.0
Maximum peak force (lb)	122	97.1	25.68	50.3	177.5
Time to peak (sec)	122	0.42	1.32	0.05	9.4
Pulse (lb/sec)	152	65.6	16.29	27.8	124.3

though they are few. Of these few reports on the effects of physical training on women, all but one (which covered only a 2-month period) showed significant improvement in cardiorespiratory function. The study by Hanson and Nedde of eight previously sedentary women showed progressive improvement in the physiologic efficiency of completing constant treadmill work loads over an 8-month period as well as overall increased ergometric work capacities.

The social acceptance of a sedentary lifestyle for women has been institutionalized in the U.S. public school system, which until enforcement of Title IX of the Civil Rights Act in 1976—77 provided minimal financial resources and encouragement for athletic activities for female students through their junior and senior high school years.

TABLE 6

Maximum Work Load (30 U.S. College Women)[17]

	Maximum ventilation (ℓ/min ± 1 SD)[a]	Oxygen uptake (ℓ/min)
Swedish	76.2	2.23
U.S.		
Test 1	41.9 ± 9.9	2.10 ± 0.12
Test 2	45.2 ± 3.7	2.00 ± 0.22

[a] Standard deviation.

Even the most affluent communities, which supported extensive intra- and intermural sports programs for boys to compete in wrestling, football, and basketball, confined their financial support for girls to a few cheerleaders. The systematic exclusion of women from sports programs continued into the college years until Title IX requirements completely altered the social climate and attitudes of young women and men toward physical activity. The sedentary woman may not remain the norm much longer. It seems possible that in the U.S. a new wave of women with maximum physical capacity somewhat in excess of that shown by their older sisters and mothers when they entered the work force is soon likely to appear. Although predictions of this nature must by their very nature be uncertain, it is all the more necessary to develop a good research climate in the U.S. for studies of physical conditioning and maximum work capacity of women.

The major source of data on women has come from Scandinavia[18,19] where the attitude toward physical activity differs markedly from that in the U.S. It is of interest then that Hanson and Nedde noted significant psychologic alterations in the American subjects. Self-satisfaction and self-acceptance increased, perception of physical self improved, sense of personal worth and adequacy increased, adequacy in social interaction improved, and the overall level of self-esteem and self-confidence increased over the 8-month period of training. Work testing with a bicycle ergometer showed that work capacity prior to reaching a pulse rate of 170 per minute increased 19% after the first 4 months of training, in addition to a 31% increase in minute volume of ventilation, 33% increase in oxygen uptake, and 24% increase in carbon dioxide production. Minute volume of ventilation and oxygen uptake were also increased at 50% and 25% of the work load at a pulse rate of 170 per minute. Treadmill walking improved markedly in 4 months so that all subjects could complete the 12-degree treadmill walk at a group mean heart rate of 163 per minute compared to 171 per minute for the pretraining 8-degree walk.

The greater research interest in Sweden and Norway on work capacity of women has lead to comparisons with U.S. women. Michael and Horvath[20] tested 30 American college students who participated in "normal college activities and recreational sports, but were not involved in any strenuous physical conditioning programs," a modest description of the expectations concerning physical activity for U.S. women of the mid-sixties. When compared with Swedish women, also untrained, the U.S. college women reached average maximal heart rate levels of 184 beats per minute, a value comparable to other studies of women in Sweden and the U.S. However, their average maximal ventilation was considerably lower (Table 6) and oxygen uptake was also less. One explanation suggested by Michael and Horvath was that the American women were unaccustomed to hyperventilation and therefore psychological factors could be just as important as physiological constraints in affecting maximum work capacity.

The ventilatory equivalent, i.e., ventilation in liters per minute per liters of oxygen per minute, was considerably less in U.S. women (27 vs. 34 in Swedish women), which may indicate that the U.S. women were more efficient at their maximal levels or that they did not ever reach their true maximal physical capacity. When body weight was taken into account, earlier observations by Buskirk and Taylor[21] were confirmed, that in sedentary persons oxygen uptake per kilogram body weight is not an indicator of maximal oxygen uptake. The Michael and Horvath study had an important limitation in that no submaximal ventilatory measurements were made, so that predictions of maximal work capacity were not certain.[20] Therefore, their observation that low maximal oxygen uptake measurements in sedentary women were the result of less movement of air into the lungs is not conclusive. However, it is well known that hyperventilation in trained subjects, e.g., swimmers, runners, and gymnasts, is a far more psychologically acceptable maneuver than it is for sedentary individuals.

Astrand has shown that after 12 years of age the oxygen requirement per kilogram body weight at submaximal exercise is similar for men and women[18] For maximal effort, however, the oxygen requirement per kilogram body weight in women was lower by 17% than that in men. The maximal heart rate of both sexes at a given age is similar, but during submaximal work the heart rate of women is considerably higher.

Bar-or and Buskirk note that there has been far less emphasis placed on research into the circulatory responses of women to exercise when compared with the research on men.[22] Astrand's extensive studies on Swedish women over a long time period have not be emulated in the U.S., except for the many unpublished and often inacessible master's theses which have described discrete studies of physical activity in women.

Dhesi and Firebaugh have recorded heart rates during various stages of making chapatis, the flat unleavened bread eaten in India. They are made two or three times a day in Indian homes and the process may take 30 to 90 min with the woman in the squatting position.[23] However, Dhesi's study was done in the U.S. observing five Indian women in a laboratory setting. The heart rate was significantly increased in three stages of the work which involved a change from the normal squatting position. Postural changes occurred during the process of chapati making and were measured by angles of body position. Knee bending significantly affected the heart rate, due to pressure on blood vessels and nerves in the posterior part of the leg. It is evident from Dhesi's study that ill-defined domestic and other work tasks can be readily examined in terms of heart rate, a potentially useful approach to evaluation of women's work.

A good example of collaboration between a nutritionist and an anthropologist is the more sophisticated study of technological change and caloric cost in Brazilian sisal agriculture.[24] The extent to which the projected minimal daily caloric requirement could be met was estimated from direct household observation of food intake and work activity. In two households, both parents needs were being met, but for the children only a little over one half of the minimum daily caloric requirement was available. The development of further studies of comparable quality in other parts of the world would be of considerable use in understanding relationships between work activity and caloric intake in a variety of environments and economic contexts.

III. MENSTRUATION AND PHYSICAL ACTIVITY

There has been much general commentary on changes in physical performance during menstruation but only a few formal published studies on patterns of maximum efficiency during the menstrual cycle. The topic appears to have been popular among master's degree candidates in schools of education where theses unfortunately do not frequently reach publication. An early study by Hollingsworth showed no recurring patterns of maximum efficiency during the menstrual cycle and she concluded that variability in performance was not attributable to physiological changes.[25] The use of pulse rate as a measure of physical efficiency, although better standardized by Astrand in the fifties, was a reliable indicator for the development of the Tuttle Pulse Ratio test.[26] Scott and Tuttle tested 100 women at different periods of time in the menstrual cycle: (1) premenstrual, 3 days before the onset of flow; (2) menstrual, the second day of the flow; (3) postmenstrual, 3 days following the cessation of flow; and (4) intermenstrual, 12 days following cessation of flow. They concluded, on the basis of no observed significant fluctuations in pulse rate between the four stages measured, that there was no cyclic pattern of physical efficiency associated with the menstrual cycle. Other indicators were examined by Phillips who measured steadiness, reaction and movement times, blood pressure, and heart rate during the period before menstrual flow, after menstrual flow, and during the intermenstrual period.[27] There were no significant differences between the test periods in 24 subjects who had a history of normal menstruation. Phillips also evaluated heart rate during and following strenuous physical activity throughout the menstrual cycle.[25] Twenty-eight subjects rode a bicycle ergometer for 5 min at the same time of day. There was no statistically significant difference in heart rate changes during and following strenuous activity throughout the menstrual cycle. A wider array of tests which included a step test, maximum grip strength, pull-ups, Sargent Jump Test, and a 100-yard shuttle run were related to the menstrual and intermenstrual period in 54 women by Rockwell.[28] The Sargent Jump Test and the 100-yard run scores showed higher values, which were statistically significant during the intermenstrual period. However, the variability of test scores for each individual precluded a specific conclusion concerning differences during the menstrual cycle.

Other measures used have been static balance, leg lift strength, back lift strength, and explosive power. Auster's study of 32 college women with a history of normal menstruation showed greater stability in performance during the menstrual phase when compared with the intermenstrual phase.[29] There appeared to be an increase in measures of grip strength, and leg and back lift strength during the intermenstrual phase, but the differences were not statistically significant. There were no observed differences in balancing or explosive power tests. Doolittle and Engebretsen[30] found no statistically significant variation among standard physical fitness tests in terms of skill or speed in any phase of the menstrual cycle. Wearing et al.,[31] however, reported postmenstrual improvement in performance for a variety of tests involving stationary steadiness, total body movement time, and strength tests. Hunter[32] has reviewed additional studies concerned with reaction time and its possible relationship to performance decrement and concluded that these studies were also in conflict.

The conflicting evidence coming from many reports indicates that physical performance and efficiency probably do not fluctuate markedly with different stages of the menstrual cycle, though it must be acknowledged that it is difficult to establish the sensitivity of the studies reported and the biases which may have been introduced. Sommer,[33] in a recent review of the literature, concluded that most objective measures of performance in athletics or those using reasoning tests do not show an impairment associated with the menstrual cycle. Ruble's study in 1977[34] of psychosocial factors provides evidence that may explain some of the uncertainty which stems from apparently conflicting results. She concluded that psychosocial factors can influence menstrual related symptoms so that data derived from self-report questionnaires are likely to be biased. She was able to separate experimentally women's perceptions of their cycle phase from the actual cycle phase and identified an exaggeration of naturally fluctuating bodily states, e.g., discomfort and water retention when a woman believed

TABLE 7

Mean Duration of 40% Maximum Voluntary Contraction During the Menstrual Cycle in 7 Women[33]

	Number of women	Preovulatory phase (sec)	Luteal phase (sec)
Oral contraceptive use	3	200	168
No oral contraceptive use	4	117	114

she was premenstrual. The importance of psychosocial factors in a woman's perception of her menstrual cycle must be more closely evaluated when the physiological basis for menstrual related changes is being examined.

The effect of oral contraceptives on isometric strength and endurance has been examined by Petrofsky et al.[35] A series of five fatiguing isometric contractions at a tension of 40% of maximum voluntary contraction was measured in seven healthy young women, three of whom had been taking oral contraceptives. The isometric endurance in the women not taking oral contraceptives varied sinusoidally during the menstrual cycle, with peak endurance midway through the ovulatory phase and the lowest endurance midway through the luteal phase. In contrast, for women taking oral contraceptives the isometric endurance did not vary during their menstrual cycle. There is no readily obvious explanation for the fluctuations observed in the former group, particularly when the response became hyperbolic with the maximal endurance at the beginning and end of the cycle when there was stabilization of muscle temperature by immersion of the forearm in water at 37°C. The authors concluded that at least two factors must influence isometric endurance during the menstrual cycle in women not taking oral contraceptives. Of these two factors, one may be dominant over the influence of muscle temperature which is affected by the variations in core temperature and thermoregulatory function during the menstrual cycle.[34] Isometric strength was unaltered during the menstrual cycle in both groups. The design of this study developed out of earlier observations by Petrofsky et al.[37] on men and women from 20 to 60 years of age. They reported that young women (20 to 29 years old) show less strength but greater endurance than men of the same age and also experience less cardiovascular response to fatiguing static effort. By about 60 years of age the differences in strength and endurance are more pronounced and are particularly evident in women after menopause. Fluctuations in sex hormone levels might therefore be expected to influence muscular performance. The observation is therefore of some interest that isometric endurance of women taking oral contraceptives did not vary either under conditions when forearm temperature varied as a function of the ambient temperature or when stabilized by immersion of the forearm in water at 37°C. The endurance of those taking oral contraceptives was considerably less than those who did not, though the difference was modified when the forearm was immersed in water at 37°C (Table 7).

Athletic performance of women has been of more research interest to European physiologists and Noack has commented on the history of "functional" gynecology and its relationship to sport from the early part of the century and the participation of women athletes in the Olympic Games, beginning in 1928.[38] He showed that there was a clear premenstrual minimum for ball tossing and weight lifting in 21 women who were tested 4 days before menses, on the second menstrual day, and 4 days later. Similar responses were seen in 15 rowers who depend more on large muscle masses. Performance improved during menstruation and further following menstruation. Runners (100 and 600 m) showed a different pattern which appeared to be related to their physical training. In highly trained runners the worst performance was during menstruation, but for those not specially trained the worst performance occurred during the postmenstrual phase.

It is evident from all the studies that any fluctuations in physical efficiency during the menstrual cycle must be quite modest and the best indicators may be highly trained athletes in whom slight differences may be discernible and sufficient for establishing the presence of a true effect.

Bausenwein has reported observations on well-trained athletes at the Helsinki Olympic Games in 1952, particularly in relation to modified menstrual cycles and age of menarche.[39] Swimmers and gymnasts developed irregular cycles during training as did most of the very active athletes, but few had any menstrual discomfort. Harris recently commented on these changes in a national woman's sports magazine and there was a widespread response from women in training for a variety of sports also identifying cessation of menses when there was low body fat and high physical activity.[40]

Bausenwein also noted that mean menarcheal age was considerably later in physically trained adolescents.[39] The mean menarcheal age in competitive swimmers was 14.98 and 19% of them experienced menarche between 16 and 18. It is well known that menarcheal age has decreased for many years in America. The change has been attributed largely to improved nutritional status. It is possible that reduced physical activity during adolescence over the past 30 or 40 years could be a contributing factor and with the return to higher physical activity rates in young women the trend could change. In that the phenomenon of a relationship between physical activity and modifications in the menstrual cycle has received such little attention from gynecologists, physiologists, and endocrinologists, we have no knowledge concerning the possibility that changes might affect subsequent reproduction adversely, advantageously, or not at all.

The entry of women into physically demanding jobs could also result in reports of menstrual cycle changes, though it seems that only a few physically demanding occupations such as some forms of waitressing, airline work, nursing, and manufacturing would provide sufficient physical stress to result in some extreme physical conditioning.

At least one menstrual myth has been recently put to rest. Miller has explored a North American folktale which "holds that the odor of human menses excites stallions, making them aggressive and even violent."[41] He questioned eight women experienced in the handling of breeding stallions and was satisfied from their responses to his questions that there was no evidence at all to support the belief. Given the inherent danger of the jobs associated with the care of breeding stallions and the improved opportunities for women to work with horses, Miller's report is positive and appropriate.

IV. EFFECTS OF PHYSICAL ACTIVITY ON PREGNANCY

Efforts of the Children's Bureau to ameliorate maternal and infant mortality in the U.S. from 1912 to the mid-twenties lead to reports of the effects of employment of the mother on infant mortality, but little comment on the maternal experience itself.[42,43] Baetjer summarized the available literature to 1944 and noted only a few conflicting reports on the different pregnancy experience and outcome for those standing or sitting at work, all of them associated with the textile industry, a notoriously adverse environment for maintenance of health, whether pregnant or not.[44] Indeed there appears to be no substantive historical source of information on the effects of well-described physical activity at work on pregnancy outcome in situations where there are no other adverse associated conditions.

The most extreme physical stress is experienced by Olympic participants, and there has always been an interest in the relationship between high physical performance and its effects on pregnancy and childbirth. Zaharieva has described the experience in Bulgaria of Olympic participants from 1952 (when Bulgarian women first entered the Olympic Games) to 1972.[44] A total of 150 athletes were followed during the first phase of pregnancy, at delivery, and postpartum and included 27 Olympic participants and finalists for selection. The comparisons were made with 59 "masters of sports" and 64 "first-grade" athletes. It is apparent that demanding sports activity and childbearing are compatible. Of those who married, 94% had children before or after their participation in the Olympic Games and often in association with active training programs. Eighty-five percent became pregnant during the first 2 years of marriage and there were no miscarriages due to training. The period of delivery was shorter for all athletes compared with nonathletes, particularly the second stage of labor. More perineal rupture was found among the Olympic athletes (47%). No complications in the separation of the placenta were observed. Mastitis in the postpartum period was noted in 22.2% of the Olympic participants, a much higher prevalence than in the other athletes. Lactation continued for 7 to 9 months after delivery and during regular training. One effect of training appeared to be a reduction in lactation in 18.5% of the Olympians, comparable to earlier observations on other athletes. Resumption of competitive sports was usual within the 8 months following delivery. The Olympic athletes, with the exception of only one individual, all improved in physical fitness, increased stamina, and improved technical skill following childbirth. Zaharieva's observations on a highly selected, healthy group of women support the view that physical activity, even when extreme, does not itself jeopardize women's childbearing capacities when nutrition and medical care are adequate.

Dahlstrom and Irhman have dealt extensively with the physical work capacity of pregnant women and disagree with earlier reports claiming that the capacity for physical work diminishes during pregnancy.[46] Indeed, Irhman of that team suggests that the circulatory adjustment during pregnancy resembles in some respects the changes during physical training, with increases in the total amount of hemoglobin, the total blood volume, and the heart volume.[47] Dahlstrom and Irhman examined pulse frequency and cardiopulmonary reactions as indicators of work capacity in 50 pregnant women during the course of a year and reviewed the earlier literature comparing pregnant and nonpregnant women. They concluded that although studies in the thirties, usually using modified step tests, reported diminished capacity for physical work, more reliable results came from later studies which used measurements during work. When the bicycle ergometer was used, reduced physical working capacity was not confirmed. Dahlstrom and Irhman, using the bicycle ergometer, showed that at rest the pulse frequency was about 10 beats per minute higher than the mean value throughout the year for nonpregnant women, and during pregnancy there was a slight increase in pulse frequency, with a decrease after delivery. Their measure of physical work capacity using the bicycle ergometer showed values considerably higher in the 36th week of pregnancy when compared with earlier pregnancy, with a reduction a few days after delivery but a return to early pregnancy levels 2 months after delivery. However, the authors state that the physical work capacity overall remains fairly constant during pregnancy, with constant pulse and respiratory frequencies at rest and during work.[46] They noted that there was no decrease in physical working capacity with age in their pregnant women, the values being unchanged or increasing. Their explanation was based on physical conditioning of older women due to their walking and bicycling practices in earlier years. Associated with this experience was an increase in body weight, total amount of hemoglobin, total blood volume, and heart volume with age, which they viewed as improved physical fitness with increasing age during the child-bearing years. It should be emphasized that the women were studied in the late 1950s and were living in the far north of Sweden where winters are severe. They showed a seasonal variation in physical working capacity with a maximum in June/July (summer) and a minimum in December/January (winter) in both pregnant and nonpregnant women, which could reflect the increased physical activity of the summer months.

Arterial blood pressure during pregnancy has been studied since the 19th century with a variety of conclusions concerning its stability. Ihrman reviewed in detail the studies up to 1960 and noted the problem of defining the range of variation in order to establish a reliable guide to increases in arterial blood pressure for the diagnosis of toxemia.[48] In the course of these studies, information has accumulated on the experience many women have of being unable to adapt their circulation to the change of conditions from supine to upright posture. The orthostatic reaction is seen as an increased pulse frequency, a decrease in systolic blood pressure, an increase in diastolic pressure, reduced cardiac output, and reduced stroke volume. Symptoms of dizziness, fatigue, loss of color, and threat of fainting are not infrequent experiences when pregnant women stand up from a resting position. Dahlstrom and Irhman in their studies of 100 pregnant women stated that about 30% of the women during the first trimester of pregnancy exhibited some of the clinical characteristics of the orthostatic reaction.[46] In examining arterial blood pressure throughout pregnancy, they found both systolic and diastolic blood pressure to be within the limits for nonpregnant women of fertile age. More detailed analysis showed that during the first half of pregnancy there were no changes in systolic and diastolic pressures, but during the second half there was a slight but significant increase. At the puerperium, both systolic and diastolic pressures decreased with a return to the normal range after 2 months. These observations were in agreement with many earlier studies of blood pressure during pregnancy. The pulse pressure showed no variation and remained unchanged from the approximately 50 mm Hg found in the nonpregnant state.

During the orthostatic tests, Ihrman found a slight decrease in the systolic and a slight increase in the diastolic blood pressures when compared with blood pressures measured in the supine position in both nonpregnant and pregnant women.[48] Pulse frequency in the orthostatic tests increased over the pulse frequency at rest in both groups. Nonpregnant women throughout the year experienced an average increase of 18 beats per minute when changing from the recumbent to a standing position. In a total of 72 measures (each of 12 nonpregnant women tested six times) there were 12 who showed an increase in pulse frequency of over 27 beats per minute, which is considered to be the limit for a normal reaction. This response could be interpreted as an increased orthostatic reaction in 17% of the tests in nonpregnant women. Among women in the 11th week of pregnancy, 7 out of 50 women could not complete the orthostatic test because of nausea, dizziness, and threatened fainting. In an additional 10 women, the pulse frequency increased by more than 27 beats per minute making a total of 17 or 34% of the pregnant women who had an increased orthostatic reaction. By the 36th week, only 10% of the women showed an increased orthostatic reaction and all could complete the test. In the week following delivery, 50% of the women had an increased pulse frequency of more than 27 beats per minute although all but one could complete the test, and by 2 months post delivery 19% of the women showed increased orthostatic reactions, that is comparable to the frequency in nonpregnant women. We can conclude that many nonpregnant women experience an increased orthostatic reaction and that in the first trimester of pregnancy considerably more women are affected. However, by the 36th week of pregnancy, the proportion of affected women is lower than in the nonpregnant population.

For many years in some countries, particularly Scandinavia, Australia, and New Zealand, moderate physical training during pregnancy has been recommended and Ihrman attempted to evaluate this recommendation in physiological terms.[47] He examined the effect of supervised physical training on 26 pregnant women over a period of 10 weeks from the 20th to the 30th week and compared them with 50 pregnant women with no such training. The arterial blood pressure at rest and in the orthostatic test was the same in both groups at every examination and the orthostatic reaction did not differ. The pulse frequency at rest, in the orthostatic test, and during work tests was also the same in both groups. The vital capacity did not change during pregnancy or after delivery in either group and the maximal breathing capacity increased to the same extent in each group. The hemoglobin concentration, hematocrit, mean corpuscular hemoglobin concentration, total amount of hemoglobin, and total blood volume changed comparably in both groups. However, the heart volume increased from the 20th to the 36th week by 67 mℓ in the physical training group and 43 mℓ in the control group, a difference which was statistically significant at the 0.001 level (p value). The volume was the same in the two groups 2 months after delivery. The conclusion was that the circulatory adjustment that occurs during pregnancy does not appear to be markedly influenced by physical training during the 20th to 30th week of pregnancy, although the author was careful to point out the advantages of physical fitness, relaxation, and breathing exercises on painless and uncomplicated delivery.

Seitchik commented on the apparent fatigue of pregnant women at term, particularly when climbing stairs, a task which contrasts markedly with the intense skeletal muscle tetany occurring intermittently during the second stage of labor with severe demands on energy reserves.[49] He measured oxygen uptake during rest, while exercising on a bicycle ergometer with less than maximal effort, and during recovery in 133 pregnant women, 34 nonpregnant women, and 28 postpartum women. At rest the mean energy expenditure rate of the pregnant women increased with gestation time, although the metabolic rate per unit weight of fat-free mass remained unchanged. In terms of the total energy cost, Seitchik concluded that pregnant women were just as efficient as nonpregnant women during exercise on a bicycle ergometer. In addition, the women 24 to 35 weeks pregnant were the most efficient in terms of caloric cost for the exercise when compared with those of earlier or later gestation, which Seitchik explained in terms of the known maximal values for cardiac output and blood volume at that time in pregnancy. This finding supports Dahlstrom and Ihrman's observation of "higher physical working capacity" at the 36th week when compared with earlier pregnancy.[46] It should only be very late in pregnancy when the physiologic alterations of pregnancy are returning to the nonpregnant state that a pregnant woman could experience a limitation of her exercise tolerance, i.e., more fatigue for the same effort. The exercise in Seitchik's study was at a submaximal work load level and all patients were able to complete the activity. The subjective observation was made that in the last 4 weeks of pregnancy the women were closer to their maximal work tolerance. Posture changes and increased abdominal size were probably the prime influencing factors, particularly as this was an unselected group in terms of their activity levels and physical conditioning. Guzman and Caplan also showed, in a study of eight pregnant women, that "the rate of increase in ventilation and cardiac output with increasing work loads are the same throughout pregnancy as in the nonpregnant state, implying that the physiologic response to mild and moderate exercise is the same in both states."[50] Knuttgen and Emerson came to a similar conclusion after observing 13 subjects throughout most of their pregnancies to the postpartum period, though their conclusion was more restrictive in terms of the increased body and fetus weight.[51] They stated that "activities not involving walking, weight bearing, and lifting of the body should not be expected to involve significant increases in energy cost or physiological stress to the pregnant woman.'' Their conclusion was based on the observation that there was an increase in oxygen cost of treadmill grade walking during pregnancy, but not in cycle ergometer exercise. The heart rate decrease from prepartum levels for treadmill exercise to postpartum levels was also in accord with the increased oxygen cost during pregnancy. Observations of pulmonary volumes and their subdivisions prepartum and postpartum were similar to those reported by others and showed three major changes — a decrease in functional residual capacity, an increase in inspiratory capacity, and an increase in vital capacity. There was no change in total lung capacity. The hyperventilation in pregnancy was attributable solely to tidal volume at rest as well as during exercise, and the increase in the size of the abdominal contents did not impair ventilation during pregnancy under exercising conditions.

More recently, Pernoll et al. have measured the efficiency of pregnant women, defined as the work performed divided by the oxygen consumption in the steady state when the work was performed under standardized conditions.[52] In contrast to Seitchik[49] and Knuttgen et al.,[51] who concluded that there was no change in oxygen consumption during pregnancy, Pernoll et al. confirmed the results of Ueland et al. that oxygen cost increased during pregnancy in the steady state of gas exchange under standard exercise conditions on the bicycle ergometer.[53] An additional important observation was the significant increase during pregnancy in the oxygen debt resulting from a standard amount of exercise. The increase in oxygen consumption during exercise and in oxygen debt in late pregnancy was compared with the postpartum values in the same individuals. After accounting for the oxygen demands of increased respiratory and myocardial work, Pernoll et al. concluded that the efficiency of performing mild muscular exercise declines during pregnancy, though they could not provide an explanation for their finding. An extension of these studies on the same 12 individuals allowed a more detailed examination of the phenomenon of hyperventilation.[54] Relative hyperventilation is characteristic of the progesterone-dominated phase of each normal menstrual cycle and continues to increase in the pregnant woman at rest. Hormonal influence of the respiratory center is probably the reason, and the result is a decreased alveolar partial pressure of carbon dioxide and a greater volume of air ventilated for each liter of oxygen used, particularly during late pregnancy. As reported by others, Pernoll et al. found a nearly linear increase during pregnancy in expiratory minute volume at rest and during exercise. The resting respiratory minute volume at 39 to 42 weeks of pregnancy was 50% greater than it was at 12 to 14 weeks postpartum. There was an almost continuous increase during exercise from the 19th week of pregnancy until delivery, 38% greater at 39 to 42 weeks of pregnancy than at 12 to 14 weeks postpartum. In contrast, respiratory frequency scarcely changed during pregnancy at rest and not significantly during exercise (when compared with the nonpregnant state). Tidal volume was found to be greater at rest throughout pregnancy and 2 to 4 weeks postpartum when compared to the 12- to 14-week postpartum period, and at 39 to 42 weeks gestation was 44% greater than 12 to 14 weeks postpartum. During exercise it was only 23% greater for the same comparison periods. When compared with the 12- to 14-week postpartum period, production of carbon dioxide increased from 19 weeks of pregnancy to 2 to 4 weeks postpartum with a 38% greater production at 39 to 42 weeks at rest, but only 14% during exercise (Table 8). Ventilatory equivalent for oxygen is expressed as ventilatory volume divided by oxygen consumption and increased at rest after the 35th week of pregnancy. However, during exercise the ventilatory equivalent was significantly greater throughout pregnancy. From these observations, it could be calculated that at rest there was relative alveolar hyperventilation during pregnancy, averaging 7.4 ℓ/min during pregnancy compared to 5.1 ℓ/min at

TABLE 8

Percentage Change in Lung Function Parameters at 39—42 Weeks Gestation
(Compared with 12 to 14 Weeks Postpartum)[52]

	At rest	During exercise
Respiratory frequency	Little or no change	Little or no change
Expiratory minute volume	50% increase	38% increase
Tidal volume	44% increase	23% increase
Carbon dioxide production	38% increase	14% increase
Alveolar hyperventilation	45% increase	36% increase

12 weeks postpartum — a 45% increase. During exercise late in pregnancy, the average of 27.0 ℓ/min can be compared with 19.9 ℓ/min postpartum, a 36% increase, when end-tidal carbon dioxide concentration is assumed to represent mean alveolar carbon dioxide concentration. Carbon dioxide production is significantly increased throughout pregnancy, yet the end-tidal carbon dioxide partial pressure is lower both at rest and during exercise. Pernoll et al. concluded that during pregnancy changes in lung function keep carbon dioxide partial pressure low even during moderate exercise, with the additional energy expenditure resulting from respiratory muscle activity. Also, it appears that respiratory center sensitivity to carbon dioxide increases progressively during pregnancy whether calculations are based on observations of changes at rest or during exercise. Hyperventilation certainly is a physiologic characteristic of pregnancy at rest and during exercise, though accurate quantitative determination of the change is difficult. Pernoll et al. used several different assumptions to calculate the changes in alveolar hyperventilation and concluded that they are not as large as the changes in expiratory minute volume would indicate, most probably due to increase in the volume of the physiologic dead space. In part, this change can be explained by the findings of Gee at al., that airway resistance to air flow decreases during pregnancy which is evidence that the conducting airways have increased diameters.[55]

These changes in lung function during pregnancy are of considerable significance in evaluation of inhalation exposure and the potential uptake of toxic substances by inhalation (see Chapter 4).

Overall we can conclude that the physiologic adaptations of pregnancy are sufficient for a woman to maintain her prepregnancy range of physical activity with a possible need to acknowledge increased fatigue levels in the last weeks of gestation as body size becomes burdensome.

V. EFFECT OF MATERNAL PHYSICAL ACTIVITY ON THE FETUS

The relationship between physical activity and physical conditioning to subsequent reproduction has seldom been examined in the U.S., although the Europeans have published some studies of athletes.[56] In relation to pregnancy itself, interest in Europe has traditionally been more directed to physical conditioning than in the U.S., e.g., ". . . pregnancy far from being an illness should be considered an intensive, day and night, nine-month period of physical conditioning because of the increased demands upon metabolism and the entire cardiovascular system."[57]

Pomerance et al. used Darling's definition of physical fitness — "Physical fitness consists of the ability of the organism to maintain the various internal equilibria as closely as possible to the resting state during strenuous exertion and to restore promptly after exercise any (equilibria) which have been disturbed."[58] They examined physical fitness in the pregnant woman in relation to the well-being of the fetus. The variables they examined in the babies of 41 women were length of gestation, length of labor, birth weight, length and head circumferences, and 1-min Apgar scores. The only statistically significant association was between physical fitness score and length of labor in multiparas. The study pointed out several difficulties, particularly in estimating maximum oxygen uptake from heart rate response to submaximal work loads. The Astrand method calculations, used by Pomerance, are based on nonpregnant women, and with a standard error of as much as 15%, the evaluation of physical fitness in pregnant women is far from satisfactory.

In a further study of 54 women, Pomerance et al. have attempted to identify distressed fetuses and infants by screening mothers for uteroplacental insufficiency.[59] Responses to a short exercise test on a bicycle ergometer at approximately 36 weeks gestation were measured in a low-risk homogeneous population of pregnant women. Eleven babies were born with fetal distress, of which six had compromised umbilical cord circulation and one had no apparent cause for the distress. Four had uteroplacental insufficiency diagnosed on the basis of fetal bradycardia (fetal heart rate less than 120), meconium-stained amniotic fluid, or 1-min Apgar score less than 7. In these four mothers the exercise test at 36 weeks had resulted in a change in fetal heart rate of more than 16 beats per minute. The authors consider this measure to be a readily available indicator of potential fetal stress predicting the need for close monitoring during labor and delivery. Strenuous activity by the woman approaching term would also be contraindicated. A physical fitness score was established for each woman in the Pomerance study, but could not be considered a good indicator of the true condition of physical conditioning, on the basis of the indirect method described for assessment. The conclusion by the authors that a high degree of maternal physical fitness does not decrease the incidence of uteroplacental insufficiency does not appear to be justified on the basis of the data they present on five women.

Stembera and Hodr have also shown that exercise test differences can be found in the phonocardiogram of healthy fetuses and of potentially distressed ones.[60] The study population was divided into four groups:

1. Healthy fetuses after a physiological course of pregnancy
2. Fetuses whose mothers showed pathologic conditions, but in whom no signs of hypoxia appeared during or after birth.
3. Fetuses with clinical symptoms of hypoxia during delivery, but in whom all signs of sustained intrauterine hypoxia receded up to one minute after birth
4. Hypoxic newborns

The prenatal records of fetal heart rates showed differences that indicated a greater incidence of extreme variations in those with the higher potential fetal distress, more towards tachycardia than bradycardia. The exercise load of the mother was associated with far more pronounced differences in the variability of fetal heart rates in healthy fetuses when compared with those with potential hypoxia. In Group 1 (healthy fetuses) there was very little change in variations in heart rates. In Group 2 there was a marked shift toward tachycardia. Group 3 showed a shift both towards tachycardia and bradycardia, and Group 4 showed a marked shift towards bradycardia. It is interesting to note that the average heart rate evaluated for the whole time interval of 10 min after maternal exercise load does not show any marked differences and varies as before the exercise load in all groups in the range of 140 to 148 beats per minute. However, for the fetus in hypoxic distress, bradycardia appears immediately after the exercise load of the mother, though it may only last for a very short time. These observations suggest that the higher vulnerability of some fetuses may be identifiable by their response to maternal exercise, though we cannot conclude that there is causal relationship.

It is still unclear whether perfusion of the placenta during physical exercise is affected by the physical fitness of the mother. It does appear however that for the compromised fetus it's response to physical activity in the mother can be monitored even though the maternal activity itself has not necessarily been the cause of the uteroplacental insufficiency. Abruption, hemorrhage, or infarction, which can seriously compromise the fetus, are conditions less likely to be directly associated with maternal activity itself. During exercise there is a reduction in the high resistance to blood flow found in resting voluntary muscle. A relatively low resistance shunt in parallel with the placenta results when large muscle masses are exercised which could be expected to a decrease in effective uteroplacental blood flow could then be expected.

Placental "respiratory reserve" may change in relation to fetal requirements, particularly when pregnancy is close to termination. A greater stress on the fetus about to be born could then result from any diversion of uterine blood flow.

VI. NUTRITION AND WORK CAPACITY OF PREGNANT WOMEN

The physiology of pregnancy in relation to maternal nutrition under adequate living conditions is fairly well understood, and in industrialized countries depressed socioeconomic conditions are associated with higher than average maternal and infant mortality.

Cross-cultural review of the reproductive experience of women provides some useful information on the variability of nutritional status, particularly in terms of food taboos, prohibitions,and privileges. Rosenburg has described the widespread character of sex-differential diets and commented on the lack of attention given by earlier workers to the nutritional impact of food deprivation on women and their offspring.[61] The many examples of food replenishment experiences, both natural and purposeful, which have occurred across the world have established the positive advantage for pregnancy outcome and maternal health.

However, we find only sparse references in the anthropological literature to the physical activity of women. Do conditions of work in the form of physical labor change with the progress of pregnancy? There certainly appear to be fewer seclusion practices related to pregnancy itself when compared to menstruation and childbirth periods. One can gain a general impression that work goes on during pregnancy — work in the fields, carrying water, walking, and collecting food.

The success of pregnancy under marginal subsistence conditions is dependent primarily on the nutritional quality of the woman's environment from her conception to the completion of her childbearing. Her physical activity must affect the nutritional safety margin in terms of the caloric demands for the work performed. However, work and exercise can also result in physical conditioning and possible benefit for the experience of childbearing itself.

Very few studies on the physical capacity of pregnant women have been done. It seems unlikely that we will be getting more in the immediate future. Restrictions on the use of human subjects have become more rigorous and a double standard is applied to research on pregnant women for a variety of rational and irrational reasons. In our society we are unable to answer the questions that come from workers from unions, industry, and insurance companies — on the vulnerability of the pregnant women under conditions of hard physical labor.

The severe data gap comes from the lack of reports on the work activity of women.

TABLE 9

Nutritional Adequacy and Physical Activity

	Adequate nutrition	Physical activity
Southwest Africa	+	+
Java, West New Guinea	−	+
U.S. inner city	−	−
U.S. suburban	+	−

Note: + denotes adequate for health and optimal performance.
− denotes inadequate for health and optimal performance.

Under what circumstances in primitive or industrial societies do women reach maximal work loads? Does physical conditioning either for workers or athletes markedly alter the physiological character of pregnancy? Do all pregnant women automatically reduce their work loads as pregnancy progresses? Is their nutritional status affected?

Cross-cultural studies could be useful in examining the relationship between nutritional status, physical activity, and pregnancy outcome. There are societies where nutritional status and physical activity are in good balance for healthy survival, e.g., the Bushmen of Southwest Africa.[62] Physical activity may be high and nutritional status low as had been observed and studied in western New Guinea and Java.[63,64] Physical activity may be low and nutritional status low as in the case of long-term famine and under certain socioeconomic conditions such as those found among poor inner city populations in the U.S. Physical activity may be low and nutritional status high — the usual experience for middle class American women (Table 9).

There is little information to provide objective physiological evaluation of the physical capacity of fertile women for childbearing in relation to their food intake. One study by Baumslag and Petering provides a clinical picture of the reproductive experience of the 'Kung who live in the northwestern region of the Kalahari Desert.[65] They are nomads subsisting on wild game, berries, and bulbs; since 1957, they have been using iron cooking pots. Hematologic data were gathered for 160 adults — 38 men and 122 women. Hemoglobin, hematocrit values, serum iron, serum B_{12}, and serum folic acid levels were measured. Hair samples were obtained from 38 women (12 young, nonpregnant, 11 lactating, 15 postmenopausal) and 8 men. Contents of trace metals in the hair were analyzed to establish the levels of zinc, copper, and iron. There was no evidence of clinical anemia and no sex difference in hemoglobin, hematocrit, or mean corpuscular hemoglobin concentration, though hair analysis for zinc and iron content showed lowest values in lactating women and highest values in men. The 'Kung are able to maintain adequate maternal nutrition without supplementation. Iron deficiency anemia was not encountered and there was no evidence of iron, vitamin B_{12}, or folic acid deficiency. Although mothers had been lactating for some time, some up to 4 years, they still maintained high nutritional status. A comparison group of Bantu mothers was studied and both iron deficiency and folic acid deficiency were found. The Bantu could be regarded as urban dwellers with a sedentary life style when compared with the 'Kung. Comparisons were made with inner city nonlactating mothers from Cincinnati, Ohio in the same study and their hair levels for iron and other elements were the lowest, 16% were anemic and yet all were supposed to be receiving iron supplementation and vitamins. Observations on the cycle of physical activity for these women would be an invaluable supplement to the nutrition reports.

In contrast, in East Java near Jogjakarta, long-term malnutrition results in a high prevalence of hunger edema.[63] The general appearance of the population is "sturdy" despite the obviously poor hygienic, dietary, and agricultural conditions. Men and women both bear burdens of cassava, bananas, and wood up to 60 and 40 kg, respectively, for long distances. Their "subsistence" nutrition is dominated by one of the cheapest and worst staple foods, cassava. It has been claimed that the protein intake is the poorest in the world, quantitatively as well as qualitatively. However, it is not reported whether pregnant and lactating women modify their physical activity to balance their nutritional needs during pregnancy. It seems possible that the demands of the infant could be satisfied at the expense of the mother. To what extent do these women in Java modify the effect of pregnancy and lactation demands by changes in their work activity? What advantage does good physical conditioning provide? Does the physical conditioning of Javanese women have any impact on the adverse effects of malnutrition on pregnancy, childbirth, and infant survival? The childbearing experience itself involves episodes of intense but intermittent skeletal muscle tetany to produce the expulsive effort of the second stage of labor. There are few other physical activities which make such extreme demands on the human body — for men or women.

Field survey methods have been well developed for nutritional studies and many societies have been examined in detail, without a comparable analysis of activity patterns.There is a need for a more systematic methodology in improving the quality of such observations — not just in the case of pregnancy, but for all participants in the community. For example, we know from studies of adolescent changes in size and physical performance that cultural factors determine the motor performance of adolescent girls. It might be expected in societies where girls become sedentary at puberty (as has been the dominant tendency in the U.S.) that their later working capacity will be affected, whether pregnant or not.[66]

The economic contribution of the healthy fertile (and potentially pregnant) woman in terms of work load must be taken into account in tribal societies, and developing and industrialized countries. Social sanctions and women's expectations are influenced by the pregnancy experience itself (for example, ease or difficulty of childbirth), the social and economic value of the women (maternal mortality and morbidity may become unacceptable), and demographic changes (declining or increasing population).

The relationship of physical activity and nutrition to pregnancy outcome varies markedly throughout the world and needs more intense examination as we recognize the complex demands a woman faces in any society where she contributes her work.

REFERENCES

1. **Dukes-Dubos, F. N.**, The place of ergonomics in science and industry, *Am. Ind. Hyg. Assoc. J.,* 31, 565, 1970.
2. **Henschel, A.**, Women in Industry — The Difference, Trans. 33rd Meeting, Am. Conf. Gov. Indust. Hyg., Toronto, 1971, 73.
3. **Chaffin, D. B.**, Human strength capability and low-back pain, *J. Occup. Med.,* 16, 248, 1974.
4. **Chaffin, D. B., Herrin, G. D., Keyserling, W. M., and Foulke, J. R.**, Pre-employment strength testing: an update position, *J. Occup. Med.,* 20, 403, 1978.
5. **Chaffin, D. B., Herrin, G. D., Keyserling, W. M., and Foulke, J. A.**, Pre-employment Strength Testing in Selecting Workers for Materials Handling Jobs, Center for Disease Control, U.S. Department of Health, Education and Welfare, Washington, D.C., 99, 74, 62, 1977.
6. **Assmussen, E. and Heelboll-Nielsen, K.**, Isometric muscle strength of adult men and women, Communications from the Danish National Association for Infantile Paralysis, No. 11, Hellerup, Denmark, 1961.

7. Troupe, J. D. G. and Chapman, A. E., The strength of the flexor and extensor muscles of the trunk, *J. Biomech.*, 2, 49, 1969.

8. Nordgren, B., Anthropometric measures and muscle strength in young women, *Scand. J. Rehab. Med.*, 4, 165, 1972.

9. Snook, S. H. and Ciriello, V. M., Maximum weights and work loads acceptable to female workers, *J. Occup. Med.*, 16, 527, 1974.

10. American Industrial Hygiene Association, Guide to manual lifting, *Am. Ind. Hyg. Assoc. J.*, 31, 511, 1970.

11. Brown, J. R., Factors contributing to the development of low back pain in industrial workers, *Am. Ind. Hyg. Assoc. J.*, 36, 26, 1975.

12. Kelsey, J., An epidemiological study of the relationship between occupations and acute herniated intervertebral discs, *Int. J. Epidemiol.*, 4, 197, 1975.

13. Kelsey, J., Greenberg, R. A., Hardy, R. J., and Johnson, M. E., Pregnancy and the syndrome of herniated lumbar intervertebral disc. An epidemiological study, *Yale J. Biol. Med.*, 48, 361, 1975.

14. Diddle, A. W., Gravid women at work. Fetal and maternal morbidity. Employment policy and medico-legal aspects, *J. Occup. Med.*, 12, 10, 1970.

15. Reynolds, H. M. and Allgood, M. A., Functional strength of commercial-airline stewardesses, FAA-AM-75-2, U.S. Department of Transportation, Washington, D.C., 1975.

16. Snyder, R. G., The sex ratio of offspring of high performance military aircraft pilots, *Hum. Biol.*, 33, 1, 1961.

17. Hanson, J. S. and Nedde, W. H., Long-term physical training effect in sedentary females, *J. Appl. Physiol.*, 37, 112, 1974.

18. Astrand, P. O., Human physical fitness with special reference to sex and age, *Physiol. Rev.*, 36, 307, 1956.

19. Kilborn, A., Physical training in women, *Scand. J. Clin. Lab. Invest. Suppl.*, 119, 1, 1971.

20. Michael, E. D. and Horvath, S. M., Physical capacity of college women, *J. Appl. Physiol.*, 20, 263, 1965.

21. Buskirk, E. R. and Taylor, H. L., Maximal oxygen intake and its relation to body composition with special reference to chronic physical activity and obesity, *J. Appl. Physiol.*, 11, 72, 1957.

22. Bar-or, O. and Buskirk, E. R., The cardiovascular system and exercise, in *Science and Medicine of Exercise and Sport*, Johnson, W. R. and Buskirk, E. R., Eds., Harper & Row, New York, 1974, 121.

23. Dhesi, J. K. and Firebaugh, F. M., The effects of stages of chapati making and angles of body position on heart rate, *Ergonomics*, 16, 811, 1973.

24. Gross, D. and Underwood, B. A., Technological change and caloric cost on northeastern Brazilian sisal plantations, *Am. Anthropol.*, 73, 725, 1971.

25. Hollingsworth, L. S., Functional Periodicity. An Experimental Study of the Mental and Motor Abilities of Women during Menstruation in *Contributions to Education*, Vol. 69, New York Teachers College, Columbia University, 1914, 1—99.

26. Scott, G. and Tuttle, W. W., The periodic fluctuation in physical efficiency during the menstrual cycle, *Res. Q. Am. Assoc. Health Phys. Educ. Recreat*, 3, 137, 1932.

27. Phillips, M., The effect of the menstrual cycle on selected measures of steadiness, reaction and movement time, blood pressure and heart rate; the effect of the menstrual cycle on the heart rate during and following strenuous exercise, Papers read at the Research Section, National Convention of the American Association for Health, Physical Education, and Recreation, Minneapolis, 1962 and 1963.

28. Rockwell, M. H., The effect of the menstrual cycle on cardiovascular and muscle efficiency of college women, Masters Thesis, The Pennsylvania State University, University Park, 1962, 49.

29. Auster, M., The menstrual function of college women, Masters thesis, The Pennsylvania State University, University Park, 1944.

30. Doolittle, T. L. and Engebretsen, J., Performance variations during the menstrual cycle, *J. Sports Med. Phys. Fitness*, 12, 54, 1972.

31. Wearing, M. P., Yohosz, M. D., Campbell, R. and Love, E. J., Effect of the menstrual cycle on tests of physical fitness, *J. Sports Med. Phys. Fitness*, 12, 38, 1972.

32. Hunter, S., The relationship of total estrogen concentrations and menstrual cycle phase to the performance of three reaction time tests, Masters thesis, The Pennsylvania State University, University Park, 1976.

33. Sommer, B. The effect of menstruation on cognitive and perceptual motor behavior, *Psychosom. Med.*, 55, 515, 1973.

34. Ruble, D. N., Premenstrual symptoms. A reinterpretation, *Science*, 197, 291, 1977.

35. Petrofsky, J. S., Le Donne, D. M., Rinehart, J. S., and Lind., A. R., Isometric strength and endurance during the menstrual cycle, *Eur. J. Appl. Physiol.*, 35, 1, 1976.

36. **Senay, L. C.,** Body fluids and temperature responses of heat exposed women before and after ovulation with and without rehydration, *J. Physiol. (London),* 232, 209. 1973.
37. **Petrofsky, J. S., Burse, R. L. and Lind, A. R.** Comparison of physiological response of women and men to isometric exercise, *J. Appl. Physiol.,* 39, 639, 1975.
38. **Noack, H.,** Die sportliche Leistungefahigkeit der Frau in Menstrual Zyklus, *Dtsch. Med. Wochenschr.,* 79, 1523, 1954.
39. **Bausenwein, I.,** Zur Frage Sport und Menstruation, *Offizielles Wissenschaftliches Organ des Deutschen Sportarztebundes, Stuttgart,* 2, 1530, 1954.
40. **Harris, D.,** personal communicaton, 1978.
41. **Miller, R. M.,** Observations of the reactions of mature stallions to the presence of menstruating women, *Vet. Med. Small Anim. Clin.,* 71, 678, 1976.
42. Infant Mortality, Results of Field Study in Johnstown, Pa., Publ. No. 9, Children's Bureau, U.S. Department of Labor, Washington, D. C., 1915.
43. Infant Mortality, Results of Field Study in Gary, Ind., Publ. No. 112, Children's Bureau, U.S. Department of Labor, Washington, D.C., 1923.
44. **Baetjer, A. M.,** *Women in Industry. Their Health and Efficiency,* W. B. Saunders, Philadelphia, 1946.
45. **Zaharieva, E.,** Olympic participation by women, *JAMA,* 221, 992, 1972.
46. **Dahlstrom, H. and Ihrman, K.,** A clinical and physiological study of pregnancy in a material from Northern Sweden. V. The results of work tests during and after pregnancy, *Acta Soc. Med. Ups.,* 65, 305, 1960.
47. **Ihrman, K.,** A clinical and physiological study of pregnancy in a material from Northern Sweden. VIII. The effect of physical training during pregnancy on the circulatory adjustment, *Acta Soc. Med. Ups.* 65, 335, 1960.
48. **Ihrman, K.,** A clinical and physiological study of pregnancy in a material from Northern Sweden. VII. The arterial blood pressures at rest and in orthostatic tests during and after pregnancy, *Acta, Soc. Med. Ups.* 65, 315, 1960.
49. **Seitchik, J.,** Body composition and energy expenditure during rest and work in pregnancy, *Am. J. Obstet. Gynecol.,* 97, 701, 1967.
50. **Guzman, C. A. and Caplan, R.,** Cardiorespiratory response to exercise during pregnancy, *Am. J. Obstet. Gynecol.,* 108, 600, 1970.
51. **Knuttgen, H. G. and Emerson, K.,** Physiological response to pregnancy at rest and during exercise, *J. Appl. Physiol.,* 36, 549, 1974.
52. **Pernoll, M. L., Metcalfe, J., Schlenker, T. L., Welch, J. E., and Matsomoto, J.,** Oxygen consumption at rest and during exercise in pregnancy, *Respir. Physiol.,* 25, 285, 1975.
53. **Ueland, K., Novy, M. J., and Metcalfe, J.,** Cardiorespiratory response to pregnancy and exercise in normal women and patients with heart disease, *Am. J. Obstet. Gynecol.,* 115, 4, 1973.
54. **Pernoll, M. L., Metcalfe, J., Kovach, P. A., Wachtel, R., and Dunham, M. J.,** Ventilation during rest and exercise in pregnancy and post partum, *Respir. Physiol.,* 25, 295, 1975.
55. **Gee, J. B. L., Packer, B. S. and Milten, J. E.,** Pulmonary mechanics during pregnancy, *J. Clin. Invest.,* 46, 945, 1967.
56. **Zaharieva, E.,** Our data about motherhood of sportswomen, *Medizina i fizkultura, Sofia,* 221, 1963.
57. **Klaus, K.,** On maternal mortality in Czechoslovakia, *Dtsch. Gesundheitswes.,* 16, 374, 1961.
58. **Pomerance, J. J., Gluck, L., and Lynch, V. A.,** Maternal exercise as a screening test for uteroplacental insufficiency, *Obstet. Gynecol.,* 44, 383, 1974.
59. **Pomerance, J. J., Gluck, L., and Lynch, V. A.,** Physical fitness in pregnancy: its effect on pregnancy outcome, *Am. J. Obstet. Gynecol.,* 119, 867, 1974.
60. **Stembera, Z. J. and Hodr, J.,** The "exercise test" as early diagnostic aid for foetal distress, in *Intrauterine Dangers to The Fetus,* Horsky, J. and Stembera, Z. K., Eds., Excerpta Medica, New York, 1967, 349.
61. **Rosenberg, E.,** Ecological effects of sex differential in nutrition, in Abstracts, 72nd Ann. Meet., American Anthropological Association, New Orleans, 1973.
62. **Frisch, R.,** Menarche and fatness. Re-examination of the critical body composition hypothesis, *Science,* 200, 1506, 1978.
63. **Bailey, K. V.,** Rural nutrition studies in Indonesia. IV. Oedema in lactating women in the cassava areas, *Trop. Geogr. Med.,* 13, 303, 1961.
64. **Bailey, K. V.,** Nutritional status of West New Guinea populations, *Trop. Geogr. Med.,* 15, 389, 1963.
65. **Baumslag, N. and Petering, H. G.,** Trace elements in Bushman hair, *Arch. Environ. Health,* 31, 254, 1976.
66. **Malina, R.,** Adolescent changes in size, build, body composition and performance, *Hum. Biol.,* 46, 117, 1974.

Chapter 3

THE PHYSICAL ENVIRONMENT

I. INTRODUCTION

Research on the adverse effects of physical hazards such as ionizing radiation, microwaves, heat, and noise has included women in the populations studied. A better evaluation is possible of the effect of extreme conditions on women workers and their reproduction than is the case for most toxic chemical exposures. This chapter also includes a review of the biological responses of women which result from changes in the human circadian rhythm due to shift work and transmeridian flights.

II. IONIZING RADIATION*

An evaluation of radiation exposure and protection in the occupational health setting provides a marked contrast with exposure to other hazards of chemical, biological, or physical origin. The differences strongly suggest that the philosophy of protection of workers from the vast range of industrial hazards is far from being a unitary concept. Particularly, hazards in the work place which can affect human reproduction are perceived differently for women and men.

A short summary of the history of the human experience with ionizing radiation is useful because the level of conscious concern has been higher and more sophisticated than for any other occupational hazard. The discovery of the physical principles of ionizing radiation at the end of the 19th century by the Curies and Becquerel initiated an immediate development of new medical, scientific, and industrial uses with proliferation of inventions using X-rays and subsequently radioisotopes throughout the world. Almost immediately, adverse effects of X-rays were recognized. Serious burns and ulceration of the skin became evident within a year and malignancies were being documented by 1911. The victims were physicists and chemists, radiologists, laboratory assistants, technicians, and nurses. By the time radiography was coming into industrial use, the need for protection by shielding and controlled exposure had been recognized. However, the protection itself was slow in coming and not universally used, even though the efficacy of lead shielding was known by 1903. The disfigurement, chronic illness, severe anemias, and terminal cancers of health professionals and scientists in the early part of the century were in marked contrast to the expectant public view that X-rays provided remarkable diagnoses and miraculous cures.[1]

The accumulated experience came into focus in the mid-20s with the identification of necrosis of the jaw among workers using luminous paint in New Jersey. The dental profession had played an important role in controlling other occupational diseases where oral pathology was severe through prophylactic and preventive dentistry. They now found that more extensive medical care and hospitalization was necessary for "radium necrosis." Dentists in New Jersey refused to extract teeth from the women who were radium dial painters because of the severe and frequently fatal sequelae.[2] This unique, widely publicized American experience was the first recognized evidence

---

* From Hunt, V., Occupational radiation exposure of women workers, *Prev. Med.,* 7, 1978. With permission.

that radioisotopes such as radium, when internally ingested, could remain in the body indefinitely and cause serious illness and death. The deceased (by means of exhumed remains) and living radium dial painters have been and are still being intensively studied to establish the level of radioactivity associated with cancer and other changes in the skeleton and soft tissues.[3] These data have been part of the research base to establish maximum permissible standards for all workers exposed to radiation. However, it is difficult to understand why virtually no useful information has been reported on their reproductive experience. Belated attempts are now being made with the result that detailed, accurate information on menstrual changes, fetal deaths, miscarriages, and congenital abnormalities is now virtually impossible to obtain. Similarly, there is no reproductive information available for those working with external radiation — X-ray technicians, for example.

It is probable that the radium dial painters' experience contributed to the identification by other countries of potential sources of industrial poisoning from radioactive chemicals and X-rays.

In 1928, the International Commission on Radiological Protection (ICRP) was formed as a voluntary organization of radiologists attending the 2nd International Congress of Radiology in Stockholm and proceeded to develop recommendations for X-ray and radium protection. It is worth noting that voluntary nongovernment organizations outside the normal lawmaking institutions have been primarily responsible for the development of radiation protection standards in most of the world. The National Council on Radiation Protection and Measurements (NCRP) is the U.S. counterpart of ICRP and is a nonprofit corporation chartered by Congress.[4] It recently published *Review of the Current State of Radiation Protection Philosophy*, which analyzed the reports published since 1970 by the ICRP, NCRP, and The National Academy of Sciences of the U.S. This is the continuation of a process of reevaluation that has gone on for more than 30 years.[5]

The current guiding principle of the NCRP, which undergoes continual review and which has most strongly influenced federal agencies in the setting of numerical radiation protection guides or dose limits for occupational exposure, is that the "lowest practicable radiation level" is the concept basic to the establishment of radiation standards. In addition, the working assumption is made that there is no dose threshold below which radiation damage cannot occur. In other words, numerical radiation protection guides or dose limits for the exposure of radiation workers are provided only as upper limits, with the expectation that all exposures will be kept to a practicable minimum, far below what is allowable.

The appendix to the Nuclear Regulatory Commission Regulatory Guide 8.13 applies to workers employed in facilities licensed under the U.S. Atomic Energy Act and stems from an amendment to Section 19.12, 10CFR Part 19; it requires NRC licensees to instruct all workers about the biological risks to embryos or fetuses exposed to ionizing radiation, and, to advise women employed in jobs involving radiation exposure, that the intent is to minimize exposure to and possible adverse effect on embryos or fetuses.[6] The amendment also states that licensees should make particular efforts to keep the radiation exposure of an embryo or fetus to the very lowest practicable level during the entire gestation period.

The recent concern arises from a recommendation made several years ago by the NCRP[7] that during the entire gestation period the maximum permissible dose equivalent to the fetus from occupational exposure of the expectant mother should not exceed 0.5 rem, i.e., one tenth the maximum permissible dose allowed the worker — 5 rem. The following is the comment that went with the recommendation:

The need to minimize exposure of the embryo and fetus is paramount. It becomes the controlling factor in the occupational exposure of fertile women. In effect, this implies that such women *should* be employed only in situations where the annual dose accumulation is unlikely to exceed 2 or 3 rems and is acquired at a more or less steady rate. In such cases, the probability of the dose to a fetus exceeding 0.5 rem before a pregnancy is recognized is negligible. Once a pregnancy is known, the actual approximate dose can be reviewed to see if work can be continued within the framework of the limit set above...the method of application (of the recommendation) is speculative and needs to be tested for practicality in a wide range of occupational circumstances. For conceptual purposes, the chosen dose limit essentially functions to treat the unborn child as a member of the public involuntarily brought into controlled areas. The NCRP recommends vigorous efforts to keep exposure of an embryo or fetus to the very lowest practicable level.

On March 1, 1977 the NCRP confirmed this recommendation of 1971 in *Review of NCRP Radiation Dose Limit for Embryo and Fetus in Occupationally Exposed Women.*[8] The latest report analyzes the most recent information on health risks of occupational radiation exposure of the embryo-fetus and provides a useful review of the English language literature. The conclusions and recommendations are

A. On the basis of the current review, the NCRP has decided to make no change in the current recommendation of its radiation dose limit to the unborn. The NCRP recommendation is restated here as follows: During the entire gestation period, the maximum permissible dose equivalent to the embryo-fetus from occupational exposure of the expectant mother should be 0.5 rem.
B. The basic reason for the identity of position in 1977 and 1971 with respect to the recommendation that the radiation dose limit should be 0.5 rem is that since the preparation of the 1971 report there has been no new evidence concerning teratogenic or carcinogenic effects of irradiation of the embryo-fetus that would justify a change in the limit in either direction.
C. It is implicit in this position and recommendation that women who can reasonably be expected to be pregnant should not, in certain instances, be exposed to the same radiation environment as women who are not considered fertile or as men. This applies particularly to conditions where radiation workers can receive dose equivalents of 0.5 rem or more in short periods. However, any special restrictions that need to be imposed on potentially pregnant women depend on a number of circumstances. These include the amount and temporal distribution of radiation exposure and such matters as whether female employees agree to or are asked to disclose pregnancy to management, and how soon after conception a pregnancy can be recognized. Because of these variables, and perhaps others of a legal nature as well, it appears impracticable for NCRP to make detailed recommendations concerning modes of practical implementation of the recommended dose limits.
D. The recommendations of the NCRP are directed at protection of the embryo-fetus as being involuntarily subjected to the radiation exposure as a consequence of the occupational exposure of the expectant mother.

From the first recommendation on X-ray and radium protection in 1931 and 1934, NCRP recommendations have always been accepted by U.S. federal and state regulatory agencies as the best knowledge and evaluation available at the time and have served as the basis for establishing and promulgating standards. It is evident from the above recommendations that the NCRP is providing a biological evaluation and accepts no responsibility for the social conditions which might influence implementation of their recommendation. However, their discussion of these probable influences shows considerable insight for a committee of this type, far more than has been evident for other industrial hazards.

Although individual monitoring for radiation exposure in industry has been a regular procedure for many years, it is only very recently that hospital administrators have started to become more responsible in their checking of exposure records. They are still irresponsible in their lack of instructional programs for employees regarding occupational hazards. The National Institute of Occupational Safety and Health (NIOSH) study on hospital occupational health services showed that in the hospitals reporting, 89% of the small hospitals, 74% of the medium hospitals, and 57% of the large hospitals had no routine inservice training programs for the control of radiation exposure.[9] Many of these institutions are not NRC licensees, but are now under the jurisdiction of OSHA. Less than 2% of the more than 5000 responding hospitals replied that pregnancy received any emphasis in their safety and health education programs. Better work practices are going to have to be demanded of health professionals as is currently expected of NRC licensees. It is ironic that epidemiologic studies of the longevity, morbidity, and mortality of radiologists (usually excluding the few who were female) have been going on for 20 years — but there are no U.S. studies of X-ray technicians, nuclear medicine technologists, or nurses dealing with radiation therapy.

Estimates of exposure rates from secondary radiation to persons manually restraining patients during radiographic procedures are reported in a recent publication of the National Council on Radiological Protection and Measurements which deals with radiation protection for medical and allied personnel.[10] The exposure at eye level, dependent on X-ray machine specifications and operation, can range from 15 to 75 mR/mAsec. These ranges represent ideal conditions with leakage radiation less than 1% of the useful beam.

The NCRP has also developed exposure rates surrounding the bed of a patient containing 100 mg of radium, (^{226}Ra), 200 mCi of gold (^{198}Au), or 300 mCi of iodine (^{131}I). They range from 200 mR/hr in close proximity to the patient to 50 mR/hr 2 to 3 ft from the bedside to 10 mR/hr at 7 ft. The precautions currently expected in the nursing of patients with radioactive inserts are quite rigorous in comparison with the past. Film badges are now worn; there is minimum patient contact compatible with adequate nursing care, rotation of nursing personnel, and strict isolation of the patient with controlled disposal of all excreta. These procedures are in marked contrast with the attitude of inevitable acceptance of risk which prevailed up to about 1970.

A survey of medical radium installations in Wisconsin was made from 1968 to 1970. The conclusion was that the majority of registrants (that is medical radium installations) were unable to demonstrate that personnel exposure aspects of radium use met acceptable standards "simply because personnel monitoring was not performed on all or even most of the individuals exposed to radiation from the use of radium.

"Survey findings show that personnel monitoring was provided to at least one individual during radium use at about 50% of the installations. At these installations the individual monitored was usually the radiologist who wore a film badge as a matter of routine. Other exposed individuals (anesthesiologists, gynecologists, surgery room nurses or technicians, floor nurses, or aides) were very infrequently monitored. At the remaining installations personnel monitoring was not provided for any individual during radium treatments..."[11]

In the survey of 20 hospitals, film badges were distributed for whole body monitoring and the results are shown in Table 1. These values included five high doses received by three physicians and two nurses with individual doses of 600, 1130, 1220, 1240, and 1360 mrem per individual per quarter, respectively, making aides the most highly exposed group on the average. These doses would result from the frequent and extended care given the patient directly at the bedside.

The weekly maximum permissible standard for occupational exposure is 5 rem/yr or 100 mrem/week, which allows 1 hr/week for bedside care of radium patients.[10] Extrapolation from the survey results in Wisconsin, shown in Table 1, indicated that the 93 mrem average exposure to aides represented about 1 hr of bedside care per week.

Blum and Liuzzi[13] have made measurements of thyroid ^{131}I in medical and paramedical personnel exposed to radioactive iodine in both diagnostic and therapeutic settings. Table 2 shows the range of values observed. In the extreme case among the technicians (if 18,131 pCi was the constant burden — a rather unlikely occurrence), the annual dose could be as high as 3840 mrad. The maximum permissible value for annual oc-

TABLE 1

Radiation Dose by Job Category (per person)

Job category	Number of persons	%	Total dose accumulated (mrem)	Av. dose/person (mrem)	Range of person doses/quarter[a] (mrem)
Physician	30	14	5,150	172	20—1360
Aide	27	13	2,480	92	10—320
Nurse	78	38	6,560	84	10—1220
Unspecified female	69	27	3,450	50	10—190
Unspecified male	5	2.5	200	40	10—120
Other	5	2.5	150	30	10—40
Technician	7	3	180	26	20—50
Total	221	100	18,170	—	—
Overall	—	—	—	82	10—1360

[a] A calendar quarter was the maximum interval. Some individuals were monitored for one month or one treatment, then rotated to a different department of the hospital.

From the Survey of Medical Radium Installations in Wisconsin, Rep. No. 8022, U.S. Department of Health, Education and Welfare, Washington, D.C., 1975.

TABLE 2

Thyroid ^{131}I Burdens

	Number of subjects	Thyroid Burden (pCi)	Range (pCi)	Inferred average annual dose (mrads)
Unexposed controls	62	12.3±20.4	0—58	2.7
Clinical laboratory supervisory physicians and physicists	11	92.1±89.1	22—343	20
Clinical laboratory technicians	25	2,373.8±4,432	35—18,131	503
Physicians administering therapy	4		74—1,827	14 mrad/patient
Nurses — 24 hr after therapy	6	262±153	98—441	7 mrad/patient

[a] Mean ± ISD

From Blum, M. and Liuzzi, A., *JAMA,* 200, 992, 1967.

cupational exposure to radioactive iodine as recommended by the Federal Radiation Council in 1960 was 30,000 mrad. This level was established as a limit with little if any consideration given at that time to the possibility that technicians could be pregnant. Lombardi et al. substantiates the view of Blum and Liuzzi that there is wide variation in laboratory practices from one technician to another.[14] In reviewing the use of technetium - 99m, which provides the highest hand dose received by nuclear medicine technologists, they concluded that with the relatively large quantities of ra-

TABLE 3

Some Comparisons of Annual Radiation Doses

Category	Number of individuals	Man-rems Total	Man-rems Individual
Diagnostic X-ray	366×10^3	60×10^3	0.165
Nuclear medicine	$25—33 \times 10^3$	9×10^3	0.27—0.35
Ra-Rn therapy	$20—40 \times 10^3$	35×10^3	0.9—1.8
Industrial radiography (radioactive material)	$5—7 \times 10^3$	7×10^3	1—1.4

From The Survey of Medical Radium Installations in Wisconsin, Rep. No. 8022, U.S. Department of Health, Education and Welfare, Washington, D.C., 1975.

dioactive isotopes being used routinely in hospitals, standardization of routine scanning procedures is urgently needed to minimize patient and personnel exposures.

A comparison of average annual doses for individuals in various job categories involving medical irradiation has been compiled from a number of surveys in the U.S. (Table 3), and the authors noted that occupational exposure of brachytherapy personnel has been a "long neglected facet of public health", a conclusion also reached by Gerusky et al. for Pennsylvania.[11,15] A more recent compilation of available U.S. surveys of occupational doses among medical workers shows a wide range of exposures observed in the early 1970s. Those involved in radium treatments and nuclear medicine appear to have the highest annual average dose, between 0.5 and 0.6 rad compared with those in diagnostic and therapeutic medical and dental radiology whose annual average dose was given as 0.32 rad. Other countries reported annual average doses that were considerably lower — Canada - 0.20 rad, Switzerland - 0.15 rad, and Denmark - 0.30 rad. In Denmark, Australia, and Germany brachytherapy was found to be the procedure presenting the highest annual average exposure to medical workers, comparable to that seen in the U.S.[16]

The major contribution to occupational radiation exposure of working women comes from the medical sector — hospitals and private offices of dentists, physicians, and chiropractors. It should be kept in mind that women in the health field are distributed in subprofessional categories as nurses aides and untrained assistants, as well as nurses, X-ray technicians, nuclear technologists, physicians, and dentists. Many nurses aides in past years have repeatedly held patients during diagnostic X-ray procedures, a practice that probably has not yet been eliminated completely. Untrained assistants throughout the U.S. are given responsibility for carrying out diagnostic X-rays in private dental and medical offices. In contrast there are far fewer women exposed to industrial sources (a recent increase has occurred with airport baggage inspection) such as X-ray diffraction and spectrographic equipment. Users of analytical X-ray equipment comprise almost 2% of the users of ionizing radiation in one industrialized state, Pennsylvania.[17] However, they present a radiation protection problem because of the higher rate of acute accidental exposure despite their small number.

The use of film badges and other dosimeters to monitor exposure in itself produces a marked improvement in general operating procedures with the secondary result of reduced exposure. Most workers are now kept well within the allowable occupational exposure standard of 5 rem/year (1.25 rem per quarter) in well-controlled situations. Unfortunately, the effects of careless technique and use of untrained personnel are difficult to assess. More importantly, the lack of epidemiologic studies on the occupational groups exposed to ionizing radiation under controlled or uncontrolled conditions leaves a serious gap in the biological base for risk assessment. Today epidemiologic studies of groups with known high exposure in the nonoccupational setting have to suffice.

A. Epidemiology of Breast Cancer

Observations of breast cancer in association with radiation exposure of women in the Japanese bombings lead us to a concern for women occupationally exposed in hospitals, laboratories, and industry. The radium dial painters are the only group of occupationally exposed women to have been definitively studied. However, their exposure was the result of internal emitters — radium, mesothorium, and daughters deposited in the skeleton and unlikely to have a direct impact on breast tissue. The far larger number of women who have been occupationally exposed to external irradiation in this century have never been examined to quantitatively establish their breast cancer prevalence.

The United Nations Scientific Committee on the Effects of Atomic Radiation (UNSCEAR) has made extrapolations to predicted numbers of cases per million persons exposed per year per rad from high radiation doses (generally over 100 rad) experienced by Japanese survivors and women in the U.S., Canada, and Sweden who have had therapeutic irradiation.[16] In contrast, the dose accumulated over a woman's working life would be likely to be less than 20 rad under current hospital and industry working conditions, although the allowable 5 rem/year could result in a higher work-life dose under circumstances where routine radiations protection procedures were ignored.

UNSCEAR has estimated that for a period of 25 to 30 years after exposure the breast cancer total risk rates per rad (unit of absorbed dose) to adults would be about 50×10^{-6} based on studies of the Japanese bomb victims and 200×10^{-6} based on the therapeutic radiation experience in Western countries. The mortality risk rates are approximately 10×10^{-6} for the Japanese experience and approximately 60×10^{-6} from therapeutic irradiation data.

The continuing detailed study of the survivors of the Japanese bombing has shown that until 1972 no women who had been under 10 years of age at the time of the explosion had died of breast cancer. Among those aged 10 to 19 at the time, there had been 10 deaths from breast cancer recorded, vs. 0.4 expected with no statistically significant excess for older ages of women with a dose of 10 rad or more. The comparison was made to mortality among those with less than 1 rad exposure. A more detailed analysis of morbidity showed that an increased incidence did not appear within 5 years after exposure but probably did between 5 and 10 years. 20 years after the explosion the group exposed when they were from 10 to 19 years of age showed an excess beyond that experienced by the older groups indicating that those under age 20 may be at higher risk for the same radiation dose. The mean latency period of approximately 18 years is independent of dose for the age groups under 30 years of age when exposed and the incident rate is estimated to be approximately $2.5 \times 10^{-6} \times yr^{-1} \times rad^{-1}$. Histologically the majority of tumors of the bomb victims are infiltrating ductal carcinomas which progress slowly and have a high cure rate. Other types occur in proportions comparable to the experience in the unexposed Japanese population.[16]

The survival of Western women exposed to therapeutic irradiation has been more adverse when compared with the Japanese women. Mackenzie[18] first reported increased prevalence of breast cancer in Canadian patients treated for pulmonary tuberculosis by artifical pneumothorax. Subsequent studies of the same population[19] indicated an excess cancer incidence rate of 30 to $140 \times 10^{-6} \times rad^{-1}$ (90% confidence limits

20 to 200 × 10^{-6} × rad^{-1}) over the 20 years since exposure. The calculated rate may be an underestimate for this population due to problems of incomplete ascertainment. There does appear to be a higher risk for those under 30 years when exposed. Among Massachusetts women with similar treatment protocol for pulmonary tuberculosis, there was an estimated mean dose to the breast of 150 rad with an annual risk rate of 6.2 × 10^{-6} × rad^{-1} (90% confidence limits 2.8 to 10.7), when compared with New York State health statistics.[20] As with the earlier studies, age at exposure appears to be important and most of the observed excess was in women between the ages of 13 and 20 at time of treatment. The latency period was about 7 years. The major uncertainty in these studies was the estimate of dose to the breast itself. In other studies where the patients were not facing the X-ray tube, excess breast cancer was not observed though the radiation dose to the patient per examination seemed comparable.[21]

Treatment of post-partum mastitis by breast irradiation is also associated with subsequent development of breast cancer.[22] In a well-controlled American study that examined two groups of post-partum mastitis patients, only one of which experienced X-ray therapy, breast cancer incidence increased after 12 to 15 years in the exposed group. The population of 571 with a control group of their sisters has been followed for a mean period of 25.2 years and the risk of cancer induction has been calculated to be 7.3 × 10^{-6} × year^{-1} × rad^{-1} for those aged 15 to 29 years and 12.0 × 10^{-6} × year^{-1} × rad^{-1} for those over 30 years of age at exposure. The younger age group in this study did not share the relatively higher risk seen in the Japanese studies and in the pneumothorax cases. However, a larger Swedish study of X-ray treatment of benign breast diseases showed a marked age gradient, even taking into account possible biases related to ascertainment, with an apparent increased sensitivity of the breast to irradiation at younger ages. In the follow-up period since treatment the total excess number of cancers when examined by age group was seen in the 20- to 29-year age group as an excess rate per breast of 308 × 10^{-6} × rad^{-1} compared with 89 × 10^{-6} × rad^{-1} for the 30- to 39-year age group and 40 × 10^{-6} × rad^{-1} for the 40- to 49-year age group. Incomplete ascertainment of the experience of women in each age group could be affecting these rates but probably does not completely explain the marked excess seen in the under-30-year age group.[16]

In the Japanese women 25% of the diagnosed cases have resulted in death in contrast with 45% in the therapeutic radiation cases among Western women. In addition, the discrepancy in the "spontaneous" occurrence and histological type of breast cancer between Japan and Western countries is marked so that direct comparisons are not appropriate. It is evident, however, that the effect of ionizing radiation on breast tissue is confirmed by studies on both populations.

The concern that arises from these studies, which have only been recently evaluated in the context presented here, is that young women experience training and work in hospitals with varying radiation protection practices. Radiology departments may be well controlled while operating rooms and other areas of the hospital using portable equipment and brachytherapy are not. More precautionary use of lead aprons, closer monitoring of film badges, and more refined operating practices are necessary to maintain exposure to the breast as low as possible.

B. Epidemiology of Thyroid Cancer

The susceptibility of the thyroid gland to radiation-induced, neoplastic change is sufficient to direct attention to the occupational exposure experience. The increased prevalence of thyroid cancer among persons therapeutically exposed during childhood and Japanese survivors under 20 years of age at the time of the explosion again leads us to a concern for the exposure of young workers occupationally exposed. The doses from both external X-ray exposure and deposition of iodine radioisotopes in thyroid tissue appear to be comparably effective. Fortunately, the well-differentiated histologic characteristics of thyroid cancer are usually associated with slow benign growth so that the cure rate is high.[16] Although appearing at a lower rate in older people, their thyroid cancers tend to be more malignant. Overall, human epidemiologic studies where high doses at high dose rate have been experienced show those under 20 years of age to be at high risk, i.e., over 1000 rads result in 100% cancer induction though most cancers are benign. Unfortunately, there is little comparable information for low dose rates. The apparent age effect may not be real if the latency period for adults is considerably longer than it is for those under 20 years.

An important observation in epidemiologic studies of populations exposed to external radiation (the Japanese survivors) and to internal irradiation from radioactive fallout (the Marshall Islanders) has been the higher rate of cancer induction in women when compared with men. In the Marshall Islanders, all the seven thyroid cancers occurred in the 130 exposed women, a rate of 5.4 (2.5 to 10.2)% with none occurring in the 113 exposed men nor in those who were children at the time. However, thyroid cancer resulting from childhood therapeutic X-ray exposure is also seen to have a high ratio of females to males for cancer induction — over 2 in the U.S. and Israel.[10] There is no evidence that *in utero* exposure to X-rays results in subsequent development of thyroid cancer.

UNSCEAR's estimate of the lifetime risk of death from radiation-induced thyroid cancer is 5 to $15 \times 10^{-6} \times$ rad^{-1} assuming a 3% fatality risk, although the morbidity risk is considerably higher, particularly in children and in the women of the Marshall Islands.

The therapeutic dosage of ^{131}I has diminished markedly in recent years and more careful nursing practices are in effect. However, we do not know what the experience of nurses, nuclear technologists, and X-ray technicians has been.

C. Genetic Effects

Examination of the genetic effects on human populations of exposure to low levels of ionizing radiation has been under review since the 1956 Biological Effects of Atomic Radiation (BEAR) report of the National Academy of Sciences.[23] The recommendation then was that the general population should not receive "an average of more than 10 roentgens, in addition to background, of ionizing radiation as a total accumulated dose to the reproductive cells from conception to age 30." The subsequent 1972 Biological Effects of Ionizing Radiation (BEIR) report in making a comparison with the earlier report noted that medical radiation is still the major contribution to the genetic risk.[24] The earlier genetic risk assessment still the major contribution to the genetic risk.[24] The earlier genetic risk assessment was judged to be possibly too high, so that 10 roentgens was a conservative suggestion, particularly in light of more recent studies showing that radiation at low dose rates is much less effective than at high dose rates and that mouse oocytes throughout life seem very resistant to radiation induced mutations.

The contribution of occupational exposure for those risk estimates was averaged as the genetically significant dose to the total population and has not been considered as the effect on a discrete group within the total population.

Spermatogonia and oocytes are our present and future human resource. Their integrity ensures the viability and subsequent development of the fertilized ovum into a normal embryo, fetus, live-born child, and independent adult and the relative importance of each of these stages from germ cell to adulthood changes in relation to the hazards in the immediate environment. In the radiation environment sperm and ova become the critical stage in this scheme.

TABLE 4

Induction of Gene Mutations and Chromosome Aberrations By Ionizing Radiation

	Paternal	Maternal
Recessive mutations	60×10^{-6} per gamete × rad^{-1}	?
Dominant mutations	20×10^{-6} conceptions × rad^{-1}	?
Reciprocal translocations		
Congenitally malformed (live born)	$2—10 \times 10^{-6}$ conceptions × rad^{-1}	Very low
Recognizable abortions	$10—50 \times 10^{-6}$ conceptions × rad^{-1}	Very low
Losses at early embryonic stage	$20—100 \times 10^{-6}$ conceptions × rad^{-1}	?

From Sources and Effects of Ionizing Radiation, United Nations Scientific Committee on the Effect of Atomic Radiation, United Nations, New York, 1977.

Large populations of mice have been intensively examined for genetic effects of radiation and extrapolation to human germ cells is the most reliable and convenient method available to us for estimating human genetic risks. More meager information is available from human populations and primates to provide some additional check points.

Paternal irradiation can produce approximately 60×10^{-6} per gamete × rad^{-1} recessive mutations, but a far lesser effect with apparent resistance to mutation is observed from maternal irradiation. There is little evidence to indicate that the human ovary differs markedly from the mouse ovary in its response to ionizing radiation and, on the basis of this assumption, the risk of dominant mutations from low dose irradiation of females at low dose rates is considered to be also very slight.[16] In contrast, for paternal irradiation the overall estimate of induction of mutations resulting in dominant effects is 20×10^{-6} conceptions × rad^{-1}. There are more data from primates and human studies for estimates of risk of chromosomes aberration induction. Reciprocal translocations of chromosomes resulting in adverse pregnancy outcome are estimated to be per million conceptuses per rad of paternal exposure — 2 to 10 for congenitally malformed live-born children, 10 to 50 recognizable abortions, and 20 to 100 losses at the early embryonic stage. As in the case of gene mutations, maternal irradiation from all the animal and human evidence available presents a risk too low to be reliably quantified, though a conservative approach could be to assume the risk to be comparable. However, it is apparent that the known effects of paternal irradiation are primarily effects on the father (Table 4) and, therefore, there clearly can be an effect on the mother of adverse pregnancy outcome resulting from the occupational exposure of the father if his germ cells have been affected.

Although there are reservations noted in relying on extrapolations from the female mouse to human beings, there is a consistency of biological effect seen as a resistance of the female germ cells to killing. In addition, sensitivity to mutation is very low and much lower than in the male for both low dose and low dose rate, i.e., chronic irradiation.

In human epidemiological studies Alberman et al.[25] have shown more abnormal karyotypes in spontaneous abortuses among human mothers with a preconception history of medical irradiation. They had experienced a higher mean gonadal dose than mothers of abortuses with normal karyotypes and of live-born controls. The mean gonadal doses were quite low ranging from 0.18 rad for mothers of 45,X abortuses to 0.74 rad for mothers of triploid abortuses. The abnormal karyotypes observed are rarely found in the live born and the abnormal conceptus is most likely to be an early pregnancy loss. As there appeared to be a cumulative dose effect in this study, it seems possible that a maternal age effect was also present.

In contrast Kinlen and Acheson[26] in a retrospective study compared the radiation history of mothers who had spontaneously aborted or who had delivered malformed children with a control group and found no significant difference. Graham et al. in a case control study of 319 children with leukemia found that maternal radiation prior to conception carried a relative risk 1.6 times that of other children, an observation that also has implications for the occupationally exposed fertile woman. Paternal preconception radiation also carried a small excess risk of 1.31 of borderline significance.[36] The human data and analysis do not provide a consistent picture for direct application to the occupational setting, which again highlights the disadvantages of never having systematically examined the reproductive experience of workers exposed to ionizing radiation.

D. Irradiation *in Utero*

Many uncertainties are associated with the evaluation of the effects of radiation exposure to the developing embryo and fetus *in utero*. In addition to the common epidemiologic limitations of inadequate numbers of cases for observation and unavailability of appropriate control groups it is usually impossible to establish the exact stage of development of the embryo at the time of irradiation. The absorbed dose to the whole body is difficult to estimate and malformations or growth disturbances are not necessarily observable at birth but may become apparent in later life.

Malformations that result from irradiation of the embryo show no particular characteristics that differ from the effects of other teratogenic agents such as toxic chemicals. Certainly more precise evaluation of radiation effects has been possible experimentally because the dose can be well controlled in place and time in contrast to administration of chemical agents which must cross the placenta.

The human preimplantation period covers the first 8 days postconception and the adverse effects of irradiation during this period are not likely to be recognized. On the basis of extensive animal exposures it is certain that if preimplantation damage occurs, implantation itself usually fails so that survivors can proceed through subsequent stages to birth with little apparent effect. Body growth does not appear to be impaired and the induction of malformation is of low probability, indicating that damage at the preimplantation stage is more likely to result in death than impaired survival.

In contrast, postimplantation irradiation is associated with more prenatal, neonatal, and postnatal death.

In human epidemiologic studies it has been well established that the pattern of survival and congenital malformations parallels that seen in animal experiments in terms of relative gestational age at irradiation.[27] Dekeban showed that in a series of 200 cases of therapeutic pelvic irradiation where doses to the human embryo were all above 250 rad that irradiation between 4 and 11 weeks caused a variety of malformations with the central nervous system being particularly vulnerable and microcephaly a common finding. Even following organogenesis, irradiation of the fetus (from 12 to 19 weeks) results in microcephaly, stunted growth, and mental retardation with lesser effects apparent in the latter few weeks. From 20 weeks only minor effects on hemopoiesis and the skin are seen. The risk applied only to high acute doses over 50 rad and is given as 10^{-3} rad^{-1}. In the Japanese children who survived the atomic bombing *in utero* and were examined at 19 years of age, the gestational age at 6 to 15 weeks appeared to be the most sensitive for subsequent microcephaly and mental retardation.

A prospective study of 20,000 children exposed *in utero* when their mothers experienced diagnostic abdominal irradiation has now provided data on malformations.[28] According to trimester, for both sexes and for black and white children the irradiated children had a slightly higher incidence of abnormalities than the controls. The effect of irradiation on mortality differed markedly for black and white children, with mortality in irradiated white children almost twice that of controls although no differences in mortality between irradiated and control black children were observed.

Epidemiologic studies of *in utero* exposure must of necessity rely primarily on women undergoing medically necessary X-ray diagnosis and more attention is now being given to the possible influence of the mother's medical condition on the pregnancy outcome.[29] There appears to be a strong probability that women experiencing irradiation for diagnostic purposes are themselves quite different from women who have had routine irradiation for no medical reason and that these differences may explain some of the excess adverse pregnancy outcome observed in the former. Extrapolations from studies of diagnostic exposures to the exposure experience of a healthy group of workers would appear then to provide an overestimate of the potential danger.

The confirmation of Stewart's observation in 1961 of the relationship between X-irradiation *in utero* for diagnostic purposes and subsequent development of childhood cancers has resulted in a sophisticated body of epidemiologic studies.[28,30-32] Stewart has suggested plausible reasons for the observations that prospective studies of X-rayed fetuses appear to show a low incidence of childhood cancers and that retrospective studies of these diseases show a high incidence of prenatal irradiation. One explanation is that preleukemic children are at high risk of premature death before diagnosis of the disease so that detection of the small number of leukemia cases of radiogenic origin becomes far less likely in prospective studies. In contrast, all retrospective studies have shown excess deaths among children irradiated *in utero.* The relative risk of various childhood cancers following intrauterine exposure to diagnostic radiation has been found to be from 1.4 to 1.6, and somewhat higher for leukemia.[32,33] Large populations are necessary to detect such a relative risk because of the low disease incidence. The Oxford Survey's childhood leukemia cases numbered 1820 in 1963 after a collection period of 10 years.[34] The aim is to be able to distinguish between a standard risk for leukemia of 1 in 3000 and a risk of 1 in 2150 for the exposed population. If the risk of errors of the first and second kind are set at 5% and 10%, respectively, a total of 950,000 individuals would have to be followed for 10 years each. Even with comparison to a standard nonexposed group with known leukemia incidence, 250,000 exposed subjects would have to be followed.[34] Stewart made extrapolations from the MacMahon study and estimated that for the total U.S. population born during the years 1947 to 1954 about 500 leukemia deaths by 1960 could be attributed to antenatal diagnostic radiology. She emphasized that the number of lives saved because of the diagnostic procedures was probably greater although that view provides little excuse for not improving X-ray procedures and eliminating unnecessary examinations, as she clearly points out.[34] The problem of estimation of the whole-body radiation dose to the fetus has not been resolved in any of the epidemiological studies examining the relationship of prenatal irradiation to childhood cancers. Stewart was able to develop a dose estimate from the number of films used and showed an increasing relative risk from 1.3 at 200 to 250 mrad to 1.6 for 1200 to 1389 mrad. However, the radiation dose estimates are far from accurate and can only be regarded as a general guide.[34,35] Stewart estimated that the low radiation dose used in diagnostic obstetric radiology possibly may have caused 5% of childhood cancers, which supports the likelihood of many causative factors in the etiology of childhood cancers.

Fetuses of occupationally exposed women, accumulating comparable doses, could share the same risk seen in patients, if indeed the latter are not a specially selected population with confounding characteristics that lead to the need for diagnostic X-rays.

E. Internal Emitting Isotopes

Studies of the reproductive effects of internally deposited radioisotopes have been virtually confined to animals except for the relatively ineffectual efforts to obtain information from the radium dial painters. Plutonium [239] (as citrate solution) intravenously injected into mice is deposited almost completely within the intertubular spaces of the testes and in the surrounding peritubular tissues.[37] With the short path length of alpha particles, the spermatogonial stem cells become the critical target cells for the high-energy alpha radiation and the dose to these cells is considerably higher than for the testes as a whole. Further reproductive studies by Luning and Frolen[38] showed a significant excess of intrauterine mortality when females were mated to males intravenously injected with [239]Pu nitrate solution. The intrauterine mortality increased from 9% in the animals conceived the first week following injection to 12 to 13% in the animals conceived the fifth week following injection, after which mortality dropped. During the first 5 weeks of fertilization of ova, the sperm used were those in post- and perimeiotic stages at the time of injection so that the effect of alpha irradiation on that stage of spermatogenesis was induction of dominant lethality. In addition, F_1 males sired by [239]Pu injected fathers sustained the dominant lethal effect, seen as an increase in intrauterine mortality in mated females over controls.[38]

Dominant lethals were induced in both male and female mice fed tritiated water,[39,40] with the most marked effect being observed when both parents or the mother only were exposed.

The effects of internal emitters on the gonads and germ cells have not been adequately examined to date in animals or working populations so that any satisfactory extrapolation to a particular work setting is uncertain.

Costa and Cottino[41] have shown that human fetuses 6 and 7.8 cm (presumably 70 to 77 days old) did not absorb the radioiodine administered to the mother but the 9.5 cm fetus (presumably 80 days old) and those older exhibited radioiodine uptake and the presence of stable iodine in the thyroid gland. At about the third month of gestation, the total stable iodine content of the fetal thyroid is tenfold between the sixth month and birth. The iodine content of the thyroid increases at a faster rate than its weight, so that the iodine content per gram of gland increases as pregnancy progresses. "Hormonogenesis" is complete in the 3½ month (16 cm) fetus and radioiodine accumulation in the fetal thyroid can be as much as ten times that in the maternal thyroid, weight for weight.

There have been a number of published case studies showing radioiodine damage to the fetal thyroid gland from millicurie therapeutic doses, in addition to studies reporting no untoward effects. These cases are reviewed by Pfannensteil et al.[42] and they report induced congenital hypothyroidism which apparently occurred during the tenth week of embryonic life. Diagnostic administration of ^{59}Fe to 700 pregnant women with a dose to the fetus of 5 to 15 rad was not found to be associated with additional malformations when compared with a control population.[43]

F. Maternal Irradiation and Fetal Malformations

The UNSCEAR report in the chapter on mechanisms of radiation teratogenesis raised an issue of particular concern to the evaluation of female reproduction in relation to the radiation environment.

"One issue concerning mechanisms which has attracted much attention, particularly in the older literature, is the influence that the irradiated maternal organism might have on the appearance of foetal abnormalities. The reasons for such a continued interest can hardly be explained, since it stems mainly from experiments of doubtful significance..."[16]

Brent et al. in experiments in mice showed that by a series of organ-shielding procedures they could establish that irradiation of the mother and shielding of the embryo resulted in no increase in resorptions.[44,45] Irradiation of the placenta while the mother and conceptus were shielded was not associated with any adverse effects on the fetus. In none of the experiments were malformations increased so that it is unlikely that irradiation to the mother herself can result in malformations in the embryo or fetus. High doses of irradiation of the mother sufficient to have an adverse effect on her, of course, could indirectly affect the viability of the embryo or fetus.

G. Conclusion

It seems likely that, as in the past the evaluation of radiation protection will proceed as a continuous process to ensure that new information will be incorporated into the risk estimate process.

The methodology of making risk estimates of the effects of ionizing radiation is now well established largely due to the extensive animal experimentation and observations of human populations over a long period of time. The benefits of diagnostic and therapeutic irradiation can, therefore, be balanced against the hazards that ionizing radiation presents.

Women who work in a radiation environment are likely to be in health-related jobs. The industrial sector is now also employing more women where they may work with, or in the vicinity of, industrial X-ray machines, accelerators, radium sources, radionuclides, and power reactors. Manufacturing and distribution of radionuclides and research activities must also be taken into account as we evaluate the reproductive integrity of both male and female workers.

The serious deficiency at this time appears to be the inadequate evaluation of breast and thyroid cancer prevalence among women occupationally exposed to ionizing radiation from their young adult years through 20 or more years of employment. In addition, the lack of information on the reproductive experience of wives of men occupationally exposed is serious in light of the risk estimates of the radiation effects on sperm integrity. Adverse pregnancy outcome can be a dangerous medical hazard for the mother herself, an indirect impact on her of her husband's occupational hazard. Finally, the evaluation of the reproductive experience of the woman worker herself in relation to her radiation environment needs attention from epidemiologists.

III. NONIONIZING RADIATION

The expanding use of nonionizing radiant energy, which includes ultraviolet, infrared, visible light, microwaves, radio-frequency waves, and coherent light sources (lasers) occurred during a time when the research emphasis was being placed on ionizing radiation. Biological effects of microwave radiation are belatedly under closer scrutiny in part because of the reevaluation of the occupational exposure standard of 10 mW/cm² for an 8-hr work day. A power density in excess of 10 mW/cm² should not occur for a period any longer than 6 min. The performance standard for microwave ovens specifies a maximum level of 1 mW/cm² at 5 cm from the external surface of the oven at manufacture and a maximum of 5 mW/cm² at 5 cm from the external surface of the oven throughout the life of the product. Microwave ovens are extensively used in restaurants, during drying procedures for a wide variety of manufacturing procedures, and more recently in the home kitchen.

Standards in Eastern Europe are considerably more stringent on the basis of general malaise reported among workers at far lower occupational exposure levels than the U.S. standard. The symptoms reported include weakness, fatigue, vague feelings of discomfort, headache, drowsiness, palpitations, faintness, and memory loss.[46]

There is a serious deficiency of information on the biological effects of microwaves with suggestive evidence indicating adverse human reproductive effects. Absorbed energy of microwaves is transformed into increased kinetic energy of the absorbing molecules so that heating of the tissue results. Microwaves can penetrate to deep tissues with potential disruption of normal cell growth and development. Lancranjan et al. examined 31 young men with long-term exposure to microwaves and found alterations of spermatogenesis in 74% of them. There was a statistically significant difference when compared with a control population in the number of spermatozoa, number of normal sperm, and number of motile sperm per ejaculate. The conclusion was that there was probably a direct effect of microwaves on the germinal epithelium of male gonads in that no evidence of an influence on the testes endocrine function was found.[47] Unfortunately, no studies on the reproductive experience of the wives of these workers were reported.

In mice, Rugh et al. have produced anomalies in fetuses using high levels of microwaves — 2450 MHz for 5 min at an estimated power density of 125 mW/cm^2. Gross hemorrhage, resorption, exencephaly, stunting, and fetal death were observed.[48] Human case studies have been few. A women irradiated during the first 59 days of pregnancy aborted on the 67th day and three patients who conceived within 3 months of microwave therapy delivered normal infants at term.[49] Microwave heating of the uterine wall during parturition is an accepted clinical procedure with recognition that large doses could increase the temperature of the fetus and the amniotic fluid, though adverse effects have not been reported.[50]

The NIOSH guide to occupational diseases included a review of the Eastern Europe literature in which there are reports of changes in menstrual patterns, retarded fetal development, congenital effects in newborn babies, decreased lactation in nursing mothers, and an increased prevalence of miscarriages for women working with microwaves.[51]

Many manufacturing operations where women work use microwaves during drying and sealing processes, e.g., wood working and furniture assembly; glass fiber drying; paper drying and heating; plastic heat sealing in packaging, which is a particularly female-intensive occupation; rubber processing; and yarn drying in the textile industry.[51]

IV. NOISE AND VIBRATION

There is no doubt that noise is associated with adverse human effects. There are numerous reports in the literature showing that noise can cause permanent and temporary hearing impairment, interfere with speech communications, hinder performance on certain tasks, and be a source of annoyance.

A. Animal Studies

Animal studies provide us with most of the information available concerning the effects of sound on the reproductive process. The laboratory animal most frequently used was the female rat. Mice, guinea pigs, and rabbits were used occasionally. Singh notes that relatively more is known about the reproductive system and controlling mechanisms in the rat than in any other laboratory animal and enough data are available to estimate the effects of auditory stimuli on their reproductive process.[52]

Auditory stimuli produce irregularities in the estrus cycles of rats. Arvay, using multiple stimuli, noted more days of estrus than normal during the first 10 or 12 days of exposure.[53] The number of days between each estrus lengthened with the cycle becoming irregular until the majority of rats showed a constant diestrous pattern of vaginal smears at 42 days. Zondek and Tamari found increased ovarian weights in rats exposed to sound stimuli,[54] while Sackler et al. noted decreased ovarian weights.[55] Neither the nature nor the duration of the sound stimuli were comparable in these experiments.

After 2 months of auditory stimulation, Zondek and Tamari reported that the ovaries of the rats were composed essentially of corpora lutea.[54] Arvay noted two distinct phases in the ovaries of rats following sound stimulation.[53] During the early phase there was accelerated maturation of the follicles with some follicles showing well-defined degenerative changes. The late phase was characterized by atretic follicles dominated by mature or atretic corpora lutea. Singh and Rao observed different changes in the ovaries with the early phase, the ovaries showing only follicles and/or corpora lutea. After prolonged exposure to sound, persistent estrus occurred and the ovaries showed cystic follicles but no corpora lutea.[56]

There are few studies available regarding the function of the ovaries in sound-exposed animals. Zondek and Tamari concluded that sound stimuli had a stimulating effect on the ovaries because the ovaries in sound-exposed rats resembled those of rats receiving gonadotropins.[54] Singh comments that biochemical and endocrine studies are necessary to answer important questions relating hormonal levels, ovarian function, and sex behavior and mating in rats.

Morphological studies of the nongravid uterus also show contradictory results. Zondek and Tamari have reported increased uterine weights in rats subjected to auditory stress.[54] On the contrary, Sackler et al. observed decreased uterine weights and atrophy of the uteri in sound-exposed rats.[55] Characteristics of the stimuli used in each of the studies were different.

Singh states that there is some evidence that there is a drop in the fertility index of sound-exposed rats, as defined by the number of pregnancies over the number of females mated, and a drop in productivity.[52] The early period of gestation appears to be the most vulnerable to the insults of auditory stress. Zondek and Tamari are of the opinion that auditory stimuli have no effect on embryonic development if the fertilized ova is well established in the endometrium.[54] Geber found that multiple stimuli produce multiple malformations in the young, delayed conception, and increased stillbirths and neonatal deaths.[57]

B. Human Studies

There is scant information in the literature with regard to the effect of sound on the human reproductive system.

Sound is composed of audible vibrations and vibration studies may, therefore, provide us with some information concerning the effects of sound on the reproductive process that are not initiated by auditory pathways. Glowacki has noted that vibration exerts an adverse effect on the female generative tract.[58] Low frequency vibrations are the most detrimental because they may lead to resonance of internal organs. In addition, sound is often accompanied by vibration in an industrial setting. If any adverse effect to the reproductive process is observed in an industry where noise is present, then the vibrational characteristics of the situation should also be considered.

The cardiovascular system is known to respond to noise by vasoconstrictions and fluctuations in arterial blood pressure. In a review of the literature on the extra-auditory effects of noise, Anticaglia states that vasoconstriction of the small arterioles occurs with noise exposures of only 70 dB.[59] It is possible that noise has a secondary

TABLE 5

Fertility in Families of Female Textile Workers and Male Machinists

Group	Number of families	Childless	1 Child	2 Children	More than 2 children	Total
Textile	220	22%	42%	28%	3%	95%
Machine	110	21.8%	57.2%	20%	1%	100%
Controls	200	10%	21%	42%	27%	100%

From Carosi, L. and Calabro, F., Folia Med. (Index Medicus Serial), 51, 264, 1968.

effect on the reproductive process. Dunbar suggests that certain stresses may disturb uterine circulation sufficiently to bring about detachment of the placenta, thus causing abortion.[60]

Kalicinski et al. measured arterial blood pressure and electrocardiograms (ECG) in 140 women who had worked for a long time under exposure to industrial noise.[61] The noise was characterized as having a sound pressure level between 95 and 105 dB and frequencies between 32 and 16,000 Hz. The incidence of hypertension and ECG signs of ischemia among the women increased relative to the duration of work exposure to noise.

Griefahn also investigated vasoconstriction in women, but under laboratory conditions.[62] She exposed 17- to 39-year old women to white noise at 95 dB(A) for five periods of 2-min duration. During the experiments pulse rate, finger pulse amplitudes, and respiration frequency were measured. She found greater vasoconstriction in women with small pulse rate and small cardiac output in contrast to women with high pulse rate and great cardiac output during noise exposure. The degree of vasoconstriction was greater during the follicle of the menstral cycle phase than during the corpus luteum phase and this appeared to be dependent upon the level and duration of the vibration.

Frolova investigated the effect of vibration on the blood supply to the true pelvis at different periods of the menstrual cycle of female tractor drivers.[63] The women were exposed to vibration at 4 Hz frequency and 123 dB sound pressure level. The vibration caused development of venous congestion which was most pronounced during the menstruation phase. The degree of venous congestion was dependent upon the level and duration of the vibration.

Menstrual anomalies have been associated with the vibrational insults from motor vehicles. Bohm compared two groups of women with respect to gynecological complaints.[64] One group of women consisted of 1000 vehicle personnel and the other consisted of 1000 polyclinic workers. The vehicle drivers had significantly more complications of pregnancies and menstrual anomalies. These results are questionable because of the sampling method that was used. The vehicular personnel were not selected for nonpregnant gynecological complaints, whereas this bias did exist in the polyclinic women.

Pramaterov and Balev examined the vibrational characteristics of various transportation vehicles and investigated menstrual anomalies in the women operators.[65] They found that the loss of capacity for work was directly related to the vibrational characteristics of the vehicle operated. The greater the amplitude and acceleration of the vibration, the greater the loss of capacity for work. No comparison was made with other types of female workers in regard to the amount of time lost from work as a result of menstrual disorders.

There is some indication that productivity is lowered in workers exposed to noise.

Carosi and Calabro studied spouses working in two industrial plants.[66] In a textile plant the workers were almost all female and in a machine shop the workers were exclusively male. He compared the number of offspring in these families to families in which neither spouse was exposed to industrial noise. Birth control was not practiced in most of the families. No explanation is offered for the 5% missing in the textile group. The data in Table 5 seem to suggest that those families exposed to noise had smaller families (none or one child) while the control group had larger families (2 or more children).

Some studies have shown noise and vibration to be associated with pregnancy complications. Japanese studies reported by Welch and Welch of the reproductive histories of families living near an airport showed that there was an increased rate of premature births in these families.[67]

Tzetkov identified factors in the textile industry which he believed to have an unfavorable effect on pregnancy. These factors include horizontal and vertical vibration, excessive heat, strained body position, incessant walking, and lifting weights.[68] He also noted that nonoccupational factors such as maternal constitution, diseases of the mother, and first pregnancy would affect the pregnancy outcome. Of 618 women studied, 8.6% reported spontaneous abortions and 6.08% reported premature deliveries. The number of spontaneous abortions was reported in the abstract to be greater than the expected prevalence.

Gratsianskaya et al. investigated the reproductive histories of female concrete layers who were exposed to high-frequency vibrations. This group had a higher prevalence of menstrual disturbances than other female occupational groups for which data were available. Some of the effects observed were a high rate of abnormal labor, an increased frequency of asphyxial complications in the neonates, and an elevated perinatal mortality.[69]

It remains to be established whether environmental stimuli have any effect on fetal sensory development and subsequent behavior. Omerod states that by the 24th week of intrauterine life the cochlea and the sensory end organs have completed development.[70] Premature infants of only 28 weeks gestation are known to react to sound stimuli. In order to assess whether external stimuli affect the fetus, it is necessary to know the sound characteristics of the uterine environment, the extent to which external sound and vibration contribute to this sound energy, and the nature of the fetal response to externally produced sound.

In an attempt to measure intrauterine sound pressure levels, Bench placed a microphone at the cervix of one woman in labor.[71] The internal background noise was rhythmic and averaged 72 dB. He attributed the intrauterine sound level to pulsations of uterine blood. However, this method underestimated the true sound pressure level within the uterus because the microphone was located in the vagina at the cervix rather than within the uterus.[72,73]

Although the information on intrauterine sound level and maternal tissue attenuation of sound is relatively recent, researchers have long been interested in fetal response to external sound stimuli.[74] Peiper examined women in late pregnancy and found that the sudden honking of an automobile horn within a few feet of the mother's abdomen could cause easily distinguishable movements of the fetus.[75] Forbes and Forbes cite several cases in which the mother reported fetal movement immediately after sound stimulation.[76] On the basis of these observations they concluded that the human fetus has the ability to respond with sudden movements to a loud sound originating outside the body of the mother 4 or 5 weeks prior to birth. It could not be determined whether this was a response initiated by the auditory system or a response elicited by tactile organs in the fetal skin.

Sontag and Wallace observed movements of the fetus in response to sound stimuli provided by an ordinary doorbell buzzer whose knocker was made to strike a small wooden disk on the abdomen of the subjects.[77] Observations ranged from 127 to 1 day before birth. The results of this experiment were as follows: (1) a reliable increase in detectable fetal movements following the sound stimulus; (2) responses beginning at about 31 weeks gestation; and (3) an increase in the frequency of the response as the fetus neared term. It was their opinion that such a response might furnish some index of the development and maturity of the fetus.

Bernard and Sontag presented tonal stimulation to 4 gravida during the last 2½ months of pregnancy.[78] The frequencies used ranged from 20 to 20,000 Hz and were varied systematically. Fetal heart rate was used as a measure of the fetal reactivity. Results showed a significant cardioacceleration of the fetus following tonal stimulation. The rapidity of the response eliminated the possibility that the response was the result of a maternal humoral change transmitted secondarily to the fetus. Cardioacceleratory responses of the fetus appeared to be direct responses to the tonal stimulations. It was not establised whether the perception of the tone was accomplished by means of the fetal auditory organs or vibratory perception of other parts of the body. Fleischer graphically registered the movement of fetuses following tonal stimulation.[79] All fetuses had reached 24 weeks of gestation. Murphy and Smyth reported that fetal heart rates increased significantly after pure tones of 50 and 4000 Hz were transduced through the maternal abdominal wall.[80] They ruled out the possibility that the response was due to uterine contraction by using a tocodynamometer.

Dwornicka et al. measured fetal heart rate in 32 women in the last month of pregnancy after the presentation of auditory stimulation.[81] The stimulation consisted of a 1000 or 2000 Hz tone at 100 dB for a duration of 5 sec. At 1000 Hz, the fetal heart rate increased an average of 7 beats per min; at 2000 Hz, the increase was an average of 11 beats per min. Maternal heart rate was also measured following tonal stimulation. The absence of any maternal cardioacceleration ruled out the possibility that the response was due to an excitation of the maternal cardiovascular system. Johansson used tonal stimulation with frequencies above 1500 Hz to exclude the possibility that the fetal reaction was due to vibration.[73] He found significant increases of fetal heart rate in 9 of 12 fetuses tested.

The findings of Bench and Vass do not support the earlier studies.[82] They presented tones at frequencies of 500 and 4000 Hz at 100 dB for a duration of 15 sec. No significant increases in fetal heart rate were measured. They felt that earlier work such as that of Murphy and Smyth[80] and Dwornicka were weakened by a lack of adequate control data. Some problems which they noted were control periods different in duration from stimulus periods and the measurement of spontaneous, rather than induced, increases in fetal heart rates. They noted that their failure to find a significant increase in fetal heart rate might be due to poor transduction of sound energy into the maternal tissues in an air coupled system. Grimwade et al. felt that the inability of Bench and Vass to measure increases in fetal heart rates was the result of an inadequate intrauterine sound pressure level.[83] Since the intrauterine sound pressure level produced by Bench and Vass was approximately 61 dB at 500 Hz and less than 40 dB at 4000 Hz,[82] the normal intrauterine sound pressure level would mask the externally produced noise in such an instance.

Grimwade et al. delivered both tonal and vibrational stimuli to gravida at frequencies ranging from 20 to 5000 Hz.[74] The intrauterine sound pressure level of the tonal stimulation that the subjects received was 70 to 90 dB; from the vibrational stimuli (20 to 100 Hz), the sound pressure level was 95 to 110 dB. They concluded that the responses were initiated by the fetal nervous system since 78% of the increases in fetal heart rate began within 5 sec of the introduction of the stimulus.

Grimwade et al. reported the most thorough study on the response of the fetus to sound and vibrational stimulation.[83] Stimuli were presented only when the fetal heart rate had maintained a baseline value for 3 min. This procedure reduced the chance that any measured increase in fetal heart rate was spontaneous. The stimulus consisted of a pure tone sound between 55 and 1000 Hz which produced an intrauterine sound pressure level of 80 dB. The study supports the claims that the fetus does respond to tonal and vibrational stimulation by means of increased movement and accelerated heart rate.

With the aid of a probe microphone Walker et al. were able to obtain more accurate measurements of the intrauterine noise level.[72] A microphone was passed through the cervical canal to lie beside the head of the fetus in 16 women at term and in 7 nonpregnant women. Although there was no significant difference between the mean intrauterine sound levels of the two groups, the sound detected in the pregnant uterus was of greater magnitude in the higher frequencies when compared to the nonpregnant uterus. Greater turbulence of the intrauterine blood probably explains the higher sound pressure levels in the pregnant uterus at high frequencies.

The sound pressure level of the fetal environment will consist of the maternal intrauterine sound level plus any noise which passes through the maternal abdominal wall from the external environment. Thus to estimate the total sound environment of the fetus, it is necessary to know the amount of sound that passes through the maternal abdominal wall. Johansson et al. measured the attenuation of sound through the maternal abdominal wall by inserting a microphone into the uterus of four women who had just given birth.[73] He reported that the attenuation of sound is essentially the same between 1000 and 3000 Hz but he did not offer a value for this attenuation. Bench notes that results obtained by Johansson et al. are not reliable because of the absence of uterine contraction and amniotic fluid.[71,73] He presented pure tones at the maternal abdominal wall and measured the sound pressure level of these tones at the cervix. He found the attenuation of the tones to increase with frequency. The tones underwent the following attenuation of sound pressure: 19 dB at 200 Hz; 24 dB at 500 Hz; 38 dB at 1000 Hz; and 48 dB at 2000 and 4000 Hz. The values at 2000 and 4000 Hz cannot be regarded as true since the strength of the signal was not loud enough to overcome the internal background noise. These results are in conflict with Johansson et al.[73] who found the attenuation to be linear between 1000 and 3000 Hz. This is probably due to the condition of the uterus and the place of measurement being different in each of the studies.

Grimwade et al. passed a microphone into the uterus adjacent to the fetal head in order to obtain precise measurements of the maternal attenuation of sound.[74] They found, as did Bench, that attenuation increased with frequency. The attenuation ranged from 39 dB at 500 Hz to 85 dB at 3000 Hz. They concluded that high-frequency sound in the external environment would not contribute significantly to the sound pressure level in the uterus.

It is interesting to note that the attenuation values reported by Grimwade et al. are much higher than the values reported by Bench. Bench felt that his results were probably an overestimation of the maternal attenuation since the microphone was located in the vagina at the cervix rather than within the uterus. It appears, however, that he underestimated the attenuation by not taking adequate precautions to prevent sound from reaching the microphone via the vagina. Walker et al. used the same procedure as Grimwade and colleagues to measure attenuation of sound but corrected the attenuation values for microphone impedence error. Their results agree with earlier studies in that they found attenuation to increase with frequency. They concluded, "The attenuation is such that there will rarely be an integral value for an environmentally generated noise level that will exceed the intrauterine noise level at any particular frequency, and the external sound can then be said to be masked...The great attenuation suffered by frequencies above 1000 Hz and the low level of these in most environmental situations makes it unlikely that the fetus normally receives sound of this nature."[72] However, it is possible that the fetus will be exposed to additional noise of low frequency if the fetus is in a subway, close to an aircraft, or in an industrial setting with high noise levels.

Ando and Hattori have now supplemented earlier epidemiologic studies that had shown an increase the prevalence of low-birth-weight babies in a population living near an international airport.[84] Human placental lactogen levels in the serum of pregnant women and the birth weights of their infants were determined.[85] One group of 343 women lived in the district surrounding a jet airport and 112 women lived in a commercial and industrial area with comparable atmospheric pollution, population density, standard of living, weather, and living conditions. After the 32nd week of pregnancy the human placental lactogen (HPL) serum levels of more than 40% of the subjects in the noise area had fallen to more than one standard deviation below the mean. By the 36th week of pregnancy, the difference between the two groups was statistically significant. There were 45% of the women in the noise area after the 35th week of pregnancy who had HPL serum levels lower than 4 μg/mℓ, considered to be the fetal danger level compared with 9% of the women living in the quiet area. The decrease in HPL levels was also associated with lower birth-weight babies and, for those in the noise area, the birth weights associated with HPL more than 6 μg/mℓ were significantly higher than those with HPL levels 4 μg/mℓ or less. The incidence of birth weights below 3000 g was 23% for the higher HPL values and 73% for the lower values. The difference was statistically significant. Although the results as presented show clear differences, the use of HPL as an indicator has some disadvantages. Significant fluctuations occur within any 24-hr period and variations have not been shown to follow a systematic pattern, and indeed may exceed the methodological error.[86] Single samples from an individual patient may be misleading and it is not clear how Ando and Hattori controlled the sampling procedures during their observations.

C. Overview

From the animal studies it is evident that sound stimulation affects the onset of sexual maturation, is associated with abnormalities of estrus and lower productivity, and can be teratogenic in combination with other stimuli. The standard cautions with respect to all data of this type are in order. It is impossible to predict the likelihood and the degree to which results from animal experiments will be manifested in humans. Furthermore, it should be realized that exposure conditions in these experiments were different from normal occupational or environmental exposures.

Human studies are seriously lacking in all aspects of the problem. The information that does exist suggests that noise exposure may have a deleterious effect on the human reproductive process. These effects can be grouped into three areas: (1) effects on the male and female reproductive systems, (2) effects on the gravida which affect pregnancy outcome, and (3) effects on the fetus which have an impact on postnatal life.

Much more is known about the effect of noise on the female reproductive system than the male system. Laboratory studies have demonstrated stimulation of ovarian function and vasoconstriction as a result of noise exposure. Menstrual anomalies were observed in females who operated motor vehicles. These workers were exposed to vibrational as well as noise insults. In males sexual dysfunction was reported by workers with a history of noise exposures. Families of men and women exposed to industrial noise were generally smaller than families in which neither spouse was exposed to noise in their occupational environment.

Some of the pregnancy effects observed were spontaneous abortion, premature delivery, and a high rate of abnormal labors. It is yet to be determined whether exposure during the first 3 months of pregnancy is related to these disorders as is the case with chemical teratogens and ionizing radiation. Animal studies indicate that once the fetus is implanted, noise has no effect on physiological development of the fetus.

Evidence that the fetus can respond to sensory stimulation has stirred interest in the possible effects that externally produced sound might have on the fetus. Maternal attenuation studies demonstrate that low-frequency sounds reach the fetus more frequently than high-frequency sounds that rarely, if ever, transduce the maternal abdominal wall. Postnatal adaption to sound has been associated with fetal exposure to aircraft noise.

Although many of the human studies are in no way conclusive regarding the effect of noise, they do raise suspicions as to the safety of occupational and environmental noise with respect to the reproductive process. The scarcity of human studies makes evaluation of the problem difficult. Epidemiological studies should be performed on the impact of industrial and environmental noise on the reproductive process. Information is needed on the reproductive effects on the male worker, on the pregnant and nonpregnant female worker, and on the wives of male workers exposed to noise. Animal studies are also needed to assess the effect of sound and vibration on spermatogenesis.

V. TEMPERATURE — HEAT AND COLD STRESS

The consideration of women in studies of heat and cold tolerance has been more consistent than in other areas of environmental stress and can be partially attributed to the influence of Hardy and Dubois.[87] In 1940 they read a paper before the National Academy of Sciences and noted that there had been "a large number of publications dealing with the reactions of men to changes of environmental temperature, but very few studies with women. Just why there has been such a neglect of half our population is not clear. Air conditioning is theoretically based on physiological studies and politeness alone would demand more consideration of the ladies."

A. Physiological Response to Heat

In 1934 Mason had concluded that the basal metabolism of European women in South India was 5% lower in tropical India than it was in the temperate zone.[88] With the newly available calorimeter Hardy and Dubois began studies on women which set the pattern for their inclusion up to the present. They found that under cold conditions the heat loss for seven women when motionless was about 10% lower than that of the men because of their lower skin temperature and subcutaneous adipose tissue. Under hot conditions, 30 to 32°C, the metabolism of most of the women was 14 to 20% lower than that of the men. Men began to sweat at 29°C and women did not start until 34 to 36°C had been reached. The conclusion was that in adjusting to changes in the thermal environment women had a physiological advantage. For women, the comfort zone in which the heat loss and heat production were equal extended over a 6° range but only 2 to 3° for men.[87]

Senay has studied women who had not been acclimated and who did not participate in any physical activities beyond their normal daily routine.[101] The aim was to examine changes within the body that might explain the lower sweating experienced by women and their higher body temperature when compared with men under the same heat stress. Constituents and contents of the vascular volume of resting women under heat stress were examined before and after ovulation and under conditions of dehydration and rehydration. The unacclimated women failed to expand their circulatory blood volume when exposed to heat in contrast to the change that occurs in men. The resulting hemodilution in men appears to be dependent upon dilation of the cutaneous vascular bed and although the response is the same for women, the transfer to or retention of fluid in the vascular space is not maintained. The ratio of skin-surface area to blood volume is greater in women, so that they already have a larger proportion of the plasma volume in the cutaneous capillary bed. Additionally, the ratio of total body water to body weight is smaller in women. On this basis when a 50 kg woman whose total body water equals 50% of her body weight loses 0.24 ℓ as sweat (0.5% of her body weight) in 1 hr of heat exposure, she has lost 1% of her total body water, in contrast to only 0.83% loss for a 60 kg man under the same conditions.

Senay and Fortney extended these studies to untrained women under conditions of submaximal exercise and heat to examine the effects on body fluids.[100] The previous observation of reduced hemodilution was confirmed with a 12% increase in hematocrit and a 12.7% reduction in plasma volume. Exercise causes an increase of protein in the vascular volume but, for the untrained and unacclimated women working in hot conditions, the protein and accompanying water are not retained but are lost to the cutaneous interstitial spaces. Resulting fluid shifts are influenced by the characteristics of the dilated, cutaneous vascular bed and can be markedly moderated by physical conditioning and heat acclimation. All women in this study experienced signs of onset of thermoregulatory stress with dry skin, circumoral pallor, and heart rates in excess of 180 beats/min at an exercise level of 30% of maximum oxygen uptake for 45 min at 45°C and 28% relative humidity. Most parameters returned to control values within 25 min post exercise.

Henschel et al. have examined elderly women and men under hot conditions and increasing work loads.[102] Thermal balance was achieved and physiological strain was no more evident than for young people. In addition, measurable amounts of natural heat acclimation developed during the summer months. The more important change with age is the reduced ability to tolerate hard physical work.

Kamon and Avellini have reexamined the estimates of physiologic limits to work which they developed for a male heat-acclimated population and repeated the study on ten heat-acclimated women.[103] When ambient water vapor increases in a hot environment, physiologic limits are reached at a lower temperature for the same air movement. For a relative work load of 30% of maximum oxygen uptake, which is close to the limit of continuous work during an 8-hr shift, Kamon and Avellini have defined a safe limit of heat exposure taking ambient water vapor pressure into account. Under tolerable conditions of high temperature when ambient vapor pressure is not high, increases in rectal temperature, mean skin temperature, and heart rate as physiological responses to work reach a steady state. Body core temperature increases more rapidly when thermal ambient conditions are nearing physiological limits but ordinarily equilibrates at levels proportional to the metabolic rate. In these studies the upper limit of ambient vapor pressure was established at eight levels of air temperature ranging from 30 to 52°C. The vapor pressure was increased at each temperature for each individual under standard work conditions until the increasing rectal temperature showed an inflection that deviated markedly from the increased rectal temperature already established for the ambient temperature under subcritical conditions. The coefficient that described the safe-limit line was found for all practical purposes to be applicable to both men and women who were in a state of full acclimation. When the air temperature was 36°C, the female subjects had a mean skin temperature of about 35.5°C which was higher than male subjects for the same conditions. The rectal temperature at a work level equivalent to 30% maximum oxygen uptake with the water vapor pressure at a subcritical level equilibrated at about 37.65°C for men and about 37.82°C for women. The ovulatory cycle appeared to have no marked effect on the rectal temperature, but it is likely that a change could not be observed within the temperature increase resulting from exercise and heat exposure.

B. Occupational Exposure to Heat

Human limits of comfort and tolerance to work under hot conditions are related to air temperature, water vapor pressure, and air movement. Physiologic characteristics that become limiting factors for an individual's comfort and tolerance are increased core body temperature, mean skin temperature and heart rate, limited sweating capacity, and cutaneous vasodilation. Previous and recent heat acclimation affect these responses. Women as a group react more markedly when introduced initially to severe heat. The level of acclimation for women and men is eventually comparable though women take longer to reach physiological balance with the hot environment. Once acclimated, temperature and circulatory response of women and men are similar, though women continue to sweat less.[104]

In women the lower sweat production is though to be due to fewer active sweat glands during the heat exposure, even though the total number of sweat glands and the number per unit area of skin surface is greater in women.[105]

For a woman working in heat without acclimation there is a balance between the degree of sweating, her body temperature, and her rate of work. When compared with men, she is likely to sweat less and have a higher temperature. The ovulatory cycle does not markedly affect the stimulation of sweating although body temperature post-ovulation is higher in some women at rest.[101]

An acclimation procedure based on industrial experience has been recommended by NIOSH.[106] A period of 1 week is recommended for new workers to become acclimated, with work on the first day reduced by one half, followed by a gradual work increase of 10% daily. For workers who have been absent for 10 or more days, the daily increase in workload can be 20% after the first day so that only 4 days are needed for acclimation. A worker's deep body temperature must not exceed 100.4°F if heat stress is to be avoided. The NIOSH recommendation for women is an environment where the combination of air temperature, humidity, radiation, and windspeed does not exceed 70°F WBGT, 3°F below that recommended for men, due to the higher body temperatures and heart rates for identical work in heat for women. Warning signs are necessary when climatic heat exceeds 86°F WBGT in that a worker could collapse before being able to leave that environment if she is already close to her endurance limit. At rest the maximum endurable body temperature is the same in both sexes but women, under experimental conditions, have found the stress intolerable earlier. The effects of work load and physical conditioning may be quite different from one individual to another in terms of response to heat stress.

In many female-intensive occupations with sweatshop conditions, there is little likelihood of recommended preplacement and regular medical examinations. Self-selection certainly occurs but for women in canneries, laundries, and some manufacturing jobs, economic necessity overrides their physiologic comfort and well-being.

C. Epidemiologic Studies

Extensive analyses of mortality rates during episodes of extreme heat in a number of U.S. cities have established that excess mortality does occur.[107,108] The seriousness of excessive heat as a primary or contributing cause of death has been well recognized by clinicians but appears to be little recognized by the lay public today, particularly with the advent of air conditioning for those who can afford it. Although Ellis' review of the national experience from 1952 to 1967 showed that for heat-related deaths men outnumbered women. Schuman's more detailed comparison of mortality in St. Louis and New York during the severe heat wave of late June and mid-July of 1966 showed the largest increase in deaths among women in both cities, white females in New York — 56%, and nonwhite women in St. Louis — 140%.[108]

There are severe heat conditions, particularly in the first hot summer days or during subsequent heat waves, where women in jewelry factories (invariably old buildings with little ventilation) and laundries, to cite only two extreme possibilities, have repetitive experience of excessive heat as part of their work environment.

Ellis believed he noted a slight excess of maternal deaths in July and August over the years 1952 to 1967 from complications of pregnancy, childbirth, and the puerperium, though the numbers were small and he derived his data from state vital statistics.[107]

Unfortunately the accuracy and analysis of vital statistics in relation to heat waves has not been particularly sophisticated in the past and it is difficult to draw firm conclusions from much of the available data. Morbidity has been even less examined but it is generally agreed that incapacitating heat disorders may have long term sequelae, particularly cardiovascular and neurologic effects.

D. Reproductive Effects

The effect of heat on fertilization has long been observed in domestic animals — cows, sheep, and rabbits. Breeding failures have been attributed to early embryonic death, which is known to occur in ewes.[109] Extended estrous cycles may be associated with early embryonic death and stimulation of corpus luteal activity with delayed luteolysis and delayed onset of the next estrus period. In cows the sequence of estrous cycle events is not affected by heat stress but the duration of estrus is much reduced and fertility is reduced. Uhlberg and Burfening have examined embryonic death in sheep and cattle under heat-stress conditions by use of embryo transfer experiments.[110] They conclude that a slight increase in temperature even for a short period is sufficient to affect the spermatozoa before fertilization or the ovum immediately after fertilization resulting in death of the resulting embryo. There is little substantive information on the effects of heat stress on preconception ova and none that provides an evaluation of the human experience. Significant reduction in fertility is known to occur in heat stressed Holstein-Friesian cows in Arizona.[111] The number of live calves born per number of breedings may drop below 20% in the hot months in contrast to 80% in cool weather. Some studies have shown residual reduced fertility for several months and implicated continued circulation of progestins due to heat stress. Observations of sheep grazing in hot regions and experimentally exposed to heat stress have confirmed the effect on birth weight.[112] A marked reduction in birth weight is seen following heat stress applied during the last two thirds of pregnancy, an effect more serious than that seen in nutritional restriction. Possible influences include diversion of blood from the uterus due to thermoregulatory stress.

Little insight can be gained directly into the relationship of the human physiological changes during pregnancy and heat tolerance. Although many pregnant women consciously note their improved cold tolerance in terms of comfort, detailed observations of a scientific nature are lacking. Taggart et al. have shown that increases in skinfold thickness (a measure of subcutaneous fat) occur up to at least 30 weeks of pregnancy and decrease a considerable amount between 38 weeks of pregnancy and the first postpartum weeks.[113] Measurements of skin temperature of the fingers have shown increases after 30 min at room temperature from 17°C before pregnancy to 34°C at term, and from 20 to 27°C, respectively, for toes.[114] Hytten and Leitch believe that finger temperature in late pregnancy may be "close to the physiological maximum and is similar to the temperature reached in non-pregnant subjects when reflex vasodilatation is caused by immersing the feet in hot water. In late pregnancy little or no increase occurs with such reflex heating."[115] The basal body temperature fluctuates with the menstrual cycle with an increase of 0.3 to 0.6°C after ovulation, which in pregnancy is maintained until about mid-term when it declines to normal levels.[116]

Descriptive comment concerning laundry workers by early Department of Labor studies gave the impression that the reproductive experience was likely to be adverse.[117] However, the socioeconomic status was clearly a serious confounding factor. McDonald noted in a prospective study of 3295 working women and their pregnancies that a higher proportion of the mothers of infants with major defects had engaged in certain types of heavy work early in pregnancy, particularly in laundries. Four of the 27 laundry workers had infants with major defects — anencephalus, hydrocephalus, congenital heart defect, and hypospadias.[118]

These isolated comments on laundry workers are among the most tantalizing in the reproductive literature. The hot environment in association with hard physical work has been the most constant feature of laundry work over the past 100 years or more, but we have no accumulation of anecdotal or scientific observation to assess the effects of heat on human reproduction.

E. Cold Tolerance

The professional women skin divers in Japan have the most extreme conditions of cold and exertion so far studied.[119] In the 1960s there were 17,000 to 18,000 who collected marine plants and shellfish from reefs in water at a temperature of about 20°C. Marked physiological adaptation of the respiratory sytem and tolerance of temperature changes do not seem to have impaired their general health, though they must be a selected population. It is claimed that the obstetrical and gynecological experience is not unusual and that they are healthy women whose ages range from 20 to 50 years.

VI. CIRCADIAN CHANGES

Adjustment of the circadian system can be made directly by changing the usual sleeping hours to working hours and remaining in the same geographic location. Indirectly, rapid travel by air across meridians results in similar physiologic responses. In both instances light-dark changes and different social cues make individual adjustment difficult. Our individual location in time can be very much affected by work patterns, many of which are imposed on workers ill-suited to the stress.

Identification of the types and distribution of shiftwork systems have been attempted for the U.S. work force despite the inadequate data available.[120] In the U.S. the Bureau of Labor Statistics maintains the most comprehensive list of industry/occupational groups and Table 6 lists the manufacturing and service industries with the highest incidence of shiftwork, by absolute number and percentage of shiftworkers. It is evident that the female-intensive industries and those where many women are employed, such as hospitals and food processing, are likely to involve shift work as a condition of employment. However, the Bureau of Labor Statistics does not report whether the shift work is fixed or rotating. The effects of rotational work shifts can be particularly debilitating on returning to an original schedule, for example the electroencephelogram rhythm may resynchronize in 5 days while the respiratory rate rhythm may take 11 days. More research is being done on physiological rhythms and sleep patterns in contrast to the earlier emphasis on worker performance, job satisfaction, and shift preference. However, there is still a tendency to emphasize the responses of men without a comparable attention being accorded women. Most of the information on hospital workers is confined to nurses. The additional stress of household responsibilities that most women workers maintain is often mentioned but seldom evaluated quantitatively.

TABLE 6

Number and Percentage of Shift Workers in Manufacturing and Service
Industries-1965

Grouping	Number (1000s)	Shift workers (%)
Hospital	1117	36.9
Education	1115	17.0
Other transportation service	763	39.6
Food and kindred products	593	42.7
Health	572	29.9
Private household	507	40.7
Transportation equipment	498	29.9
Primary metal industries	402	37.5
Machinery except electrical	363	18.9
Printing and publishing	327	28.5
Electrical equipment and supplies	278	14.8
Postal	277	45.8
Fabricated metal products	261	23.6
Other professional services	246	17.3
Welfare	221	21.8
Textile mill products	216	34.4
Chemical and allied products	199	19.7
Railroad and railway express service	177	32.6
Paper and allied products	176	32.4
Rubber and plastic products	174	35.0
Stone, clay, and glass products	154	28.5
Lumber and wood products	130	25.4
Instruments and related products	56	12.9
Apparel and other textile products	54	5.2
Miscellaneous durable industries	49	12.0
Petroleum and coal products	42	17.7
Furniture and fixtures	33	7.7
Ordnance	29	15.1
Tobacco	20	32.8
Leather and leather products	17	7.3

From *Shift Work Practices In the United States*, National Institute for
Occupational and Environmental Health, U.S. Department of Health,
Education and Welfare, Washington, D.C., 1965.

Over 16 million workers, or close to 20% of the U.S. labor force, experience shift scheduling of some kind. The most severe social and physiological stresses are likely to be associated with rotational work shifts where workers change periodically from day to evening to night shifts. Shift work is a significant factor influencing the health of workers but epidemiological and physiological research on the relationship has not yet reached a sophisticated level. The wide variety of shift-work patterns and self-selection of workers have been serious problems in the design of reliable studies. Scheving has discussed the limitations of the research so far developed for studies of shift-work effects and has emphasized the chronobiological approach, which allows monitoring during a span of shiftwork of performance and of psychological and biochemical variables.[121] Temperature, radial pulse, systolic blood pressure, and pulmonary function are synchronized in both frequency and phase with the diurnal cycle and, overall, enough evidence has been accumulated to show that the endocrine system fluctuates rhythmically, that the flow of urine is rhythmic, and the cardiovascular, hematopoietic, respiratory, and autonomic nervous system all exhibit rhythmic patterns.

There are maximum and minimum values for the circadian rhythms of human physiological systems, many of which are synchronized with the 24-hr day by periodic factors in the environment, such as alteration of light and dark and social patterns. When the internal rhythms become desynchronized from the external environment, they also tend to become desynchronized from each other. There are marked changes in sleep patterns of workers who change shifts so that sleep disturbance is one of their most common complaints. Weitzman described a nurse on night work for 10 years for 5 days each week but who returned to nocturnal sleep and diurnal waking on weekends.[122] Her sleep pattern was markedly affected with the sleep period fragmented by long awakenings and loss of normal organization of sleep stages. Felton made a more extensive study of 39 nurses who rotated shifts around the clock by examining time of occurrence of the peak of temperature and urine cations, creatinine, and osmolality.[123] Before the change to night duty, temperature was low in the early morning and rose during the day to a maximum at 1500 hours, then began to decrease. The urinary sodium creatinine and osmolality maximum occurred at 0600 hours, then decreased during the day. Potassium reached a maximum at 1200 hours before decreasing. Change to the night shift advanced the temperature and potassium cycles 3 hr and the sodium, creatinine, and osmolality cycles returned to the original daytime activity cycle, but temperature and potassium did not return until more than 10 days following the change back to the day shift. There was a general reduction in the quantity and quality of sleep, continued fatigue, and disruption of bowel habits for a week. These changes can be viewed as desynchronization of rhythms in returning to prechange conditions. Felton believes that rotating shifts present a conflict for individuals between two tendencies in the circadian system. Social synchronizers maintain entrainment in the normal environment yet there is a need to become adjusted to the shifted work-rest cycle. Aschoff and Weaver have described the human circadian system in terms of multiple oscillators. Internal synchronization of such rhythms as activity and temperature variation have the same circadian rhythm of about 25 hr. When there is a substantially longer activity period because of shift changes, other rhythms may remain at about 25 hr. There is internal desynchronization when different rhythms may not reach a stable phase relationship but may continue to run with different frequencies. For example, two self-sustaining oscillators exist for activity and temperature rhythms and after desynchronization the degree of persistence of the oscillators mostly influencing the temperature rhythm is twelve times greater than for those oscillators mostly influencing the activity rhythm.[124]

The impact on women working under rotating shift conditions is not confined to restoration of circadian rhythms. 30-day rhythms are associated with the menstrual cycle and have been reviewed by Reinberg and Smolensky.[125]

They concluded that circatrigintan (30-day) secondary rhythms are related to hormonal changes in the menstrual cycle and provide some insight into the problem of interpreting data on the effects of shiftwork and transmeridian time changes. For example, the circadian amplitude of body temperature is greater than the circatrigintan amplitude so that experimental design in terms of standardized measurement conditions becomes far more important in evaluation of results. Use of profiles of 24-hr duration at weekly intervals throughout the menstrual cycle are suggested as a means of reducing the high noise level inherent to these studies. Despite methodological inadequacies in many studies Reinberg and Smolensky have reviewed the temporal occurrence of the crest of rhythm calculated from a vast range of reports published from 1950 to 1972. They concluded that circatrigintan menstrual rhythm can be observed for the nervous system, various characteristics of blood, plasma and serum, and for uterine cervical and endometrial physiology (Table 7). It is not surprising that efforts

TABLE 7

Crest of Circatrigintan Menstrual Rhythms

Pre-O	Pre ovulation
O	Ovulation
Post-O	Post ovulation
M	Menstrual

Characteristics of Nervous System

Reaction Time (Post-O
Optical Signals
Acoustic Signals
Depressive Mood (M)
Irritibility (M)
Eye Movement Interval (M)
Pupil Width (Pre-O)
Taste Threshold (O)
   Quinine
   Propylthiourea
Heat Pain Threshold (Pre-O)

Blood, Plasma, Serum Characteristics

Blood	Erythrocytes (Post-O)
	Hemoglobin (Post-O)
	Reticulocytes (Pre-O)
	White Blood Cells (Pre-O)
	Eosinophils (Pre-O)
	Lymphocytes (O)
	Myelocytes (M)
	Platelets (Pre-O)
	Alkali Reserve (Pre-O)
Plasma	Follicle Stimulating Hormone (Pre-O)
	Luteinizing Hormone (Pre-O)
	17-OH Progesterone (Post-O)
	Progesterone (Post-O)
	Renin Concentration (Post-O)
	Renin Activity (Post-O)
Serum	Copper Concentration (O)
	Albumin (O)
	Vitamin A (O)
	Dehydroascorbic Acid (Post-1)
	Ascorbic Acid (M)

Characteristics of Cardiovascular, Respiratory, Gastrointestinal Systems

Cardiopulmonary	Pulse (Post-O)
	Capillary permeability to fluid and protein (Post-O)
	Alveolar pCO_2 (Pre-O)
	Vital capacity (Pre-O)
Gastrointestinal	H^+ Concentration (Pre-O)
	H^+ Amount (Pre-o)
	Cl^- Concentration (Pre-O)
	Parietal Secretion (Pre-O)
Skin	Palmar sweat activity (Pre-O)
	Cutaneous reactivity to histamines (M)
	Erythema (Post-O)
Miscellaneous	Body weight (Post-O)
	Oral temperature (Post-O)

TABLE 7 (continued)

Crest of Circatrigintan Menstrual Rhythms

	Cl⁻ Concentration (Pre-O)
	Parietal Secretion (Pre-O)
Skin	Palmar sweat activity (Pre-O)
	Cutaneous reactivity to histamines (M)
	Erythema (Post-O)
Miscellaneous	Body weight (Post-O)
	Oral temperature (Post-O)
	Basal metabolic rate (Post-O)
	Mammary volume (Post-O)
	Urinary excretion - Nonprotein nitrogen (M) Uric acid (O)
	Pregnanediol (Post-O)
	Aldosterone (Post-O)
	Serotonin (Post-O)
	Melanocyte stimulating hormone (M)

Characteristics of Uterus

Cervix	Sialic acid (M)
	Total vitamin C (Post-O)
	Dehydroascorbic acid (Post-O)
	Ascorbic acid (M)
Endometrium	Zinc concentration (M)
	Alkaline phosphatase (Post-O)
	Lactic acid (Post-O)
	Lactic dehydrogenase in glands, blood vessels, stroma (Post-O)
	Succinic dehydrogenase - glands (O)
	Malic dehydrogenase (Post-O)
	B glucuronidase - glands (Pre-O)
	Acid phosphatase - glands, blood vessels, stroma (Post-O)
	Asparate amino transferase (Post-O)
	Triphosphopyridine nucleotide (Pre-O)

From Reinberg, A. and Smolensky, M. H., in *Biorhythms and Human Reproduction,* Ferin, M., Halberg, F., Richart, R. M., and Mande Wiele, R. L., Eds., John Wiley & Sons, New York, 1977, Chapter 15.

to describe the menstrual experience of airline attendants crossing time zones have not produced consistent results. Preston et al. noted that Russian studies showed that menstrual cycle length was undisturbed though menstrual discharge increased and dysmenorrhea worsened, whereas another European study showed no long-term adverse effects on any aspect of the menstrual cycle.[126]

Postponement or suppression of ovulation can result from a variety of stresses, both physical and emotional. Ovulation delay or inhibition may result from an environmental change in the preovulatory phase so that menstruation is postponed. However, menstruation will occur on time even though the change is the same but occurs in the postovulatory phase. Preston et al. had noted that British cabin crews complained of irregular cycles on initiation of long-term transmeridian flights. They issued log books to 119 flight attendants for recording menstrual cycles and although the response was low — only 29 or 24% — they concluded that a high proportion, 28%, of the women did experience irregular menstrual cycles, mostly due to prolonged cycles. No comparison group was studied. They also carried out a series of performance and physiological experiments on eight airline attendants in a controlled environment isolation unit, which allowed the imposition of time zone changes without the fatigue and stress of flying. One group of four was subjected to a time advance of 8 hr, simulating a prolonged flight east, and remained in isolation with another 8-hr advance 2 days later, with a total stay in the unit of 96 hr. A second group of four experienced no time change during their 96-hr stay in the unit. The first group experienced marked performance decrement in a series of short-term memory, vigilance, visual search, reaction time, and addition tests, which was attributed to the time-zone transition itself. However, there was also a marked decrease in daily sleep to about 5 hr which could have contributed to the poor performance.[126]

The subjective complaints of shift workers are well substantiated by research findings and it is likely there is a marked self-selection of those who can tolerate disruption in circadian rhythm. Temperature and noise stress are also better tolerated by some than others with self-selection in many industries for those who have occupational mobility. Other environments with physical stresses such as high altitude and increased atmospheric pressure occur in a few occupations, but any differential effects on women are not known.

REFERENCES

1. Hunter, D., *Diseases of Occupations,* 4th ed., Little, Brown, Boston, 1969.
2. U.S. Department of Labor, Radium poisoning, industrial poisoning from radioactive substances, *Mon. Labor Rev.,* 28, 1200, 1929.
3. Polednak, A. P., Long term effects of radium exposure in female dial workers, *Environ. Res.,* 13, 237 and 396, 1977.
4. Review of the Current State of Radiation Protection Philosophy, *NCRP Natl. Coun. Radiat. Prot. Meas. Rep.,* 43, 1975.
5. Hansen, O., Development and application of radiation protection standards, *Idaho Law Rev.,* 12, 1, 1975.
6. Nuclear Regulatory Commission, Amendments to Section 19-12, 10CFR, Part 19, Paragraph 20.1(c) of 10CFR, Part 20, *Fed. Regist.,* 40, 1975.
7. Occupational Exposure of Fertile Women, *NCRP Natl. Coun. Radiat. Prot. Meas. Rep.,* 39, 1971.
8. Review of the NCRP Radiation Dose Limit for Embryo and Fetus in Occupationally Exposed Women, *NCRP Natl. Coun. Radiat. Prot. Meas. Rep.,* 53, 1977.
9. Hospital Occupational Health Services Study, Vol. 1 and 2, National Institute for Occupational Safety and Health, U.S. Department of Health, Education and Welfare, Washington, D.C., 1972.
10. Radiation Protection for Medical and Allied Health Personnel, *NCRP Natl. Coun. Radiat. Prot. Meas. Rep.,* 48, 1976.
11. The Survey of Medical Radium Installations in Wisconsin, Rep. No. DHEW-BRH 75-8022, U.S. Department of Health, Education and Welfare, Washington, D.C., 1975.
12. Maletskos, C. J., Braun, A. G., Shanahan, M. M., and Evans, R. D., Quantitative evaluation of dose-response relationships in human beings with skeletal burdens of radium 226 and radium 228, in *Assessment of Radioactivity in Man,* Vol. 2, International Atomic Energy Agency, Vienna, 1964.
13. Blum, M. and Liuzzi, A., Thyroid [131]iodine burdens in medical and paramedical personnel, *JAMA,* 200, 992, 1967.
14. Lombardi, M. H., Beck, W. L., and Cloutier, R. J., Survey of Radiopharmaceutical Use and Safety in 69 Hospitals, Rep. No. 73-8029, Department of Health, Education and Welfare, Washington, D.C., 1972.
15. Gerusky, R. M., Lubenau, J. O., Roskopf, R., and Lieben, J., Survey of radium sources in offices of private physicians, *Public Health Rep.,* 80, 75, 1965.
16. Sources and Effects of Ionizing Radiation, United Nations Scientific Committee on the Effects of Atomic Radiation, United Nations, New York, 1977.
17. Lubenau, J. O., Davis, J. S., McDonald, D. J., and Gerusky, T. M., Analytical X-ray hazards: a continuing problem, *Health Phys.,* 16, 739, 1969.

18. **Mackenzie, I.,** Breast cancer following multiple fluoroscopies, *Br. J. Cancer,* 19, 1, 1965.
19. **Myrden, J. A. and Hiltz, T. E.,** Breast cancer following multiple fluoroscopies during pneumothorax treatment of pulmonary tuberculosis, *Can. Med. Assoc. J.,* 100, 1032, 1969.
20. **Boice, J. D. and Monson, R. R.,** Breast cancer following repeated fluoroscopic examinations of the chest, *J. Natl. Cancer Inst.,* 59, 823, 1977.
21. **Delarue, N. C., Gale, G., and Ronald, A.,** Multiple fluoroscopy of the chest: carcinogenicity for the female breast and implications for breast screening programs, *JAMA,* 112, 1405, 1975.
22. **Shore, R., Hempelmann, L., Kowaluk, E., Mansur, A. S., Pasternak, B. S., Albert, R. E., and Haughlie, G. E.,** Breast neoplasms in women treated with X-rays for acute post-partum mastitis, *J. Natl. Cancer Inst.,* 59, 813, 1977.
23. Biological Effects of Atomic Radiation, National Research Council-National Academy of Sciences, Washington D.C., 1956.
24. National Academy of Sciences, National Research Council, The Effects on Populations of Exposure to Low Levels of Ionizing Radiation, Report of the Advisory Committee on the Biological Effects of Ionizing Radiations, National Research Council-National Academy of Sciences, Washington, D.C., 1972.
25. **Alberman, E., Polani, P. E., Roberts, J. A. F., Spicer, C. C., Elliott, M., Armstrong, E., and Dhadial, R. K.,** Parental X-irradiation and chromosomal constitution in their spontaneously aborted fetuses, *Ann. Hum. Genet.,* 36, 185, 1972.
26. **Kinlen, L. J. and Acheson, E. D.,** Diagnostic irradiation, congenital malformations and spontaneous abortion, *Br. J. Radiol.,* 41, 648, 1968.
27. **Dekeban, A. S.,** Abnormalities in children exposed to X-irradiation during various stages of gestation: tentative time table for radiation injury in the human fetus. I, *J. Nucl. Med.,* 9, 471, 1968.
28. **Diamond, E. L., Schmerler, H., and Lilienfeld, A. M.,** The relationship of intra-uterine radiation to subsequent mortality and development of leukemia in children, a prospective study, *Am. J. Epidemiol.,* 97, 282, 1973.
29. **Oppenheim, B. E., Griem, M. L., and Meier, P.,** The effects of diagnostic X-ray exposure on the human fetus: an examination of the evidence, *Radiology,* 114, 529, 1975.
30. **Stewart, A.,** Etiology of childhood malignancies, *Br. Med. J.,* 1, 452, 1961.
31. **Kneale, G. W., and Stewart, A. M.,** Mantel-Haenszel analysis of Oxford data. XI. Independent effects of fetal irradiation subfactors, *J. Natl. Cancer Inst.,* 57, 1009, 1976.
32. **MacMahon, B.,** Prenatal X-ray exposure and childhood cancer, *J. Natl. Cancer Inst.,* 28, 1173, 1962.
33. **Stewart, A. and Neale, G. W.,** Role of local infections in the recognition of hemopoietic neoplasms, *Nature (London),* 223, 741, 1969.
34. **Stewart, A. and Hewitt, D.,** Leukemia incidence in children in relation to radiation exposure in early life, *Curr. Top. Radiat. Res.,* 1, 221, 1963.
35. **Stewart, A.,** The carcinogenic effects of low level radiation. A re-appraisal of epidemiology methods and observations, *Health Phys.,* 24, 223, 1973.
36. **Graham, S., Levin, M. L., Lilienfeld, A. M., Schuman, L. M., Gibson, R., Dowd, J. E., and Hempelmann, L.,** Preconception, intrauterine and post-natal irradiation as related to leukemia, *Natl. Cancer Inst. Monogr.,* 19, 347, 1966.
37. **Green, D., Howells, G. R., Humphreys, E. R., and Zenart, J.,** Location of plutonium in mouse testes, *Nature (London),* 255, 77, 1975.
38. **Luning, K. G. and Frolen, H.,** Genetic effects of ^{239}Pu salt injections in mice, *Mutat. Res.,* 34, 539, 1976.
39. **Carsten, A. O. and Commerford, S. L.,** Dominant lethal mutations in mice resulting from chronic tritiated water (HTO) ingestion, *Radiat. Res.,* 66, 609, 1976.
40. **Carsten, A. O. and Bronkite, E. P.,** Genetic and Haematopoietic Effect of Long-term Tritiated Water in Biological and Environmental Effects of Low Level Radiation, Vol. 1, International Atomic Energy Agency, Vienna, 1976, 51.
41. **Costa, A., Cottino, F., Dellapiane, M., Terraris, G. M., Lenart, L., Patrito, G., and Zappetti, G.,** Thyroid function and thyrotropin activity in mother and fetus, in *Current Topics in Thyroid Research,* Proc. 5th Int. Thyroid Conf., Cassano, C. and Andreoli, M., Eds., Academic Press, New York, 1965.
42. **Pfannenstiel, P., Andrews, G. A., and Brown, D. W.,** Congenital hypothyroidism from intra-uterine ^{131}iodine damage, in *Current Topics in Thyroid Research,* Proc. 5th Int. Thyroid Conf., Cassano, C., and Andreoli, M., Eds., Academic Press, New York, 1965.
43. **Hagstrom, R. M., Glasser S. R., Brill, A. B., and Heysgel, R. M.,** Long-term effects of radioactive iron administered during human pregnancy, *Am. J. Epidemiol.,* 90, 1, 1969.
44. **Brent, R. L. and Bolden, B. T.,** Indirect effect of X-irradiation on embryonic development. III. The contribution of ovarian irradiation, uterine irradiation, oviduct irradiation and zygote irradiation to fetal mortality and growth retardation in the rat, *Radiat. Res.,* 30, 750, 1967.

45. **Brent, R. L. and McLaughlin, M. M.,** The indirect affect of irradiation on embryonic development. I. Irradiation of the mother while shielding the embryonic site, *Am. J. Dis. Child.*, 100, 94, 1960.

46. **Michaelson, S. M.,** Standards for protection of personnel against non-ionizing radiation, *Am. Ind. Hyg. Assoc. J.*, 35, 766, 1974.

47. **Lancranjan, I., Maicanescu, M., Rafaila, E., Klepsch, I., and Popescu, H. I.,** Gonadic function in workmen with long-term exposure to microwaves, *Health Phys.*, 29, 381, 1975.

48. **Rugh, R., Ginns, E. I., Ho, H. S., and Leach, W. M.,** Are Microwaves Teratogens?, Proc. Int. Symp. Biol. Effects Health Hazards Microwave Radiat., Warsaw, Poland, 1974, 98.

49. **Rubin, A. and Erdman, W. J.,** Microwave exposure of the human pelvis during early pregnancy and prior to conception, *Am. J. Phys. Med.*, 38, 219, 1959.

50. **Daels, J.,** Microwave heating of the uterine wall during parturition, *Obstet. Gynecol.*, 42, 76, 1973.

51. Occupational Diseases, Rep. No. 181, National Institute of Occupational Safety and Health, U.S. Department of Health, Education and Welfare, Washington, D.C., 1977, 483.

52. **Singh, K. B.,** Effect of sound on the female reproductive system, *Am. J. Obstet. Gynecol.*, 112, 981, 1972.

53. **Arvay, A.,** Cortico-hypothalamic control of gonadotropic function, in *Major Problems in Neuroendocrinology,* Bajus, E. and Jasmin, G., Eds., Williams & Wilkins, Baltimore, 1964.

54. **Zondek, B. and Tamari, I.,** Effects of auditory stimuli on reproduction, in *Effect of External Stimuli on Reproduction,* Ciba Foundation Study Group No. 26, Little, Brown, Boston, 1967.

55. **Sackler, A. M., Weltman, A. S., and Jurtshuk, P.,** Endocrine aspects of auditory stress, *Aerosp. Med.*, 31, 749, 1960.

56. **Singh, K. B. and Rao, P. S.,** Studies on polycystic ovaries of rats under continuous auditory stress, *Am. J. Obstet. Gynecol.*, 108, 557, 1970.

57. **Geber, W. F.,** Cardiovascular and teratogenic effects of chronic intermittent noise stress, in *Physiological Effects of Noise,* Welch, B. L. and Welch, A. S., Eds., Plenum Press, New York, 1970.

58. **Glowacki, C.,** The effects of vibration on the female genitalia, *Ginekol. Pol.*, 37, 217, 1966.

59. **Anticaglia, J. R. and Cohen, A.,** Extra-auditory effects of noise as a health hazard, *Am. Ind. Hyg. Assoc. J.*, 31, 277, 1970.

60. **Dunbar, F.,** Emotional factors in spontaneous abortion, in *Psychosomatic Obstetrics, Gynecology, and Endocrinology,* Kroger, W. S., Ed., Charles C Thomas, Springfield, Ill., 1962.

61. **Kalicinski, A., Straczkowski, W., and Nowak, W.,** Cardiovascular changes in workers exposed to noise, *Wiad. Lek.*, 28, 1, 1975.

62. **Griefahn, B.,** Examples of noise-induced reactions of the autonomic nervous system during normal ovarian cycle, Document No. EPA 1.23/4.:600/1-75-001, Environmental Protection Agency, Washington, D.C., 1975.

63. **Frolova, T. P.,** Features specific for the effect of vibration on the blood supply to the true pelvis at different periods in the menstrual cycle, *Gig. Tr. Prof. Zabol.*, 19, 14, 1975.

64. **Bohm, F.,** The effect of vehicle vibration on the genitalia of female driving personnel, *Z. Gesamte Hyg.*, 10, 720, 1964.

65. **Pramatarov, A. and Balev, L.,** Menstrual anomalies and the influence of motor vehicle vibrations on the conductors from the city transport, *Akush. I. Ginekol. (Sofia)*, 8, 31, 1969.

66. **Carosi, L. and Calabro, F.,** Fertility of couples working in industrial noise, *Folia Medica*, 51, 264, 1968.

67. **Welch, B. L. and Welch, A. S., Eds.,** Physiological Effects of Noise, Plenum Press, New York, 1970.

68. **Tzvetkov, T.,** The conditions of work as a cause of abortion in females employed in the textile and tobacco industries, *Med. Probl. (Plovdiv)*, 24, 73, 1972.

69. **Gratsianskaya, L. N., Eroshenko, E. A., and Libertovich, A. P.,** Influence on high frequency vibration on the genital region in females, *Gig. Tr. Prof. Zabol.*, 18, 70, 1974.

70. **Omerod, F. C.,** The pathology of congenital deafness in the child, in *The Modern Educational Treatment of Deafness,* Ewing, S. A., Ed., Manchester University Press, 1960.

71. **Bench, J.,** Sound transmission to the human foetus through the maternal abdominal wall, *J. Genet. Psychol.*, 113, 85, 1968.

72. **Walker, D., Grimwade, J., and Wood, C.,** Intrauterine noise: a component of the fetal environment, *Am. J. Obstet. Gynecol.*, 109, 91, 1971.

73. **Johansson, B., Wedenberg, E., and Westin, B.,** Measurement of tone response by the human fetus, *Acta Oto-Laryngol.*, 57, 188, 1964.

74. **Grimwade, J. C., Walker, D. W., Bartlett, M., Gordon, S., and Wood, C.,** Human fetal heart rate change and movement in response to sound and vibration, *Am. J. Obstet. Gynecol.*, 109, 86, 1971.

75. **Peiper, A.,** Sinnesempfindungen des Kindes vor seiner Geburt, *Monatsschr. Kinderheilkd.*, 29, 236, 1925.

76. Forbes, H. S. and Forbes, H. B., Fetal sense reactions: hearing, *J. Comp. Psychol.*, 7, 353, 1927.

77. Sontag, L. and Wallace, R., The movement response of the human fetus to sound stimuli, *Child Dev.*, 6, 253, 1935.

78. Bernard, J. and Sontag, L., Fetal reactivity to tonal stimulation: a preliminary report, *J. Genet. Psychol.*, 70, 205, 1947.

79. Fleischer, K., Untersuchungen zur Entwicklung der Innerohrfunktion. Intrauterine Kindsbewegungen nach Schallreizen, *Z. Laryngol. Rhinol. Otol. Ihre Grenzgeb.*, 11, 733, 1955.

80. Murphy, K. P. and Smyth, C. N., Response of the fetus to auditory stimulation, *Lancet*, 1, 972, 1962.

81. Dwornicka, B., Jasienska, A., Smolarz, W., and Wawryk, R., Attempt of determining the fetal reaction to acoustic stimulation, *Acta Oto-Laryngol.*, 57, 571, 1964.

82. Bench, R. J. and Vass, A., Fetal audiometry, *Lancet*, 1, 91, 1970.

83. Grimwade, J. C., Walker, D. W., Bartlett, M., Gordon, S., and Wood, C., Human fetal heart rate change and movement in response to sound and vibration, *Am. J. Obstet. Gynecol.*, 109, 86, 1971.

84. Ando, Y. and Hattori, H., Effects of intense noise during fetal life upon postnatal adaptability (Statistical study of the reaction of babies to aircraft noise), *J. Acoust. Soc. Am.*, 47, 1128, 1970.

85. Ando, Y. and Hattori, H., Effects of noise on human placental lactogen (HPL) levels in maternal plasma, *Br. J. Obstet. Gynecol.*, 84, 115, 1977.

86. Lindberg, B. S. and Nilsson, B. A., Variations in maternal plasma levels of human placental lactogen in normal pregnancy and labour, *J. Obstet. Gynaecol. Br. Commonw.*, 80, 619, 1973.

87. Hardy, J. D. and Dubois, E. F., Differences between men and women in their response to heat and cold, *Proc. Natl. Acad. Sci. U.S.A.*, 26, 389, 1940.

88. Mason, E. D., The basal metabolism of European women in South India and the effect of change of climate on European and South Indian women, *J. Nutr.*, 8, 695, 1934.

89. Bar-Or, O., Magnusson, L., and Buskirk, E. R., Distribution of heat activated sweat glands in obese and lean men and women, *Hum. Biol.*, 40, 235, 1968.

90. Brouha, L., Smith, P. E., DeLanne, R., and Maxfield, M. E., Physiological reactions of men and women during muscular activity and recovery in various environments, *J. Appl. Physiol.*, 16, 133, 1961.

91. Drinkwater, B. L., Denton, J. E., Raven, P. B., and Horvath, S. M., Thermoregulatory response of women to intermittent work in the heat, *J. Appl. Physiol.*, 41, 57, 1976.

92. Haslag, W. M. and Hertzman, A. B., Temperature regulation in young women, *J. Appl. Physiol.*, 20, 1283, 1965.

93. Haynes, E. M., Buskirk, E. R., Hodgson, J. L., Lundegren, H. M., and Nicholas, W. C., Heat tolerance of exercising lean and heavy prepubertal girls, *J. Appl. Physiol.*, 36, 566, 1974.

94. Hertig, B. A., Belding, H. S., Kraning, K. K., Batterton, D. L., Smith, C. R., and Sargent, F., Artificial acclimatization of women to heat, *J. Appl. Physiol.*, 18, 383, 1963.

95. Hertig, B. A. and Sargent, F., Acclimatization of women during work in hot environments, *Fed. Proc.*, 22, 810, 1963.

96. Morimoto, T., Slabochova, Z., Naman, R. K., and Sargent, F., Sex differences in physiological reactions to thermal stress, *J. Appl. Physiol.*, 22, 526, 1967.

97. Sargent, F. and Weinman, K. P., A comparative study of the responses and adjustments of human female and male to hot atmospheres, *Arid Zone Res.*, 24, 157, 1964.

98. Weinman, K. P., Slabochova, Z., Bernaver, E. M., Morimoto, T., and Sargent, F., Reactions of men and women to repeated exposure to humid heat, *J. Appl. Physiol.*, 22, 533, 1967.

99. Wyndham, C. H., The physiology of exercise under heat stress, *Ann. Rev. Physiol.*, 35, 193, 1973.

100. Senay, L. C. and Fortney, S., Untrained females. Effects of submaximal exercise and heat on body fluids, *J. Appl. Physiol.*, 39, 643, 1975.

101. Senay, L. C., Body fluids and temperature responses of heat-exposed women before and after evaluation with and without rehydration, *J. Physiol.*, 232, 209, 1973.

102. Henschel, A., Cole, M. B., Lyczkowski, O., Heat tolerance of elderly persons living in a subtropical environment, *J. Gerontol.*, 23, 17, 1968.

103. Kamon, E. and Avellini, B., Physiologic limits to work in the heat and evaporative coefficient for women, *J. Appl. Physiol.*, 41, 71, 1976.

104. Wyndham, C. H., Morrison, J. F., and Williams, C. G., Heat reactions of male and female caucasians, *J. Appl. Physiol.*, 20, 357, 1965.

105. Henschel, A., Effects of age and sex on heat tolerance, in Standards for Occupational Exposures to Hot Environments, Proc. Symp. 1973, NIOSH 76-100, U.S. Department of Health, Education and Welfare, Washington, D.C., 17, 1976.

106. **Dukes-Dubas, F. N.,** Rationale and provisions of the work practices standard for work in hot environments as recommended by NIOSH, in Standards for Occupational Exposures to Hot Environments, Proc. Symp. 1973, NIOSH-76-100, U.S. Department of Health, Education and Welfare, Washington, D. C., 1976, 27.

107. **Ellis, F. P.,** Mortality from heat illness and heat aggravated illness in the U.S., *Environ. Res.,* 5, 1, 1972.

108. **Shuman, S. H.,** Patterns of urban heat-wave deaths and implications for prevention: data from New York and St. Louis during July 1966, *Environ. Res.,* 5, 59, 1972.

109. **Dutt, R. H.,** Temperature and light as factors in reproduction among farm animals, *J. Dairy Sci.,* (Suppl.) 43, 123, 1959.

110. **Ulberg, L. C. and Burfening, P. J.,** Embryo death resulting from adverse environment on spermatozia or ova, *J. Anim. Sci.,* 26, 571, 1967.

111. **Monty, D. E. and Wolff, L. K.,** Summer heat stress and reduced fertility in Holstein-Friesian cows in Arizona, *Am. J. Vet. Res.,* 35, 1495, 1974.

112. **Alexander, G.,** Birth weight of lambs: influences and consequences, in *Size at Birth,* CIBA Foundation Symposium, 27, New Series, Elsevier, New York, 1974, 215.

113. **Taggart, N. R., Holliday, R. M., and Billewicz, W. Z.,** Changes in skinfolds during pregnancy, *Br. J. Nutr.,* 21, 439, 1967.

114. **Burt, C. C.,** Peripheral skin temperature in normal pregnancy, *Lancet,* 2, 787, 1949.

115. **Hytten, F. E. and Leitch, E.,** *The Physiology of Human Pregnancy,* Blackwell, London, 1971, 103.

116. **Buxton, C. L. and Atkinson, W. B.,** Hormonal factors involved in the regulation of basal body temperature during the menstrual cycle and pregnancy, *J. Clin. Endocrin.,* 8, 544, 1948.

117. Survey of laundries and their women workers in 23 cities, Bulletin 78, U.S. Department of Labor, Women's Bureau, 1930.

118. **McDonald, H. D.,** Women at work, Maternal health and congenital defects. A prospective investigation, *N. Engl. J. Med.,* 258, 767, 1958.

119. **Kita, H.,** On the professional woman skin divers in Japan, *J. Sports Med. Phys. Fitness,* 5 (Abstr.), 43, 1965.

120. Shift Work Practices in the United States, DHEW (NIOSH) 77-148, U.S. Department of Health, Education and Welfare, National Institute for Occupational and Environmental Health, Washington, D.C., 1977.

121. **Scheving, L. E.,** Chronobiology and how it might apply to the problems of shift work: discussion 1, in Shift Work and Health, HEW/NIOSH 76-203, Department of Health, Education and Welfare, Washington, D.C., 1976, 118.

122. **Weitzman, E. D.,** Circadian Rhythms. Discussion, in Shift Work and Health, HEW/NIOSH 76-203, U.S. Department of Health, Education and Welfare, Washington, D.C., 1976, 51.

123. **Felton, G.,** Body rhythm effects on rotating work shifts, *Nurs. Dig.,* Jan/Feb, 1976, 219.

124. **Aschoff, J. and Wever, R.,** Human circadian rhythms: a multioscillatory system, *Fed. Proc. Fed. Am. Soc. Exp. Biol.,* 35, 2326, 1976.

125. **Reinberg, A. and Smolensky, M. H.,** Circatrigintan secondary rhythms related to hormonal changes in the menstrual cycle: general considerations, in *Biorhythms and Human Reproduction,* Ferin, M., Halberg, F., Richart, R. M., and Vande Wiele, R. L., Eds., John Wiley & Sons, New York, 1977, Chapter 15.

126. **Preston, F. S., Bateman, S. C., Short, R. V., and Wilkinson, R. T.,** The effects of flying and of time changes on menstrual cycle length and on performance in airline stewardesses, in *Biorhythms and Human Reproduction,* Ferin, M., Hallberg, F., Richart, R. M., and Vande Wiele, R. L., Eds., John Wiley & Sons, New York, 1977, Chapter 33.

Chapter 4

THE CHEMICAL ENVIRONMENT

I. INTRODUCTION

The exposure of women workers to chemicals has been a peculiarly ignored phenomenon. The social perception that men have held the "dirty" jobs has not taken into account those female-intensive industries where the use of chemicals is likely to be the constant and accepted experience. Laboratory technicians work in chemical and health-related laboratories with a changing array of organic solvents; nurses and other health workers are exposed to anesthetic gases and sterilizing agents. Dry cleaners and beauticians also work in a chemical environment. In the electronics and jewelry industries, to name only two, there is likely to be direct exposure to solvents and other organic and inorganic compounds; and in the textile industry, chemically treated fabric can provide a continual low-dose exposure. Cleaners and janitors have always been at high risk of exposure to waste chemicals and cleaning compounds; agricultural workers can seldom restrict their exposure to pesticides. The boot and shoe industry, rubber and paint industry, and the many manufacturing operations in small communities across the country employ women today as they did their immigrant grandmothers before them;[1] it is scarcely necessary to invoke some new rising tide of women experiencing a chemical environment markedly different from what they have always known. Alice Hamilton's *Exploring the Dangerous Trades* (now out of print and almost unavailable)[2] links this past to our present where women are still working in the jobs they have always had, many of them no different in quality of exposure from male-intensive jobs with comparable toxic hazards, albeit changing with the constant chemical innovations of modern industry. In addition, there has been the repetitive experience of one generation after another entering heavy industry during wartime. The current concern for asbestos exposure affects the many women who were shipyard workers in World War II, where unfortunately the short-term exposure may not have provided the protection it afforded from many other chemicals.

The array of occupationally induced diseases for women appears to be comparable to that experienced by men, e.g., the pneumoconioses affect workers generally in relation to the level of exposure. The exclusion of women from epidemiologic studies has, therefore, been paradoxical. If they were excluded because there were too few, it could be assumed they were thought to be different. But when cause/effect relationships are invoked, they also appear to apply to women workers or to workers of neuter gender.

It is expected that standard texts on occupational disease[3-5] can provide the basic information which relates to men and women workers. The missing information concerns the reproductive system and working conditions of female-intensive jobs. In this chapter and the next, emphasis will be on these omissions.

Occupational exposure to toxic substances includes, for most women, the conditions of their work at home. The use of chemicals for cleaning, pest control, household repair, and crafts is highly individualistic and seldom provides an opportunity for evaluation of effects on health and reproduction. There is the additional disadvantage that women workers have been inadequately examined in terms of their occupational health, so that any attempt to present a definitive overview of the effects of toxic substances on the woman worker would be misleading.[6,7] There are few data available for specific chemical environments and their effects on women as childbearing workers, so that it must be kept in mind that no evidence of an adverse effect is far more likely to be a reflection of the lack of observation ever made of those conditions in relation to women. The particular conditions and chemical environment of female-intensive industries, e.g., textiles, electronics, jewelry manufacturing, health and personal services, and agriculture had not been previously examined until Stellman[8] and Hricko[9] recently published descriptions. They have summarized the most likely chemical exposures for women workers in the context of the jobs they tend to have.

In order to make the best use of the information that is available, this chapter is based on the female reproductive system with emphasis on three better-studied areas of toxicology: toxic effects of metals, organic solvents, and organochlorinated and organophosphate pesticides. This approach should provide some introduction to the industrial toxicology of the woman worker and supplement what is usually presented in traditional texts in the neuter gender, although the data are likely to have been derived from studies of male workers.

New chemical substances of unknown biological effect come into the working environment daily in addition to those for which there is, so far, inadequate evaluation. It is unlikely that detailed toxicological or epidemiological information on each substance, or even classes of substances, will ever be adequate to deal with individual clinical needs. We can only expect to be able to draw on the experience we have, particularly in relation to reproduction, and build upon it as new substances must be evaluated and new research techniques are developed.[10] By following a developmental approach (that is, from ovum, uterine environment, and blastocyst, to placenta, embryo, fetus, and newborn, to adult), and using each stage to highlight the toxic effect of metals and/or compounds, there is an inevitable loss of specificity by chemical. However, the trade-off can be met by reference to studies of the substance of interest and when information is not available on any stages used in this scheme, the significance of the omissions can be evaluated. Sperm integrity and spermatogenesis are discussed in Chapter 6.

II. DEVELOPMENTAL TOXICOLOGY

The human reproductive system is susceptible to environmental factors which can produce a variety of adverse effects on the production of ova and viable sperm, on fertilization, and on implantation within the uterus, as well as on the growth and development of the embryo and fetus.

The modes of action of environmental contaminants like chlorinated hydrocarbons and organophosphate pesticides, chlorinated solvents such as trichloroethylene, and trace metals such as lead and cadmium are quite dissimilar, so that we may also expect that the germs cells, the uterus itself, the blastocyst, the embryo, and the fetoplacental unit will all respond to their contaminated environment in a manner particular to the insult. The complexities of dose-response relationships, interacting effects, and recovery/repair potential are virtually unknown for the human reproductive system, whatever the contaminant.

III. THE INFLUENCE OF ENVIRONMENTAL FACTORS ON ENDOMETRIAL FUNCTION

In the specific case of lead our only information on human populations comes in relation to disturbances experienced by industrially exposed workers where amenorrhea, dysmenorrhea, and menorrhagia have been repeatedly reported in environments of excessive contamination. Infertility may occur but after withdrawal from lead, normal pregnancy may follow.[11] A study by Vermande-VanEck and Meigs[12] of 11 young-adult, female Rhesus monkeys provides the only direct information on damage to the gonads from experimental poisoning. Menstration stopped in all monkeys during lead administration, and the sex skin lost its color by the end of the sixth month. After clinical signs of intoxication had been present for some months, laparotomy was performed and the right ovary removed. Lead injections were discontinued and the animals were allowed to recover. The left ovary and uterus were removed 8 months later.

Vermande-VanEck and Meigs[12] stated, "The important change in ovarian function was a depression of estrogen effect. Scarcely any indication of gonadal activity was present after 8 months. Microscopically, the ovaries showed damage to the primordial oocytes and an inhibition of follicle development; only a few follicles were growing in the ovaries and these degenerated in the early secondary stages before maturity was reached. Ovulation failed to occur."

The monkeys gradually recovered, and menstrual periods resumed 1 to 5 months after injections ceased. Sexual skin color redeveloped in 1 to 4 months. The ovaries removed after recovery appeared macroscopically normal. This was confirmed by microscopic examination which showed normal follicle growth with many follicles in development, normal oocytes, and young and old corpora lutea.

The recovery after cessation of lead administration is important in these animals because of their biological similarity to human beings. The function of monkey and human gonads is the same, that is a 28-day cycle, maturation and ovulation of one oocyte per cycle on day 11 to 13, menstrual bleeding, and a similar vaginal cycle.

These studies would indicate that there is evidence for a relationship between toxic metal metabolism and the menstrual cycle and pregnancy in the human female. Blood levels of metals are quite inadequate for estimating the risk of damage to the fertilized ovum or fetus; and so far, we have no information concerning the uterine environment and the effects of contaminant metals. Information on the concentration characteristics of metals in the endometrium during the menstrual cycle and during pregnancy is going to be necessary for a quantitative evaluation of the hazards of known toxic metals to pregnancy.

Although women are employed extensively in the electronics industry and dry-cleaning establishments, there has been no epidemiologic study of their reproductive experience. Tetrachloroethylene is used for commercial dry cleaning and metal degreasing. Teratogenic effects of tetrachloroethylene have been reported in mice, and an increased incidence of fetal resorptions has been observed in exposed rats.[13] We might conclude that under tetrachloroethylene-exposure conditions, a toxic environment develops in the pregnant uterus. The metabolism of tetrachloroethylene is still under investigation. As in the case of trichloroethylene exposure, trichloroacetic acid and trichloroethanol have been found in the urine of humans and animals. In addition, dichloracetic acid and ethylene glycol have been found in the urine of exposed animals. Frant and Westendorp[14] considered the consequences of chronic excretion of trichloroacetic acid, a strong organic acid which may be neutralized in the body by sodium or potassium and can result in the constant elimination of fixed alkali. The carbon dioxide-combining power of the blood could then be impaired.

We do not know the relative distribution of organic compounds and their metabolic products in the fat, equithelial, and glandular cells of the uterine wall and their secretion into uterine fluids. As an exocrine secretion, the latter should be partly comparable to sweat, which is known to excrete part of the tetrachloroethylene dose.[15]

For organochlorinated pesticides Chase et al.[16] have shown an association between high blood levels and reported menstrual dysfunction in migrant workers. However, the study population is small. The Eastern European literature contains far more commentary on menstruation, a condition which has been virtually disregarded outside the exercise and sports physiology areas in the U.S.

A number of studies have been made on the uterotropic activity of DDT (1,1-trichloro-2,2-bis [p-chlorophenyl] ethane. Conflicting results through the 1960s provided a confused perception of the relationship of experimental findings in rodents to field experiences with other animals, e.g., mink. Welch et al.[17] and Bitman et al.[18] were able to show that the *o,p'*-isomer of DDT possessed uterotropic properties similar to those of estradiol-17 β, thus explaining the incompatible results obtained when technical DDT (a mixture of about 80% *p,p'*-DDT and 20% *o,p'*-DDT was used. The *p,p'*-isomer appears to have little effect on reproductive function.[19] Both the studies by Bitman et al.[18] and Duby et al.[19] used castrated animals (mink and rat, respectively) and concluded that the maintenance of the uterotropic properties of *o,p'*-DDT indicated that its action was directly on the uterus, rather than by stimulation of endogenous release of estrogens. Uterine changes are though to be, in part, related to altered capillary permeability.

An analogy has been drawn between uterotropic activity of *o,p'*-DDT and diethylstilbesterol, a potent nonsteroidal estrogen. The work of Welch et al. and Bitman et al. suggests the *o,p'*-DDT or a metabolite binds to the estrogen receptors in the uterus to exert its uterotropic influence. Diethylstilbesterol has been found to accumulate in ovarian corpora lutea and the granulosa cell layer of follicles.[20] Similarly, Backstrom et al.[21] showed a high uptake of DDT and dieldrin in the corpora lutea of rats, allowing for an indirect influence on the uterine response to progesterone.

Endometrial secretions (and contaminants) play a vital role in determining the parameters of successful implantation and in providing nutrition to the developing blastocyst and embryo in the preplacental stage, yet there is limited knowledge about the nature and content of human endometrial tissue, especially the contaminants that may be present. Since menstrual fluid contains endometrial tissue and fluid, it represents a logical, easily accessible biological marker of the uterine environment.

IV. FERTILIZATION, IMPLANTATION, AND THE UTERINE ENVIRONMENT

A fertilized ovum passes through the uterotubal sphincter about 96 hr after fertilization. During its residence within the oviduct, division occurs several times to yield a mass of cells in which fluid is beginning to accumulate. The uterine environment and its secretions are an integral part of the early developmental process. Before implantation, conversion to a blastocyst occurs within the uterine cavity and takes about 1 day. The external surface of the blastocyst, the zona pellucida, is heavily coated with a secretory deposit produced by the endometrial glands.[22] The residence time of a fertilized human ovum within the uterus before implantation is between 2 and 6 days and usually at least 5, about 2.2% of gestation. For the several days before implantation, the blastocyst is metabolizing actively and its nutrients are drawn from tubal and uterine secretions.

The uterine fluid is primarily a product of the exocrine glands of the endometrium and, like other exocrine gland secretions, e.g., saliva, bile and other gastrointestinal secretions, sweat, tears, milk, and seminal fluid, foreign chemical association depends on pH of the secretions, the molecular weight, and degree of ionization of the compound.

The blastocyst becomes embedded in the stroma of the endometrium so that a recess forms with a uterine lining. As implantation proceeds, mucal glycoproteins are produced by the decidual cells which have formed from the enlarged and differentiated stromal cells. The further development of the embryo is in part dependent on the nutriment provided by the mucal glycoproteins.[23]

Normal implantation of a fertilized ovum is contingent on the precise physiological balance between many factors of a structural and functional nature. The hormonal output and balance that are mediated by the ovaries are prime influences on the cyclical changes that take place in the endometrium. Even a shift in the menstrual cycle, despite an otherwise normal endometrium, is enough to alter the attraction of the endometrial tissue for the blastocyst on the day of implantation.[24] Implantation occurs at the height of the secretory phase. For successful implantation, both the fertilized ovum and the endometrium must be in equivalent states of maturation.

An endometrium that provides an inadequate environment for the blastocyst may be a reflection of the inability of the endometrium to respond to hormonal stimulation; it may reflect insufficient progesterone production by the ovary or an estrogen-progesterone imbalance.[25] Phase defects, e.g., shortened proliferative phase with normal secretory phase, or vice versa, will also inhibit implantation of a fertilized ovum.

Estrogenic activity of organochlorine compounds or their metabolites can stimulate uterine growth and interfere with fertility and conception in rats and mice, though a comparable effect has not been found in sheep.[26] Ware[27] provides a broad generalization from the many reproductive studies on animals that DDT, for example, is estrogenic and uterotropic in mammals and that fetal implant resorption results from direct physiologic effect on the parent and appears to be species specific. It can be concluded that the endometrium is a target tissue, but we have had very little investigation of the effects of toxic substances on estrogen-sensitive uterine and ovarian factors in women.

If fertilization and consequent implantation do not occur, the endometrium will retrogress, lose fluid and decrease in thickness, with ischemic necrosis of superficial tissue resulting from compression of the spiral vessels. These events lead to hemorrhage in the uterine cavity, shedding of the tissues of the compactium and spongiosum — menstruation. Menstrual fluid thus contains the tissues, secretions, and glands which constitute much of the early uterine environment of the fertilized ovum, blastocycst, and embryo.

Some research has been directed to examining the means by which drugs and other chemicals pass from the maternal circulation into the uterine fluid and into the preimplantation blastocyst. Fabro[28] has shown that the substances listed in Table 1, when administered to rabbits, rats, and mice, can be found in significant amounts in the uterine fluid, together with some of their metabolites.

Fabro also suggests that the pregnant uterus could have metabolic capability in view of the accumulation of nicotine and its metabolite cotinine in the endometrium and their appearance in the uterine fluid. The compounds listed in Table 1 have been found in the pre- and postimplantation blastocysts of the rabbit.

The evidence that nicotine appears to be retarded in its passage across the placenta with low fetal concentrations, in contrast to secretion into the human uterine fluid, may indicate two extremely different transport processes. Fabro concluded that the conceptus is as susceptible to damage during the preimplantation stages of pregnancy as it is after the development of the placenta and that the toxicity from the presence of foreign compounds in the uterine lumen is likely to exert some effect on reproduction — a potential explanation for infertility, and spontaneous abortion of unknown etiology.

In recent years, the view that only relatively small molecules traverse the placenta has been moderated to include certain proteins (mol wt $\sim$ 30,000) and large molecules such as ferritin (mol wt $\sim$ 500,000). The chemical nature of the substance probably

TABLE 1

Some Experimental Substances Found in Uterine
Fluid[28]

(1-methyl — ^{14}C) — caffeine
G — (^{3}H) — nicotine
(7 — ^{14}C) — salicylate
(carbonyl — ^{14}C) — isoniazid
(2 — ^{14}C) — barbital
(2 — ^{14}C) — thiopental
(phenyl — ^{14}C) — DDT

governs its ability to reach the blastocyst. It is now believed that maternal blastocyst exchange mechanisms are carefully controlled by regulatory systems active at the level of the endometrium and the blastocyst. Although the concentration of the exogenous agent in the embryo may be only a small fraction of that found in the maternal blood stream, there may be a delay in the rate of clearance from the embryonic compartment, thereby providing a continuing exposure of unpredictable time periods in the growing embryo. In addition, the rapidly dividing cells of the embryo may be highly susceptible to toxic effects of chemicals.

Determination of blastocyst-uterine relationships involves an evaluation of the action of maternally transmitted, pharmacologically active substances upon the blastocyst. Lutwak-Mann has used the concept "embryo-seeking".[22] An exogenous, maternally transmitted agent can reach the embryonic cells within the blastocyst, passing from the epithelial cells of the endometrial into the endometrial secretion and then through the zona pellucida which encases the blastocyst.

V. PLACENTAL FUNCTION

A review of placental physiology shows that the nutrition of the early fetus is primarily due to trophoblastic digestion and absorption of nutrients from the endometrial decidua, diminishing in importance by the 12th week of gestation by which time nutrients are then obtained from diffusion through the placental membrane.[29] Guyton[29] stated, "In the early months of development placental permeability is relatively slight for two reasons: first, the total surface area of the placental membrane is still small at that time and second, the thickness of the membrane is great. However, as the placenta becomes older, the permeability increases progressively until the last month or so of pregnancy, when it begins to decrease again."

It is known that the placenta selectively controls the rates of transfer of a wide variety of materials. Any substance found in the maternal or fetal blood should be able to cross the placenta to some extent unless it is destroyed or altered during passage. A very low degree of permeability may slow the entry to a rate which renders a drug, for example, physiologically inactive and pharmacologically undetectable. The important consideration is not whether a given substance does or does not pass the placental barrier, but what is the rate and mechanism of transfer.[30]

There is some evidence to suggest that the concept of a lipoid barrier may apply to the transfer of drugs and chemicals across the placenta. The rate of entry is then governed principally by the fat solubility of the nonionized molecule. Other factors, such as concentration gradient and molecular size, are usually of secondary importance. Drugs with high degrees of dissociation or low lipid solubilities penetrate the placenta poorly in contrast to those that are found as fat-soluble, undissociated molecules at physiologic pH ranges and can penetrate the barrier almost instantaneously. However, the foregoing is a simplistic explanation and there is very little precise quantitative information of the kinetics of placental penetration of chemical substances. In considering molecular size, substances of low molecular weight diffuse freely across the placenta, but with increasing size the factor of lipid solubility becomes progressively more important. Drugs with molecular weight less than 600 cross relatively easily, but the placenta is virtually impermeable to compounds with molecular weights over 1000.

As gestation progresses, the placental membrane increases in surface area and decreases in thickness. At term, it is estimated that the membrane's surface area is about one fifth that of the pulmonary alveoli and is three times as thick.

The source of oxygen to the fetus is the maternal blood which also supplies the uterine musculature and supporting structures. The placental membrane separates maternal and fetal blood and allows transfer of oxygen and carbon dioxide from one to the other without allowing the two blood supplies to mix. The pattern of maternal and fetal blood flow during gas exchange is within a "counter-current" arrangement of blood vessels. The fetal and maternal blood streams flow in opposite directions during gas exchange, and the fetal blood at the end of its capillary transit is exposed to oxygen-rich maternal blood near the beginning of the maternal arterial array. Oxygen dissociates from maternal blood, diffuses through the placental membrane, and combines with fetal hemoglobin. The percent saturation of hemoglobin with oxygen is greater in fetal blood than in maternal blood, and the oxyhemoglobin dissociation curve of fetal blood lies to the left of that for maternal blood. The oxygen affinity is related to oxygen tension so that for the same hemoglobin concentrations and oxygen concentrations in maternal and fetal blood, the oxygen tension will be higher in maternal blood and enhanced gas transfer across the placental membrane results. The process of gas diffusion is continuous because the partial pressure of oxygen in blood on the maternal side of the placenta is higher than on the fetal side and the oxygen-poor umbilical arterial blood of the fetus on one side of the membrane is continually supplemented by oxygen from the arterial maternal blood on the other side. The oxygen tension gradient between maternal and fetal blood in the exchange process is magnified by oxygen consumption of placental tissue, the possibility that a fetal shunt may divert varying amounts of the umbilical blood flow, and nonhomogeneous placental perfusion by maternal or fetal blood. The rate of placental oxygen transfer may be limited by the rate of blood flow to the placenta rather than by the diffusion resistance of the membrane separating maternal and fetal blood. Compensatory mechanisms associated with the fetal and placental circulations can respond rapidly to protect fetal tissues from changes in the intrauterine environment. When threatened by asphyxia, the fetus can derive energy by anaerobic glycolysis with disposal of resulting tissue lactate via the placenta or maternal circulation. However, adequate oxygenation of maternal tissue is necessary for maintenance of maternal and fetal blood flow to the placenta.[31]

A. Carbon Monoxide

The most prevalent modifying agent of the maternal/fetal oxygen-transfer system is carbon monoxide. Its high concentration in cigarette smoke is sufficient to raise the carboxyhemoglobin concentration in the blood (percentage hemoglobin combined with carbon monoxide) from a normal range of 0.4 to 2.7% (for pregnant women) to 4 to 6%. The affinity of hemoglobin for carbon monoxide is about 200 to 250 times its affinity for oxygen, which results in a markedly reduced oxygen-carrying capacity of the blood. The oxyhemoglobin dissociation curve also shifts to the left so that tissue oxygen tensions must fall to much lower levels before oxygen is released from the oxyhemoglobin.[32] The biological half-life of carbon monoxide in sedentary adults at sea level is 4 to 5 hr. Endogenous carbon monoxide production is increased 50% or more during pregnancy and returns to nonpregnant levels by the 4th day postpartum. In part, the increase is due to fetal production of carbon monoxide as well as the increased red blood cell mass of the pregnant woman. Therefore, increased carbon monoxide exposure from smoking or occupational sources during pregnancy is of some significance in the evaluation of placental oxygen exchange. At higher risk of impairment of oxygen exchange is the smoking, pregnant worker and fetus exposed to toxic substances which lead to increased carboxyhemoglobin levels, such as methylene chloride, a widely used solvent. An air environment with increased carbon monoxide levels occurs near coke ovens and in enclosed spaces where internal combustion engines are operating, or where incomplete combustion occurs. Higher carboxyhemoglobin for individuals in the immediate area results.

B. Lead

Information on the placental transfer of lead comes from the comparisons made with strontium[90] skeletal uptake in the mid 1960s. Blanchard[33] proposed that there might be less placental discrimination against lead than against strontium on the basis of a higher ratio of [210]lead to [90]strontium per gram of calcium in the bones of three infants who were 3 days old when compared with 11 other infants ranging in age from 2 to 12 months.

The placenta also has considerable storage capacity and during the first few months of pregnancy, it grows tremendously in size while the fetus remains relatively small. Calcium, along with other substances, is stored in the placenta and is available in the later months of pregnancy for growth by the fetus. It could be expected that lead would be similarly stored, evidence for which comes from Baglan et al.[34] who have shown a mean lead level in 234 placentas from Nashville, Tenn. of 1.83 $\mu g/g$ dry weight.

An analysis follows of blood lead relationships between the mother and child who have not had lead exposure above the usual dietary and air environment sources. Umbilical cord blood lead concentration has been measured in infants of urban and suburban mothers living in Boston and the mean values were found to be 22.1 $\mu g/100$ mℓ and 18.3 $\mu g/100$ mℓ, respectively. For infants of urban smokers the mean was 24.3 $\mu g/100$ mℓ and for infants of suburban nonsmokers, 15.2 $\mu g/100$ mℓ. However, with a total sample of 27, these differences were not statistically significant. The urban range was 10 to 39 $\mu g/100$ mℓ and the suburban range was 13 to 26 $\mu g/100$ mℓ.[35] In New Haven, Harris and Holley[36] found somewhat lower values, again with no statistically different means for suburban and inner city areas: 12.3 $\mu g/100$ mℓ with a range of 10 to 20 $\mu g/100$ g. Kubasik and Volosin[37] measured capillary blood in newborns in low-lead risk and high-lead risk pediatric populations (ages 1 to 6 years). These authors also considered the different hemoglobin contents of newborns and older children, showing that for newborns the values in μg of lead per gram of hemoglobin were 0.69 compared with 1.74 for low-lead risk pediatric populations and 2.47 for those with high-lead risk. With the report of Rajegowda et al.[38] of 100 samples of cord blood with a mean value of 14.6 $\mu g/100$ g (range 10 to 30), there appears to be a fairly consistent mean value (except for Boston), though the range of values is wide for each population.

A German population of 294 mother-infant pairs also showed a mean blood level in cord blood of 15.0 $\mu g/100$ mℓ, which was significantly lower than that of the maternal blood at delivery (16.9 $\mu g/100$ mℓ), with a significant correlation between the bloods of mothers and infants (r = 0.54).[39] Other studies of maternal (during labor) and neonatal blood samples have found the correlation between mothers and corresponding infants to be high (correlation coefficient of 0.64).[40] For 98 pairs, the mean for infants was 10.0 $\mu g/100$ mℓ and for mothers, 10.3 $\mu g/100$ mℓ. The study was conducted in Shreveport, La. and maternal urban residence was found to be associated wih higher maternal- and cord-blood lead levels when compared with rural residence. In Missouri populations exposed to environmental lead, Fahim et al. showed cord, placenta, and membrane values to be consistent with the above values — 11.0 $\mu g/100$ mℓ in full-term babies in both high- and low-lead areas.[41] Mothers' blood levels were 14.3 $\mu g/$mℓ and 13.1 $\mu g/$mℓ, respectively.

Until more attention is accorded the maternal/fetal relationship, particularly in the area of mineral metabolism, we are unable to extrapolate much from the above information except that at birth there are comparable maternal and infant blood-lead concentrations. In contrast, we know little of the uptake via the placenta into fetal tissues, which proceeds from at least the 12th week of gestation.

There is storage of calcium in the placenta which can be considered to be about 25 mg/100 g of placenta at mid-pregnancy, 30 mg at 30 weeks, and 100 mg at term.[42] As the calcium content of the fetus is about 1 g at 300 g, 10 g at 1500 g, and 28 g at term, there is increasing concentration of calcium in the body from under 2 g/kg for the early fetuses to over 8 g/kg at term. Analysis of the lead content of placental calcifications in relation to blood levels in the newborn may be an approach to understanding placental transfer of lead.

The lack of critical information prevents us from identifying those maternal-fetal relationships which affect blood lead levels in the developing fetus and newborn. To base our conclusions only on the maternal blood-cord blood relationshp at birth when we know that calcium-lead relationships and placental characteristics of the previous nine months have fluctuated drastically seems unwise.

C. Mercury

Mercury has long been known to be an occupational hazard. Classic symptoms of exposure to elemental mercury vapor and/or dusts of inorganic salts include fatigue, irritability, loss of memory, loss of self-confidence, depression, insomnia, and tremors.[43] Victims of recent incidents of ingested organic mercury compounds (e.g., methyl mercury) have also shown classic symptoms of mercury poisoning, as have some of the infants born to mothers with high mercury exposures, indicating transplacental passage of some forms of mercury to the fetus.

Evidence accumulated so far in rats, mice, and hamsters, plus the known incidents of human poisoning has shown that the placenta is not a barrier to the transfer of methyl mercury compounds to the fetus. High human maternal exposures have been teratogenic and mercury is found in fetal tissue. Inorganic mercury, injected mercuric chloride being used in most studies, has been shown in mice and rats to accumulate in the placenta but not to be transferred to the fetus, the placenta being a barrier to its transfer.[44-54] Unfortunately, little work has been done specifically on elemental mercury.

One study[55] in rats compared inhaled mercury vapor with an equivalent amount of injected mercury. The mercury levels in the maternal blood were 25 times higher in the injected animals than the ones which inhaled the vapor. However, the fetal/placental unit mercury levels were about the same in both. Of those which had inhaled the vapor, one half of the mercury found in the placental/fetal unit was in the fetus whereas only 1% of the injected mercury in the unit was found in the fetus. Another study[56] also done in rats showed that the fetal mercury content from inhaled mercury vapor was more than 40 times that found after an equivalent dose of injected mercuric chloride. The result was more than ten times the mercury content from injected elemental mercury when compared to injected mercuric chloride. The ability of the placenta to discriminate against ionic mercury, but not elemental (injected), is shown by the ratio of placental mercury to fetal mercury content — 80: 1 and 23: 1, respectively. The authors cited the similarity between these results and previous studies which showed that the blood-brain barrier can discriminate against ionic mercury but allows transfer of dissolved mercury vapor.

There is evidence that elemental mercury, once in the body, is oxidized to the mercuric ion.[57,58] However, this is not an immediate process and the dissolved vapor exists in that form for more than one circulation through the body. Because elemental mercury vapor is more readily diffused through biological membranes, including the placenta, a significant portion of the mercury can be transported to the placenta and the fetus as mercury vapor. The ionic form of mercury is not easily transferred once it is in that state. Since there is time for the vapor to come in contact with the whole body through at least one circulation, the vapor may be a significant source of mercury exposure to the fetus.

The sensitivity of the fetus to inorganic compounds of mercury or elemental mercury is not known. Women may be exposed to inorganic compounds and elemental mercury as dentists or dental assistants, hospital and research laboratory workers, thermometer and scientific-glassware workers, and a variety of other manufacturing operations well described by Hamilton and Hardy.[59] Mercury accumulation in the placenta and fetal membranes of 19 dental workers and their infants has been reported by Wannag and Skjaerasen.[60] A nonexposed group of 26 was also examined. At birth, erythrocytes and plasma from both mother and babies, amniotic fluid, placentae and chorionic and amniotic membranes were collected for analysis of total mercury content. There was no difference between the values obtained from exposed and nonexposed groups for mercury content of maternal and infant erythrocytes (about 9 ng/g) or amniotic fluid (about 3.2 ng/g). In contrast, there was an approximate two-fold difference between the mercury content of the placentae, chorionic, and amniotic membranes for the exposed group when compared to those not occupationally exposed to elemental mercury (Table 2). The absence of any difference in blood levels between the exposed and unexposed women was attributed to the termination of work by 14 exposed women before delivery (median 28 days, range 1 to 72 days). The whole-body, biological half-life of inorganic mercury has been established by use of protein-bound and ionic radioactive mercury in four women and four men to be 40 to 45 days, and only 0.5% of the total body burden of inorganic mercury was found in the blood 24 hr after exposure.[61] It is unlikely, therefore, that the reported blood mercury levels in Wannag's study reflect at all the mercury exposure of the women while working. When compared with maternal and fetal blood, the placentae and chorionic membranes of both exposed and nonexposed groups had a higher mercury content. The amniotic membrane mercury content was higher than blood only for the exposed group. The evident trapping of mercury in the human placenta may provide some protection for the fetus, although Lawerys et al.[62] have shown interference with enzyme activity of red blood cells and plasma at low concentrations of elemental mercury. These findings would suggest the possibility of an effect on the placenta and membranes as mercury concentrations increase during the course of pregnancy. Wannag's observations emphasize again that maternal and fetal blood may give no indication of previous exposure to a contaminant and the level in placentae and membranes may be a better indicator of the possible effects on the fetus.

It is important to note the limitations of animal research in regard to extrapolation to humans. The placental barrier is made up of a number of layers of cells between fetal and maternal circulation. The number of layers varies with the species and the

TABLE 2

Total Mercury Content of Placentas and Membranes In Dental Workers[60]

| | ng mercury per g tissue | | Students' |
	Nonexposed (N)	Exposed (N)	t-test
Placentas	12.0 ± 0.9 (26)	24.5 ± 4.1 (19)	p = 0.001
Chorion Membrane	11.5 ± 1.3 (19)	21.6 ± 3.4 (13)	p = 0.003
Amnion Membrane	4.3 ± 0.8 (19)	14.5 ± 4.1 (13)	p = 0.013

stage of gestation, which may affect the permeability of the placenta.[63] However, this variability does not mean that animal studies are irrelevant to the understanding of the problems in human beings.

D. Organochlorinated Hydrocarbons

Placental transfer of DDT was first reported in dogs in 1949[64] and subsequently confirmed in rabbits,[65] deer,[66] and mice.[67] Denes[68] and Wasserman et al.[69] measured DDT in body fat of human stillborns and neonates; and Rappolt et al.[70] measured DDT in human placentas and umbilical cords. Curley et al.[71] analyzed ten different organ tissues of stillborns and nonsurviving neonates and cord blood in 30 normal-term babies in two Atlanta, Ga. hospitals. The mothers were identified as having "had no known special exposure to pesticides". Despite such selection there was a wide range of values for a variety of chlorinated hydrocarbons. For the nonsurvivors, o,p'-DDT and (1,1-dichloro-2,2-bis(p-chlorophenyl)ethane) p,p'-DDD in adipose tissue showed outlying high values for which no explanation was available. Cord blood from the normal-term babies was within the range of values reported for human populations at that time. Zavon et al.[72] had also reported an unexplained range of values for DDE (1,1-dichloro-2-2-bis(p-chlorophenol)ethylene) concentrations (0.08 to 8.90 ppm) in tissue samples for 52 stillborns, and it seems possible that the quality of tissue from stillborn material may present analytical problems. Zavon et al.[72] concluded that all children born in the U.S. are likely to have trace quantities of chlorinated hydrocarbon pesticides in their tissues and that placental passage does occur. O'Leary et al.[73] analyzed DDE levels in the blood of infants born prematurely and at term, assuming that p,p'-DDE as the principal metabolite of DDT was an indicator of long-term exposure, at least of the mother. Table 3 shows the mean, range, and median for 23 premature infants and 44 full-term infants, with markedly higher concentrations in the former.

The unanswered question remains — what were the pesticide residue levels in the adipose tissue and blood of their mothers? A study on dairy cattle did show some of these relationships.[74] Three treatment groups and a control group of three cows were each administered DDT during pregnancy. There was one stillborn calf in each of the low-, medium-, and high-dose groups and their body fat contained 2, 97, and 210 ppm DDT, while their dams' estimated body-fat levels at calving were 6, 247, and 331 ppm, respectively. The authors concluded that "no effects on health or reproduction could be attributed to the treatments", an example of a conclusion being based on insufficient data.

A Dade County, Fla. study also included analyses of paired maternal and cord blood obtained at the time of delivery.[75] Blood from newborns and women during late pregnancy, amniotic fluid, vernix caseosa, and placenta were also obtained. As in other studies, black women had higher blood levels of DDE. Amniotic fluid and cord-blood levels were considerably lower than maternal levels but as the vernix caseosa contained

TABLE 3

p,p'-DDE Concentrations in Whole Blood of Newborn Infants (ppb)[73]

		Mean	Range	Median
White	Term	4.9	2—13	5
	Premature	22.1	18.7—26.8	21
Black	Term	6.1	3—12	5.8
	Premature	19.0	6.6—34.4	17.0

Note: parts per billion — ppb.

much higher levels of DDE particularly, as well as DDT when compared with the placenta, it was evident that transplacental passage had occurred.

An important study from the Wasserman[76] group in Israel of extracted lipids of fetal blood and placenta, maternal blood, and uterine muscle showed a pattern of pesticide concentration which suggested quantitative differences in the ability of these tissues to metabolize and/or store organochlorine compounds.

E. Organophosphate Pesticides

Placental transfer of carbon[14]-labeled parathion has been observed in sheep after i.v. injection and confirmed in fetal tissues.[77] Administered from 90 to 110 days gestation, there was a decrease of plasma cholinesterase of 50% in the mother and 25% in the fetus.

VI. PLACENTAL METABOLISM

Juchau's[78] review of placental metabolism in relation to toxicology provides a listing of aspects of placental enzymology which are in need of further investigation to adequately determine the effects of drugs on the mother and developing embryo and fetus. These areas are

1. Enzyme-dependent mechanisms for the transport of foreign and endogenous chemicals between the maternal and fetal circulation.
2. The capacity of placental enzymes (or non-enzymatic catalysts) to alter the chemical structures of drugs and foreign compounds.
3. The effects of xenobiotics on the placental enzymes that are involved in specialized physiological functions of the placenta.

A. Cigarette Smoke

One extensively studied aspect of human placental toxicology has been in relation to women who smoke during pregnancy. The enzyme activity of the human placenta in response to exposure to 3,4 benz-pyrene (BP) has been examined by Welch et al.[79] to establish the variability between smokers and nonsmokers. Although BP and other polycyclic aromatic hydrocarbons are widely distributed in polluted city air, soil, some foods, tars, mineral oils, pitch, and soot, more concentrated amounts of BP are available for direct inhalation in tobacco smoke. Hydroxylated metabolites of BP possess little or no carcinogenic activity, so it is useful to establish the levels of metabolizing enzymes in human populations and their increase in response to long-term exposure to BP and other polycyclic hydrocarbons with carcinogenic potential. Placentae from residents of New York City with normal childbirth experience were homogenized and the metabolism of BP and 3-methyl-4-monomethylaminoazobenzene was measured.

No detectable hydroxylase activity was observed in the placentae of nonsmokers, though it was noted that low concentrations could have been below the level of detectibility of the method used. In contrast, all 17 cigarette smokers had measureable BP-hydroxylase activity with no relationship to the number of cigarettes smoked. Amino-azo dye N-demethylase activity was also found in all the placentas from cigarette smokers with little or none in those of nonsmokers. Welch et al. propose that there may be genetic differences in the inducibility of enzymes that detoxify polycyclic hydrocarbons, which would explain the 25-fold variation in the BP-hydroxylase activity in the placentae of smokers which they reported. In addition, they propose that steroid metabolism of the placenta in smokers should be explored to establish whether the endocrine function of the placenta is affected by polycyclic hydrocarbons.

Wang et al.[80] have since found the highest activity for the metabolism of BP in the microsomal fraction of the placenta of smokers, and in addition, identified metabolites, which were monophenolic derivatives, primarily 3-hydroxy-BP, diols and quinones of BP. They discuss the evidence for interaction of metabolic intermediates with cellular components resulting in cancer initiation. The detoxification process which may depend on the induction of metabolizing enzymes, at the same time increases the production of other compounds. These compounds and derivatives may then interact with cellular components, a possible pathway for transplacental carcinogenesis. However, there is, so far, no corroborative epidemiological evidence that the children of smoking mothers are at higher risk of cancer.

Oxygen consumption of placental tissue is inversely proportional to the carboxyhemoglobin in oxygen consumption in maternal blood, and among light smokers inhaling carbon monoxide, the reduction may be close to 9%. A 20% decrease in oxygen consumption may occur in those smoking more than five cigarettes a day and when maternal carboxyhemoglobin levels are greater than 7.0%. Carbon monoxide in high concentrations can interfere with enzyme function involving cytochrome oxidase, cytochrome P-450, and carbonic anhydrase, but no direct measures have been made on human placentae under these conditions.[32]

Nebert et al.[81] confirmed the higher mean hydroxylase activity in placentae of women who smoked as 5 to 25-fold greater than the amount found in placentae of nonsmokers. However, they also found significant activity in some women who did not smoke and measured none in the placentae of some smokers. One explanation was that there was a heterogeneous distribution of hydrocarbon hydroxylase activity throughout the placenta (between different segments of the same placenta activity varied as much as 35%). The inter- or intracellular distribution of hydroxylase activity is not known and the cellular structure of the placenta varies markedly throughout its various tissue components. There was no effect on placental hydroxylase activity of chronic administration of phenobarbital during pregnancy.

The metabolism of endogenous substrates and exogenous contaminants by the human placenta is significant in the control of the environment of the fetus. A toxic substance may be converted enzymatically to a nontoxic, more polar derivative within the placenta; or the opposite effect could result with the metabolizing of an inactive compound to an active teratogen, for example. However, little is known of the placental enzyme activity of the human placenta of 9 to 12 weeks when compared to the placenta at term. It seems likely that the oxidative enzyme pathways contribute to normal growth and development of the fetus by maintaining appropriate hormonal balance, particularly if the hydroxylation of polycyclic hydrocarbons and steroid hormones share some common enzyme systems.

Maternal cigarette smoking is the only source of polycyclic hydrocarbons which has been well studied epidemiologically. Prematurity, low birth weight, and fetal death are

TABLE 4

Enzyme Activity of Mitochondria from Normal and Toxemic Placentas[82]

Inhibitory Effect of Zinc, Lead, and Cadmium

	Cytochrome Oxidase		Succinic Dehydrogenase	
	Normal	Toxemic	Normal	Toxemic
Zinc	+ +[a]	+ +	+ +	+[b]
Lead	− −[c]	+ +	−[d]	+ +
Cadmium	+	+	−	−

[a]   + + Marked inhibition
[b]   + Slight inhibition
[c]   − − Stimulated activity
[d]   − No inhibition

associated with cigarette smoking during pregnancy. The question is whether placental hydroxylase activity in smokers has any influence on these pregnancy outcomes. The increased rate of hydroxylation of polycyclic aromatic hydrocarbons in the placentae of smokers can also lead to production of cytotoxic phenols and quinones and intermediary metabolites, such as reactive peroxides. Juchau[78] concludes that such compounds may be lethal to placental and decidual cells, which could be a factor in premature births and abortions. If decidual cells are more sensitive than trophoblastic cells, the case for an association with abortion would be stronger.

B. Cadmium, Lead

Dawson et al.[82] have examined the effect of trace metals, cadmium, lead, and zinc on succinic dehydrogenase and cytochrome oxidase of mitochondria isolated from human placentae at term. Lead and cadmium were chosen on the basis of an early report of the relationship of toxemia to lead availability in different parts of Britain[83] and the animal experiments of the effects of cadmium on the placenta by Parizek.[84] Dawson et al. examined placentae from both normal and toxemic women and found a marked difference in the response of mitochondrial succinic dehydrogenase and cytochrome oxidase activity to the addition of trace metals. There was no statistically significant difference between the succinic dehydrogenase activity of the normal and toxemic placentae; but with the addition of serial levels of lead ion in the form of lead chloride (0 to 173.0 μ mol), there was complete inhibition at every added level in the mitochondria enzyme activity from the toxemic placentas, but only a modest, progressive decrease in the activity of normal placental mitochondria. In contrast, for cytochrome oxidase activity of mitochondria, addition of lead ion increased the activity in normal placental mitochondria, though complete inhibition occurred in the mitochondria from toxemic placentas. Cadmium, added as cadmium chloride, appeared to show far less effect with a progressive increase in succinic dehydrogenase activity in both normal and toxemic mitochondria. For cytochrome oxidase activity there was also far less inhibitory effect than was seen for lead on mitochondria from both normal women. Zinc, added as zinc chloride, was somewhat similar to lead, inhibiting succinic dehydrogenase activity at all levels added, in both normal and toxemic mitochondria and inhibiting cytochrome oxidase activity completely in both normal and toxemic mitochondria (Table 4). The trace amounts of metal ions used in these experiments may not be indicative of the mode of action at higher levels of contamination. However, the differential effect of lead on the enzyme activity of mitochondria from normal and toxemic placentas is of interest.

As with other systems of the body when there may be impaired kidney, liver, or lung functions, the possibility of impaired placental function must be kept in mind when considering the effects of toxic environments.

The integrity of the placenta in the face of toxic insult has been examined by Parizek,[84] particularly in relation to cadmium. Under experimental conditions, small amounts of cadmium salts given to pregnant rats resulted in rapidly progressive changes in the placenta and destruction of the pars fetalis. In addition, there was a high mortality of pregnant rats given doses of cadmium cations causing selective circulatory damage in estrogen-producing organs, an hypothesis supported by the observations of severe effects of cadmium on the circulatory system of the testes leading to severe necrosis.

VII. AMNIOTIC FLUID

A. Mercury

Mercury has been found at the time of delivery in the amniotic fluid of Norwegian women who had been exposed to elemental mercury inhaled, ingested, and absorbed through the skin during their work as dental assistants.[60] A single observation of amniotic fluid during the epidemic of methylmercury poisoning in Iraq showed the presence of mercury.[85]

Amniotic fluid has been more intensively examined since amniocentesis became a common clinical procedure, and the significance of trace-element contamination has been discussed by Suzuki et al.[86] in terms of the transplacental route of entry to the fetus. In order to better understand the pharmacokinetics of inorganic and organic mercury, they made separate measurements on the amniotic fluid of 57 women, of whom 27 were at term and the others ranged from 4 to 8 months gestation. Detectable amounts of mercury were found in all samples of amniotic fluid except one, inorganic mercury in all but two samples, and organic mercury in 30 of 57 samples. The mean inorganic mercury level for all gestation groups was 6.0 nmol Hg per liter (range 1.5 to 26.0). For organic mercury the mean level for each gestation group was 2.0 nmol Hg per liter. The difference was statistically significant and there was a significant correlation between the two. There appeared to be an increase in both organic and inorganic mercury in the seventh month with a subsequent decrease. However, these values did not represent longitudinal observations of the same women so the significance of the fluctuation is unclear. Earlier studies of Japanese fish-eating populations by Suzuki, as well as reports of Swedish women who also consumed fish, and the Iraqi mercury-poisoned women have shown that human fetal erythrocytes contain about 30% more mercury than maternal erythrocytes and that the placental accumulation of mercury is greater than the accumulation in maternal and fetal blood. The question raised by Suzuki's study is the means by which inorganic mercury appears in excess of organic mercury in the amniotic fluid. It may be that metabolism of the organic form to inorganic occurs during transplacental passage. There is no evidence that biotransformation of organic mercury into an inorganic form takes place in the fetus.

B. Organochlorinated Compounds

Analyses of organochlorine compounds in maternal and fetal tissue during labor have been made by Polishuk et al.,[76] and the highest concentration of organochlorine pesticides and polychlorinated biphenyls in extracted lipids was in amniotic fluid, when compared with adipose tissue, maternal blood, fetal blood, uterine muscle, and placenta. However, only four samples were analyzed and the quantity of extracted lipid was taken into account. Presumably, the absolute amount of these contaminants in the amniotic fluid must be low.

C. Nicotine

Sensitive radioimmunoassay procedures for the detection of nicotine and a principal metabolite, cotinine, have been used by Van Vunakis et al.[87] to analyze amniotic fluid from 100 women between 14 and 20 weeks gestation. In 22 of 37 women who were smokers, nicotine was found in amniotic fluid (up to 31 ng/mℓ). Cotinine was present in the amniotic fluid of 33 of them (up to 129 ng/mℓ). In part, the different levels of nicotine and cotinine relate to their biological half-lives, which for nicotine is about one half hour in blood and for cotinine is 30 to 40 hr. Up to about 20 weeks of pregnancy there is no impediment to fluid movement in that the fetal skin has not yet developed and up to about mid-pregnancy the composition of the amniotic fluid is closely similar to that of fetal extracellular fluid. Hytten and Leitch[88] consider that at this stage the amniotic fluid may be regarded as an extension of fetal extracellular fluid. The composition of amniotic fluid changes to about 99% water in late pregnancy, by which time there is balance between urine passed by the mature fetal kidneys and amniotic fluid ingested by the fetus.

It is significant then that in both the Suzuki and Van Vunakis studies on the composition of amniotic fluid that organic and inorganic mercury, nicotine, and cotinine were present before 20 weeks when these contaminants would have been in direct contact with all fetal tissues. With the development of skin and maturing of the fetal kidney, the increase in amniotic fluid mercury concentration at 7 months and subsequent decrease to term may give some indication of the extent of the contact with fetal tissues of contaminants in amniotic fluid.

VIII. TERATOGENIC EFFECTS AND FETAL GROWTH

Developmental defects which arise during the period of cell differentiation in the embryo can result from a variety of insults. There is general agreement that chromosome aberrations cause 5 to 10% of observed malformations, recessive and dominant genes cause about 20%, ionizing radiation (therapeutic, diagnostic, nuclear, and natural) causes 1% or less, maternal infections cause 2 to 3%, and maternal disease states (excluding nutritional deficiencies) cause 2 to 3%. From 63 to 70% of developmental defects remain unaccounted for. Wilson[89] believes that although there may be interactions and combinations within the above categories, they do not explain the large group labeled "unknown". On the basis of the large numbers of drugs and industrial chemicals known to be teratogenic in the laboratory,[90] he believes that there is a strong likelihood that many of them will be identified as interacting substances. He holds a particular concern for the potentiating interaction found in rats and other laboratory animals when two or more known teratogens were used simultaneously at threshold doses and below.[91] The implication for the human embryo is the unknown effect of maternal intake of a variety of therapeutic drugs simultaneously and in association with a chemical environment usually considered safe for the adult worker. In light of the experience with thalidomide and rubella, Wilson has suggested four criteria appropriate for the identification of a new teratogenic agent:

1.   An abrupt increase in the incidence of a particular defect or association of defects

2. Coincidence of this increase with a known environmental change, e.g., widespread use of a new drug
3. Knowledge of exposure to the environmental change early in pregnancies yielding characteristically defective infants
4. Absence of other factors common to all pregnancies yielding infants with the characteristic defects

The limitations of the approach are discussed by Wilson with the recognition that it is unlikely to be a totally dependable tool for human teratogen identification. In terms of industrial exposures the problems of sample size, interaction with other causative factors, and inadequacies of documentation are even more severe. It is well to keep in mind that under the scheme of estimated proportion of causes of developmental defects, the numbers of affected infants per 1000 births is small, e.g., chromosome and genetic abnormalities affect 15 to 25 infants, maternal disease and infection 2 to 4, known drugs and environmental chemicals, less than 1. The unknown group which makes up 62 to 70% of the total observed cases of developmental defects numbers 31 to 39 infants per 1000 births.

Another view is given by Brent,[92] who attributes the cause of defects in the unknown 62 to 70% as spontaneous errors in embryogenesis or multifactorial relationships between genotype and environment. In his view, if the environment were optimal embryopathology would still occur because the reproductive and developmental processes have a built-in probability of going .[11] With some modifying comments he states that "rather than expend energy on further environmental testing, it would be far better to learn the spectrum of mechanisms involved in embryopathy and the factors essential to normal embryonic development." Despite Brent's view that it is impossible to establish an animal testing protocol that will guarantee the safety or hazard to the human of an environmental factor at a particular dosage or quantitative exposure level, such testing systems are very likely to be seriously proposed in the future for government regulatory purposes. The differences between animals and humans in genetic heterogeneity, length and rapidity of organogenesis, placental function and transfer, diet, metabolism, concurrent disease, and environmental variables are real differences but animal tests may be the only guide to examination of a potentially hazardous chemical with only limited distribution. Clinical and epidemiologic methods could well be too gross to establish the presence of a risk, if one exists.

Wilson's[90] view is that "most teratologists accept the theoretical principle that all chemical agents could, under the right conditions of dosage, developmental stage, and species selections, be shown to have adverse effects on development, . . . but there is some assurance that certain agents are unlikely to cause adverse effects within the limits of dosage ordinarily encountered."

The apparent polarization of views on some aspects of teratogenic risk to human populations will no doubt eventually lead to an intermediate position. For purposes of this discussion, identification and evaluation of teratogens must be derived from the gradual accumulation of animal and human experience. Shepard's[93] *Catalogue of Teratogenic Agents* as a continuing summary compilation is likely to be the most useful resource as more evaluation of the teratogenic effects of toxic substances is demanded.

A. Lead

A commonly repeated statement is to the effect that the "fetus is most susceptible to lead toxicity during the stage of most active growth, suggesting that the early pregnancy is most endangered and that the fetus is possibly more sensitive than the young child.''[94] However, a review of the evidence does not wholly support such an opinion but does provide some reasons why the generalizations inherent to the statement may not be reliable.

The evidence for first trimester loss is primarily from studies of acute and severe lead poisoning in women using lead salts as an abortifacient or in severe industrial-poisoning cases. The cases came to attention because of the death of the mother[95] or because of her severe poisoning. Abortions certainly occur under such conditions as the anecdotal and epidemiologic reports attest.[96] Teratogenic effects, per se, have not been observed in human fetuses and live borns who have experienced lead intoxication *in utero* throughout gestation, including the first trimester.[97,98] The weight of evidence points to toxic effects on maternal physiology as the prime cause for embryo loss in the first trimester, under conditions of high blood-lead levels in the pregnant woman (over $100\mu g/100$ mℓ). Bell[99] proposed that excessive lead first injures the chorionic epithelium of the uterus and thus indirectly injures the fetus leading to its expulsion. Hamilton and Hardy[100] stated that "expulsion of the fetus follows with or without a direct stimulating effect of lead on the uterine musculature". It is appropriate to note, in view of lead's known effect on active muscle, the considerable capacity for contraction and relaxation of the uterine musculature which is maintained throughout a woman's reproductive life, whether pregnant or not.[101] The first trimester may not be the period of highest vulnerability for the fetus itself because:

1. Specific human teratogenic effects have not been reported as a result of lead exposure. Deformities such as macrocephaly are likely to result from lead exposure throughout the gestation period, interfering with normal growth processes beyond the period of cell differentiation.
2. Probable susceptibility of uterine musculature to lead above $100 \mu g/100$ mℓ blood could result in expulsive contractions. The loss of the fetus, which certainly occurs under conditions of maternal poisoning, is more likely to result from effects on the mother and not directly on the fetus.

The remaining discussion of the identification of cumulative effects of lead contamination on the fetus throughout the gestation period proceeds on the assumption that the growing fetus is vulnerable, whatever its stage of development. For comparison there are only a few reported cases of short-term, high-lead exposures beyond the first trimester. In Denmark four pregnancies of 5 or more months duration, for which ingested lead oxide was used as the abortifacient, resulted in three normal infants, one abortion, and one postnatal death at 2 months possibly related to intrauterine toxicity.[95] In Nebraska an 8-month pregnant mother with a 2-month inhalation of battery casing fumes as her source of family lead exposure had a blood lead level of 240 $\mu g/$ 100 mℓ and delivered a normal child 1 month after a 7-day course of intravenous calcium disodium ethylene diaminetetracetate. The cord blood at the time of delivery was below 60 $\mu g/100$ mℓ. The other four children with blood concentrations similar to their mother all had symptoms ranging from hyperactivity to fatal encephalopathy. At 4 years and 3 months, a complete pediatric-neurologic examination and developmental assessment of the child born following therapy was normal. No abnormalities were found in the electroencephalogram, radiographs of the skull and long bones, urinalysis, or blood count.[94]

In contrast, examples of long-term exposure throughout gestation present more serious symptoms. Palmisano et al.[97] describe effects of long-term ingestion from untaxed (moonshine) whiskey. At age 10 weeks the child was not thriving (weight 2280 g, birthweight 1900 g), though was alert and normal in most respects except for increased muscle tone in the lower extremities, frequent and spontaneous episodes of tremulous activity of the arms and legs, and sustained ankle clonus. All deep-tendon reflexes were hyperactive. Chelation therapy resulted in high lead excretion (620 μg/ℓ of urine for the infant and 600 μg/ℓ for the mother). Blood lead levels were not obtained. Unfortunately, alcohol exposure during gestation also results in low birth weight and neurologic deficits[702] so that the maternal supply of a combination of fetal toxins, probably associated with some degree of malnutrition, complicates any evaluation of a lead-dose relationship in this case.

Toxic levels of lead contamination in men and women undoubtedly result in a high probability of reproductive loss.[11] The unraveling of the pathologic processes involved is conjectural only, but an attempt can be made by restricting the possibilities within the range of observed effects in human populatations:

1. First trimester human survivals following maternal lead exposure (acute or chronic) provide little evidence for teratogenic effects, based on Shepard's[93] definition of a teratogen.
2. Second and third trimester human survivals may show minimal physical and neurological effects when maternal exposure has been short term but after the first trimester.
3. Serious permanent sequelae in the live born result from chronic long term exposure via maternal blood, because of the accumulated body burden of lead during the period of growth and development.

We have no adequate quantitative information on human exposures to develop a dose-response relationship for these conditions during pregnancy, so that choice of a "safe" maternal blood lead level is very subjective. A maternal blood lead level above 30 μg/100 mℓ is cause for concern.

B. Mercury

Takeuchi[103] has described the effects of *in utero* exposure to organic mercury as congenital cerebral palsy, caused after formation of the placenta. There were no true malformations in the Minamata victims exposed *in utero* and there was no observed increase in the frequency of miscarriages during the period of contamination. Of the 23 infants examined in detail, all showed disturbances in mental and motor development, with speech disturbance, impairment of gait, chewing, and swallowing. There was overactivity of the tendon reflex in 82%, the primitive reflexes in 73%, the pathological reflexes in 55%, with involuntary movements in 73%, and increased salivation in 77%. Convulsions and markedly reduced brain size were also observed.

C. Chlorinated Hydrocarbons

The chlorinated dibenzo-*p*-dioxins and dibenzo furans are among the most potent teratogens known and occur as contaminants in pentachlorophenol, which is used as a wood preservative and bacteriostat and in polychlorinated biphenyls used as a plasticizer and heat exchange fluid.[104] As a trace contaminant of Agent Orange (*n*-butylesters of 2,4-D and 2,4,5-T) 2,3,7,8 tetrachlorodibenzo-*p*-dioxin was confirmed as a teratogenic agent.

An epidemic of congenital limb deformities of swine occurred in Missouri, in which nicotine in the tobacco stalks eaten by pregnant sows was implicated. However, it was noted that maleic hydrazide at 115 ppm was also a contaminant on the stalks, but due to its low toxicity in rats was disregarded as a likely cause. The authors did mention its carcinogenic and mutagenic properties, but did not consider these to be pertinent in view of the nicotine content.[105]

Another clinical report from Kentucky has also implicated tobacco-stalk ingestion during early pregnancy in the appearance of skeletal anomalies in pigs.[106] The veterinarian noted that since tobacco had been grown in central Kentucky for more than 100 years and this teratologic problem had not been recognized before it was more likley that chemicals or their combination with the plant were a likely explanation.

Although the human poisoning experience with parathion and organophosphate pesticide has been extensive throughout the world, there is a dearth of information concerning its reproductive effects. Tanimura et al.[107] mention a Japanese study where some cases of human fetal death and malformations have been related to acute poisoning resulting from an organophosphate sprinkled in a field. Fish[108] treated rats at various stages of gestation with organophosphate pesticides and found a reduction in fetal cerebral-cortical cholinesterase activity. No significant increase in resorptions or congenital anomalies was found, but there was a high stillbirth and neonatal death rate. In a number of rat and mouse studies, the administration of a variety of organophosphates did not result in any marked teratogenic effects;[109-111] however, embryotoxic effects in the form of higher mortality and decreased fetal weight have been generally found. Budreau and Singh[111] concluded that teratogenesis did not appear to be directly related to cholinesterase inhibition, but little conjecture is made by any of these authors on the embryotoxic relationship, other than the possible combined effects of transient depression of maternal food intake and direct action of the chemical and its metabolites on the embryo.

Rice[112] has noted that transplacental exposure of the human fetus to pesticides may occur either because they or their degradation products find their way into the diets of pregnant women, or because pregnant women are directly subject to percutaneous or inhalation exposure in the course of manufacture domestic, or agricultural application. An additional source is the body store of pesticide residues which virtually everybody now harbors.

The Mrak Commission in their report to the Secretary of Health, Education and Welfare in 1969 recommended that research be done on pesticides and human reproduction. "Epidemiologic data on possible effects of pesticides on human reproduction and teratology are grossly inadequate. Prospective studies on this subject are difficult to design and almost nonexistent."[113] The same recommendation could be made 10 years later.

Epidemiologic studies of human populations seldom include low birth weight as an indicator of toxic effects of environmental contamination beyond socio-economic conditions and smoking experience. There appear to have been no confirmatory studies of O'Leary's[73] observations of premature and mature infants to establish the significance of the apparent discrepancy in p,p'-DDE concentrations for these infants. (Table 3).

D. Carbon Monoxide

Reports of carbon monoxide poisoning in pregnant women go back to 1859, when illuminating gas was coming into general use. Muller and Graham[118] have reviewed 24 cases of carbon monoxide intoxication and discussed the evidence for direct poisoning of the fetus by carbon monoxide crossing the placenta vs. simple asphyxia due to lack of oxygen via the placenta from the maternal blood. Adverse effects on the fetus result in both cases. In the event of rapid acute carbon monoxide poisoning of the mother, she may die before all her cells are saturated and before diffusible carbon monoxide in the plasma reaches the placenta. The fetus dies from anoxia. Carbon monoxide which does cross the placenta can cause fetal death even when the mother survives if chronic exposure occurs. The published reports of infant survivors of maternal exposure to carbon monoxide indicate an array of long-term psychomotor disturbances and anatomic anomalies, although it is impossible to clearly differentiate the effects of maternal anoxia from carbon monoxide poisoning which also leads to fetal anoxia, but at a far slower rate. As in adults, repeated insults with cumulative permanent tissue damage to the fetus can result when there is chronic exposure to carbon monoxide, from, e.g., cigarette smoking. Mean carboxyhemoglobin levels ranging from 2.4 to 7.6% have been reported for the fetus and from 2.0 to 8.3% in mothers smoking during pregnancy, which results from the 50 to 100 ppm carbon monoxide concentrations in cigarette smoke. Low birth weights in relation to maternal smoking are well recognized and breathing irregularities and cyanosis have been observed at birth. Other contaminants in addition to carbon monoxide are present in cigarette smoke and probably contribute to the adverse effects.[32]

Interference with tissue oxygenation of the fetus leads to insufficient intracellular partial pressure of oxygen for normal enzyme activity, and provides a reasonable explanation for reduced body weight associated with carbon monoxide exposure. Ginsburg and Myers[115] used Rhesus monkeys to examine the effects of carbon monoxide inhalation on mothers and fetuses. Carboxyhemoglobin levels exceeding 60% in nine term pregnant female monkeys did not cause any clinical effects in the mothers. Severe hypoxia, detected by fetal monitoring and fetal blood sampling in utero was observed in the fetuses. Fetal hypoxia became apparent early in the exposure period with bradycardia, hypotension, and metabolic acidosis, although carboxyhemoglobin levels rose only slowly over the 1- to 3-hr exposure period. By the end of the exposure period, fetal carboxyhemoglobin was in excess of 18% when the maternal carboxyhemoglobin levels were as high as 60%. On delivery and the onset of lung breathing the fetal arterial pH, which markedly declined during exposure, returned to normal. Four of the nine infant monkeys developed normally and showed no signs of neurological abnormalities. Five animals showed severe damage and four died within 72 hr of delivery. The fifth was sacrificed. Hemorrhagic necrosis was present in the brain in all five newborns with increased cranial pressure and retinal hemorrhages. The severely affected animals had experienced arterial oxygen concentration below 2.0 ml/100 ml for up to 75 min. The marked effect observed in this study resulted from a single acute maternal exposure to carbon monoxide at levels which did not severely affect the mother. There was not time for a fetal accumulation of carbon monoxide which was only present to a small extent in fetal blood. The main impact appears to have come from the carbon monoxide-induced decrease in maternal arterial oxyhemoglobin. In view of the slow accumulation of carbon monoxide in the fetal blood, under acute exposure conditions, fetal carboxyhemoglobin appears to be related to the rate of diffusion for placental transfer of carbon monoxide rather than by the maternal or fetal blood flow.

Kline et al.[116] found almost two-fold odds of smoking during pregnancy among women with spontaneous abortions, after controlling for confounding variables. However, there were more chromosomally and morphologically normal spontaneous abortions among smokers when compared with non-smokers, which is consistent with an anoxic effect of growth impairment, rather than a mutational or teratological impact. Spontaneous abortion and low birth weight are both associated with smoking during pregnancy, which maintains a source of carbon monoxide to red blood cells of the mother and fetus.

In summary, the effects of carbon monoxide on the fetus may be severe under conditions of acute exposure due to reduced maternal oxygen supply. Under conditions of chronic exposure, both reduced oxygen supply and direct effects of carbon monoxide on efficiency of tissue oxygenation can impair the normal development of the fetus. Examination of the effects of smoking on the fetus emphasizes the probable importance of chronic carbon monoxide exposure from any source on pregnancy outcome as well as the underlying risk of the smoking pregnant worker takes with her to her job. The additional impact of any adverse occupational exposure can possibly be more severe than would be the case for the nonsmoker.

IX. EPIDEMIOLOGICAL LIMITATIONS

Although teratogenicity has been shown in one or more species of mammals for a variety of chemicals which could be encountered in the workplace, sparse evidence exists for comparable effects in human beings. The limitations of the epidemiologic method will prevent observation of adverse effects, if they exist, for many chemical agents which are likely to have limited entry into the workplace and limited worker exposure, particularly if they are known carcinogens. Oakley[121] has described the limitations of a birth-defect surveillance program in the general population, a program, however, which has not in the past emphasized parental occupational histories.

NIOSH prepares a summary of recommendations for occupational health standards four times a year.[122] Of the 74 in the October, 1977 listing, carbaryl, ethylene dibromide, polychlorinated biphenyls, tetrachloroethylene, 1,1,1-trichloroethane, and waste anesthetic gases have shown sufficient evidence of teratogenicity in animals or human beings to have employee warnings recommended. The remaining 63 chemicals included the following, for which some evidence of teratogenicity has been reported by Shephard,[93] but which were not so noted by NIOSH:

- benzene
- cadmium and compounds
- parathion
- carbon tetrachloride
- chromium compounds
- oxides of nitrogen
- cyanides
- formaldehyde
- nickel and compounds
- fluorine

Evidence sufficient for cautionary measures is frequently inadequate as has been described by Strobino et al.[119] They took into account the statistical power of epidemiologic studies of pregnancy outcome, where statistical power refers to the probability that an effect, if present, will be detected. It is affected by the frequency of the outcome variable in the unexposed population, the size of the effect expected, the acceptable level of significance, and the sample size. The difficulty of discerning an effect from an occupational hazard becomes apparent when it is realized that with the usual small relative risk, possibly 1.3 or less, for exposed vs. unexposed individuals, a large study population is needed. If an expected incidence of an event is 1 in 1000 and the risk is increased to 2 in 1000; that is, the risk is doubled in exposed individuals, 10,100 exposed individuals are required for observation in order to have a 75% probability of showing a difference significant at the 5% level using a two-tailed test. There are few if any industrial settings where such a number of pregnancies could be observed to establish the presence of teratogenic effects for a suspected agent. Strobino et al. have reviewed the few studies involving occupational exposure to anesthetic gases, vinyl chloride, polychlorinated biphenyls, and dioxin. Only in the case of two studies on exposure to anesthetic gases is the association with developmental defects at term demonstrated,[120,121] and in two other studies the evidence for an association is inconclusive.[122,123]

The widespread use of pesticides has been particularly difficult to evaluate. Exposure levels now range from the low-body burden, almost ubiquitous in the world, to higher burdens among participants and bystanders in farm work, household extermination, and pesticide manufacture and formulation. The essential linkage between monitoring of pesticide body burden and epidemiologic surveillance of the same human populations has not ever been established. Migrant workers and particularly small tenant farmers provide a clear example of inadequate examination of populations exposed to a variety of organochlorinated and organophosphate pesticide, over a 20-year period. Today we do not know if there has or has not been an effect on their child bearing in terms of teratogenicity or any other aspect of adverse reproduction.

It is difficult to establish a balance between the view that the number of established teratogens is small, or that the dispersed occurrence of congenital abnormalities defies epidemiologic surveillance. The association of ethyl alcohol and the "fetal alcohol syndrome" has now become generally accepted, although the absence of an effect in some countries must still be explained.[105,124] Although growth deficiency is the major characteristic, anatomical changes are also apparent. Both ethanol and its metabolite acetaldehyde freely cross the placenta, though as yet the etiology of the syndrome is not known. In addition, case studies have identified warfarin (used as a rodenticide and also as a therapeutic anticoagulant drug) to be associated with microcephaly and blindness, although long-term administration during pregnancy may have caused growth retardation.[125]

X. TRANSPLACENTAL CARCINOGENESIS

The unique observation (so far) of human transplacental carcinogenesis due to diethylstilbesterol (DES) is not surprising, in view of the likely necessity for enzyme-mediated metabolic conversion of most carcinogens to a chemically reactive derivative.[126] Fetal tissue usually lacks the drug-metabolizing enzymes necessary for such conversions. There is an extensive literature on transplacental carcinogenesis in animals, which has been summarized by Rice, in addition to that on experimental neonatal carcinogenesis. Published case studies in which childhood cancer is related to *in utero* exposure to a toxic substance have so far been inadequate to sustain a hypothesis of causal relationship.[127] The more likely effect of excessive exposure to a toxic chemical is teratogenesis, embryonic loss, or fetal-growth retardation. However, the conservative view is to keep in mind the DES experience, and to minimize any likelihood that maternal exposure to carcinogens might occur.

XI. CHELATION THERAPY DURING PREGNANCY

Concern has been raised that the use of chelating agents for the removal of contaminant metals in pregnant women may be harmful to the fetus.[128] One case of an 8-month pregnant woman, treated with intravenous calcium disodium ethylenediaminetetraacetate, was reported by Angle et al. Normal birth and development to 4 years of a healthy child resulted.[94] The calcium trisodium salt of diethylenetriaminepentaacetic acid (DTPA) is used for removal of various actinide elements in occupationally exposed persons in the nuclear industry. Mays et al. are recommending that zinc DTPA should replace Ca DTPA, because the recommended daily dose of 29 to 36 μmol Ca

DTPA per kilogram is within or above the range of doses, predicted from mouse and rat effects, to be fatal for the human fetus.[128] The maintenance of zinc and manganese levels when Zn DTPA is used, is thought to be a safer, more effective therapy. No significant change has been found in fetal weight, fetal mortality, or number of embryos from pregnant rats administered 1800 μmol Zn DTPA per kilogram.

XII. LACTATION

The constant production of milk during nursing is one pathway for the excretion of drugs and contaminants stored in other body tissues. The passage of drugs across the mammary barrier into milk appears to be similar to that of drugs through other biological membranes, however, there is little definite or conclusive information concerning the mechanism beyond the evidence for high-lipid synthesis activity of mammary tissue.[129] Relative concentration gradients and differential solubility are not specifically known for the wide variety of contaminants in breast milk. Because milk has a high fat and protein concentration, lipid-soluble or protein-bound contaminants pass readily to milk and are dissolved in or bound to the milk fat and protein. The blood flow to the breast is much more rapid than the rate of milk secretion so that lipid-soluble contaminants are readily available for concentration in the milk. Fat-soluble contaminants, therefore, can be expected to be in considerably higher concentrations in breast milk than in whole blood.

A. Organochlorinated Hydrocarbons

The contamination of human breast milk with DDT was reported in 1951 by Laug et al.[135] In 1961, Quimby et al.[131] reported measurements of the lipid fraction in ten individuals and found an average of 2.5 ppm DDT and 1.4 ppm DDE, in contrast to 0.08 ppm DDT and 0.04 ppm DDE in the whole milk. By 1965, when more accurate measuring techniques became available, Egan et al.[132] reported measurable amounts of heptachlor epoxide, p,p'-DDE, DDT, dieldrin, and benzenehexachloride (BHC) at levels exceeding those found in cow's milk. The extensive worldwide contamination has lead the World Health Organization (WHO) to set a limit of 0.05 ppm (1.25 ppm in milk fat) for total DDT in cow's milk and an acceptable daily intake of DDT of 0.01 mg/kg body weight.[133] In the U.S., Sweden, and Britain the WHO acceptable daily intake of DDT is likely to be exceeded by nursing infants.[134]

The more extensive studies of the 1970s have provided some additional information on characteristics of lactation, for example, that residues are significantly higher in the milk collected when the breast is nearly empty (hind milk), when compared with the milk collected when the breast is nearly full (fore milk). Concentrations also tend to be lower in the milk of older mothers, particularly those who have nursed three or more babies.[133] Their concentrations of DDT are far below the average. Kroger[134] found the highest concentrations (4.00 ppm) in milk fat of Pennsylvania mothers who were nursing their first child. Curley et al.[135] have measured both blood and milk samples from five women between 3 and 96 days post partum for DDT and residues, total BHC, heptachlor epoxide, and dieldrin, all of which varied widely.

A more extensive nationwide study has been done by Savage for the Environmental Protection Agency's National Human Monitoring Study.[136] In order to account for the variation in lipid content of breast milk in relation to time of sampling and breast fullness, all levels of pesticide and metabolites analyzed were reported as fat-adjusted levels in milk. The percent distribution of fat-adjusted levels of p,p'-DDT in 1210 whites, 37 blacks, and 42 Mexican Americans showed only 23.6% of the whites over 500 ppb, but 65% of the blacks and 74% of the Mexican Americans in excess of 500 ppb. For *o,p*-DDT 61% of whites and 38% of blacks had no measurable amounts. Adipose-tissue concentrations of DDT in blacks have been found to be generally higher by a factor of two when compared with whites,[137] so that higher concentrations in breast milk of blacks could be predicted.

Bakken and Seip[138] have analyzed 50 samples in Norway and shown that for total BHC and total DDT, colostrum samples were about 40% higher than samples taken at 9 to 16 weeks post partum, in part a reflection of the higher fat content of colostrum. For the same women providing multiple milk samples, considerable fluctuation in pesticide concentrations was observed. The explanation given was that there may be two pesticide pools in the body, one in adipose tissue and one in the blood/milk phase, so that variations in dietary intake of pesticides would contribute to the day to day variability. Egan et al.[132] have found the DDT content in body fat to be 30 times the average content of human breast milk.

Polychlorinated biphenyls (PCB) have now been identified in human breast milk and are also a worldwide pollutant.[136] The average level in the U.S. for human breast milk in 1976 was 1.8 ppm (fat-adjused level).[139] PCBs have been in commercial production for over 40 years with severe accidental exposures occurring sporadically.[140] In the Japanese incident in 1968, nine children were known to have ingested PCBs only through breast milk, having been born just after the contamination. The clinical description was enervation, lack of endurance, hypotonia, apathy, and sullen and expressionless appearance. Abnormalities have persisted in at least three of the children up to 5 or 6 years of age. In a severe hexachlorobenzene-poisoning episode in Turkey in 1957 which stemmed from ingestion of fungicide-treated seed grain, contaminated human milk was implicated in the high death rate (95% in nursing infants) over a 3-year period.[141]

These observations must be taken into account in any evaluation of occupational exposure to organic solvents in laboratories, manufacturing industries, hospitals, dry cleaning establishments, etc. For example, concentrations of benzene, trichloroethylene, and their metabolites in breast milk of women in relation to their exposure are not known. International Labour Office Convention 135 advises against exposure of nursing mothers to benzene.[142] Vozovaya et al.[143] in the U.S.S.R. have reported methylene chloride levels in breast milk of women manufacturing rubber articles. A mean value of 0.074 ± 0.046 mg/kg was found for 28 samples taken 5 to 7 hr after the start of work, with measurable amounts present in 17 of the 28 samples. Small amounts were found in the breast milk 17 hr after the termination of exposure.

For the population at large, concern has been focused on organochlorinated compounds, particularly DDT and PCBs. The tentative directive to pediatricians by government representatives has been to continue to advise breast feeding, in view of its psychological and nutritional advantages.[139] Analysis of breast milk has been advised for those who have had known high-dietary intake or occupational exposure. Adverse effects on children from contaminants in human breast milk have only been observed in severe poisoning episodes involving many people in circumscribed geographic areas. The fact that there is no evidence to indicate adverse effects for lower levels only means that a systematic evaluation has never been made. For example, the Pesticide Monitoring Study provides no medical data from the populations studied for the purposes of examining any relationship between exposure and health effects.[136]

B. Lead

The adverse effects of breast feeding by women in the lead industry were known in the last century.[144] More recently in the U.S. the average lead concentration in human milk has been found to be 0.012 ppm.[145] Higher values have been reported from Japan and Europe, in some instances such as industrialized areas, higher than cow's milk or formula milk.[146] Lead concentrations in cow's milk average 0.009 ppm, though in lead areas a range from 0.05 to 0.27 ppm has been reported.[147] Donovan[148] has shown a relationship between lead concentrations in blood and milk in cows, but no similar research has been reported on human populations.

C. Mercury

The levels of mercury in breast milk during the grain-contaminated episode in Iraq in the early 1970s were sufficient to cause clinical poisoning in infants who had not been exposed *in utero*.[85] Inorganic mercury made up 39% of the total mercury in the milk, a finding which is of interest in terms of the relative proportions of organic and inorganic mercury in amniotic fluid. In that there may be occupational exposure to organic and inorganic mercury, excretion through breast milk appears to be possible for both.[149]

XIII. TOXICOLOGICAL IMPLICATIONS RELATING TO SECONDARY SEX CHARACTERISTICS

There have been reports of differences when comparing men and nonpregnant women in their response to toxic levels of lead, beryllium, and benzene, particularly. More general epidemiologic information concerning cancer of female specific sites in certain occupations with other chemical exposures is suggestive of an additional female risk factor,[150] i.e., cancer of uterus and breast.

For lead there have been several reports noting that protoporphorin IX in erythrocytes tends to increase earlier and more rapidly in women than men for the same blood lead levels.[151,152] Wilbowo et al.[153] have examined the interaction between lead and iron metabolism and propose that the iron deficiency frequently observed in women could enhance the biochemical changes associated with lead intoxication. There appears to be little clinical information to suggest that increased hemesynthesis response to lead in women has any effect on the development of more overt symptoms of lead poisoning for the same lead exposure. The historical evidence from severe lead exposures in the 19th century does not support such a line of reasoning empirically. (See Chapter 7.) Dickens, as the Uncommercial Traveller in 1869, particularly pointed out, "..... they bear the work much better than men: some few of them have been at it for years, and the great majority of those I observed were strong and active". His inspection of white-lead manufacture in the cocklofts of 19th century England is the most perceptive an industrial hygienist can read.[154] Seppalainen has reported significant effects of lead on nerve conduction velocity and from early reports involving 8 women and 18 men suggested that there could be more of a decrement among the women at low blood lead levels than the men.[155] However, these differences were not statistically significant.

Beryllium is possibly unique in its effect on women who are not pregnant at the time of exposure. Pregnancy, even some years after termination of exposure, has resulted in exacerbation of symptoms of beryllium poisoning. Hardy[156] reported that of the 95 female deaths in the Beryllium Registry, 63 of them could be identified as having pregnancy as a likely precipitating factor. Earlier, Hardy and Stoeckle[157] had noted that, of the women with chronic respiratory disease associated with beryllium exposure who subsequently became pregnant, 40% experienced pneumonitic symptoms in conjunction with their pregnancy. The pattern of acute and chronic respiratory disease in beryllium poisoning appears to have been different for men and women, though the data have not been presented in a form that allows statistical evaluation in terms of dose. More men appear to have suffered acute episodes followed by death or chronic disease, but it is not clear if the women who died without the complications of pregnancy had exposures and a clinical course comparable to men.

The detailed clinical course of a woman chemical worker exposed to beryllium, has been described by McCallum et al.[158] In their summary they state that pregnancy was associated with relief of symptoms which persisted for some months after a normal birth. The detailed paper, however, reports that at about 4 months gestation, she experienced spontaneous pneumothorax, delivered at 8 months gestation, and died 7 months later of acute right heart failure. The onset of symptoms 2 years before pregnancy (parity not noted) was 2 years after termination of high exposure in an English laboratory with measured levels of beryllium of 2.7 $\mu g/m^3$ and other rooms with levels of over 30 $\mu g/m^3$. The present federal standard for beryllium is 2 $\mu g/m^3$ as an 8-hr time-weighted average with an acceptable ceiling concentration of 5 $\mu g/m^3$. The acceptable maximum peak is 25 $\mu g/m^3$ for a maximum of 30 minutes.[159] Severe lassitude, loss of weight, breathlessness, and radiological lung changes indicated the chronicity of the beryllium poisoning. Pregnancy itself provided some improvement of symptoms, sufficient to allow suspension of corticotropin therapy. It would be of considerable interest to compare the course of pregnancy in the women in the U.S. Beryllium Registry in detail.

The clinical observation that respiratory disease in general is not uncommon in pregnancy has been discussed by Jaffe et al.[160] High death rates have been observed among asthmatics, either during or within a year of pregnancy, and pneumonia is the second most common nonobstetric cause of maternal death. Although somewhat subjective, such information may be an indicator of the additional risk that impaired lung function imposes on the pregnant woman herself. The development of the pneumoconioses is usually protracted, and becomes severe in the post child-bearing years, so that a clinical experience has not been reported specifically for industrially related chronic lung disease and pregnancy. On the other hand, the acute toxicity of beryllium must be kept in mind, with the possibility that mobilization of body stores during pregnancy may be a precipitating event in the exacerbation of respiratory symptoms severe enough to jeopardize the woman's life.

The differential susceptibility of workers to benzene was noted in many early clinical reports under conditions of extreme exposure, in large measure because fatal anemias appeared to be unpredictable for both men and women. For women, their vulnerability was related to vaginal and post-partum hemorrhage, (see Chapter 7). Subjective comments were made early in the century that overweight workers were more susceptible. Traditionally disturbance of the hemopoietic system from chronic benzene poisoning was thought to be more severe for women than for men, though there was no supporting epidemiological data. Hamilton and Hardy[161] viewed anemia in women to be due to the demands of menstruation and pregnancy when associated with benzene exposure. Another explanation for such a difference, if indeed it exists, is the character of the body burden and the importance of fat storage of organic solvents. Under conditions of exposure in more recent years, usually below 100 ppm of air, sex differences in susceptibility to adverse effects of benzene have not been reported.

A. Effects of Body-Fat Content of Contaminants

Kinetic studies of the processes of absorption, distribution, and elimination of organic solvents which are fat soluble have shown that fat tissue markedly affects the availability of the solvent and its concentration at the site of action.[162] On the basis of Kato's[163] observations that human beings show no sex difference in the activity of drug-metabolizing enzyme systems, he attributes the higher retention of benzene in females to their body-fat distribution. In a study of five female and five male Japanese medical students exposed to 25 ppm for 2 hr, the concentration of benzene in blood and end-tidal air decreased rapidly on cessation of inhalation. After 4 hr, the concentrations were still higher in the women. However, Kato did not report any longer term follow-up in terms of differential body burden of benzene and its metabolites. It can be presumed that the Japanese medical students used in this study would not be particularly comparable in terms of their body composition with U.S. workers who are largely of other racial origins. In addition, the marked rise over the last generation in the prevalence of clinical obesity in both U.S. men and women had undoubtedly reduced some of the difference in total body fat between the sexes. The bulky distribution of body-fat tissue is now a characteristic of both sexes with implications for the development and maintenance of a body burden of an organic solvent in a large proportion of the U.S. workers.

The body burden of tetrachloroethylene in exposed workers is maintained for long periods following exposure, and excretion continues via the expired air. Gutheran and Fernedez[164] have estimated that the biologic half-life in adipose tissue is 71.5 hr so that chronic exposure in the work setting could provide a constant presence of tetrachloroethylene and its metabolites in fat. Bolanowski and Golacks[15] estimated that 25% of the inhaled tetrachloroethylene was excreted in the expired air and about 62% retained in the body and "presumably metabolized by some unknown pathway". There is, therefore, the possibility of a continual supply of a toxic substance to a target tissue, such as the germ cells, whether male or female.

In human studies, fat storage of DDT has been widely examined. By the mid 1960s, total storage of DDT and its metabolites in fat in U.S. residents had been generally quantified at about 10 ppm.[72,165-167] In contrast, for occupationally exposed men values of 35 to 1000 ppm were reported.[168] Edmundson[169] discussed the limitations of fat content as a measure of DDT storage because of variations in the chemical characteristics and content of fat in different body organs. However, these studies had shown in general that, an equilibrium develops between absorption of DDT, storage, and excretion.

The relationship between fat storage and blood levels has been difficult to establish. Surveillance programs of highly exposed pesticide workers have led to examination of blood transport and urinary excretion and efforts made to relate these measures to fat storage. (Table 2).[170]

Morgan and Roan[171] concluded that penetration of DDT into adipose tissue in men is a nonuniform process. They observed a consistent increase in adipose levels of DDT even after dosing had stopped in experimental subjects, which suggested a shifting from other storage sites into subcutaneous fat. No experimental data are available on female subjects and it is virtually impossible to extrapolate quantitatively from dosing experiments on male subjects. Fat distribution is hormone influenced and women, therefore, experience particularly marked alterations in anatomical and biochemical patterns of fat distribution from puberty through childbearing to the menopause.[172,173] The most conservative conditions in terms of DDT human adipose storage could be assumed to be those pertaining to the adult male as described by the ingestion experiments of Morgan and Roan.[171] The time course of serum and adipose saturation would be affected by these unknown redistribution effects and it is of interest to note that Morgan and Roan found that first-order curves fitted to the serum p,p'-DDT curves during dosing suggested that 95% steady-state values would be reached in about 8½ months of dosing. There was no indication, however, that steady-state concentrations in subcutaneous fat tissue were being attained over the same period. Despite these limitations, the percentage of dose stored for p,p'-DDT administered daily to two individuals at two dose levels for 183 days, was estimated to be 68% and 54%, and for

o,p'-DDT, 32% and 31%. Storage of p,p'-DDE (more likely to be of dietary origin in the population-at-large) was estimated to be 91% of the administered daily dose. It is evident that there are marked differences between storage efficiencies of the isomers and metabolites which affect our understanding of the relationship between dietary/ environmental/occupational intake and adipose storage. The time required for excretion of DDT and its metabolites from body stores was generally described by Morgan and Roan for their male subjects as being considerably slower than for monkeys, dogs, and rats. An important observation by Hayes[168] was that excretion of chlorinated hydrocarbons proceeds much more slowly from low storage levels than from high levels, and time constants for logarithmic excretion curves fall progressively with storage level. Of the chlorinated hydrocarbon pesticides, DDT has been the most extensively studied in human populations. Chemical modification and excretion of DDT in human beings is understood to proceed from initial degradation of DDT either by dehydrochlorination, yielding the unsaturated DDE (1,1-dichloro-2-2-bis p-chlorophenol ethylene) or by substitution of hydrogen for one chlorine atom, yielding the saturated DDD (1,1-dichloro-2,2-bis p-chlorophenyl ethane). DDD readily degrades further through a series of intermediates to the excretable DDA (bis p-chlorophenylacetic acid) and is rarely found as a stored metabolite in the general population. DDE apparently does not undergo further breakdown to DDA, a conclusion derived from observations of the metabolic products of p,p-DDT in the rat,[174] and the measurements in human populations showing higher tissue storage of DDE than of DDT.[165,166,171]

The propensity for human adipose storage increases from p,p'-DDD $\leqslant$ o.p'-DDT $<$ p,p'-DDT $<$ p,p'-DDE. The stability of the adipose store probably bears a similar relationship in that concentrations of the isomers and metabolites in the general populations appear to show this pattern.[168]

The conclusions concerning human contamination with DDT are far from definitive in view of the limitations of human experimentation and the paucity of data on women. It seems likely that transport in and out of fat depots is an important influence on the relationship of serum and adipose tissue concentrations in addition to chemical stability in the body and the efficiency of excretory mechanisms.

Despite the intensive evaluation of pesticide use from the agricultural viewpoint it has been difficult to identify studies of populations whose home and work environments were integrally bound to an annual cycle of pesticide use. The most extensive studies have been done in Dade County, Florida with the demographic designations being made on the basis of race and occupational exposure, due to direct contact as formulator or applicator. The occupationally exposed were all identified as men and sex designation was given for the general population group, so that no female group has been considered as being anything other than equivalent to the total female population, i.e., no female occupationally exposed group has been studied. Stratifications of tissue concentration values by age, race and sex within a population were identified in the studies of Wasserman et al.[69] in Israel, and Zavon et al.[72] in the U.S. Data from Davies et al[75] from Dade County, Florida in 1965 to 1967 show marked differences within a population for which there was no information available on occupational exposure to insecticides. The fat tissue samples were taken at necropsy from persons accidentally or violently killed in Dade County who were not necessarily residents. The age dependency was interpreted as evidence for a 5 to 10-year storage equilibrium period for human populations, under conditions of exposure in the Florida environment of the early 1960s. The analyses by Wasserman et al. in Israel[69] and Brown[175] in Canada support this estimate. The sex differences in DDT and DDE levels have also been noted in England and Israel and there is still speculation as to whether dietary, hormonal and/or occupational characteristics are the cause. In Florida, black males

TABLE 5

Organochlorinated compounds

| | Number of samples | Concentration in Extracted Lipids (ppm) Mean ± S. D.[173] | | | |
		Total DDT[a]	BHC[b]	Dieldrin	PCB[c]
Amniotic Fluid	4	91 ± 58	23 ± 13	8 ± 7	125 ± 59
Placenta	19	9 ± 5	1 ± 0.6	<1	5 ± 4
Uterine Muscle	7	12 ± 3	2 ± 0.8	<1	14 ± 3
Fetal Blood	23	11 ± 5	1 ± 0.9	12 ± 0.9	7 ± 4
Maternal Blood	26	5 ± 4	<1	<1	23 ± 2
Adipose Tissue	8	4 ± 2	<1	<1	1 ± 0.3

[a]   DDT: 1,1,1-Trichlor-2,2-*bis*(4-chlorphenyl)ethane
[b]   γ BHC: Benzene hexachloride (Lindane)
[c]   PCB: Polychlorinated biphenyls

had mean values twice those of white males and females. Black female mean values were intermediate.[75] In Israel, male mean values were higher than those for females.[69]

Although Morgan et al have concluded, on the basis of their data on male subjects, that there may be a fair correspondence between serum and lipid concentrations during periods of addition or depletion of body stores, female subjects are unlikely to show the same relationship.[171] It is entirely possible that lability of DDT isomers and metabolites differs markedly between men and women with observable changes appearing during and after pregnancy and lactation when adipose tissue changes may be extreme.

Polishuk et al. have observed 15 pregnant women and compared fat content of organochlorinated insecticides with 33 nonpregnant women accidentally killed.[173] They concluded that the statistically lower concentrations of *p,p'*-DDT, *p,p'*-DDD, o,*p'*-DDT + o,*p'*-DDD, total o,*p'*-DDT and total BHC (lindane) indicated a more active metabolism of these compounds stored in adipose tissue during pregnancy, and cited as additional evidence for this view the observations of Curley et al that plasma levels of chlorinated hydrocarbon insecticides in five pregnant women were comparable to those in non-pregnant women but in the lower range of reported values.[135] The excretion of these compounds into uterine fluid may therefore be increased markedly during early pregnancy with higher exposure to the blastocyst and embryo being possible. Lability of fat stores with accompanying endogenous exposure to the fetus of organochlorinated compounds should be taken into account in the estimates of fetal dose in relation to maternal ingestion and uptake (Table 5).

No large population of women has ever been examined to provide detailed information on their pesticide exposure despite household extermination and cleaning procedures which are part of most women's home job responsibilities.

XIV. EPIDEMIOLOGY OF OCCUPATIONAL CANCER IN WOMEN

The cancer experience of women workers has rarely been examined and then usually under conditions of obvious effect, for example, the radium dial painters. (see Chapter 8). Other exposures to carcinogenic substances most certainly have occurred but because of the pattern of practice in the field of occupational epidemiology, women have frequently been excluded from study populations. Recently, a retrospective survey of cancer has been made in relation to occupation, based on a white population served

TABLE 6

Relative Risk of Cancer by Site and Occupation (Number of Cases)[151]

Occupation	Breast Ever employed	Corpus uteri Ever employed	Cervix uteri	
			Ever employed	Employed more than 5 years
Operatives				
Apparel industry	1.37 (24)	2.18 (8)[a]	4.41 (39)[b]	7.41 (23)
Food industry	0.74 (50)	1.00 (14)	1.27 (43)	1.41 (16)
Leather industry	1.19 (20)	0.73 (3)	2.03 (16)[a]	0.32 (1)
Lumber and wood industries except furniture	0.53 (4)	—	2.97 (13)[b]	—
Miscellaneous manufacturing	0.60 (70)[b]	0.49 (10)	1.67 (106)[b]	1.73 (27)
Fabricated metal	0.50 (13)[a]	0.83 (4)	1.47 (20)	3.17 (7)
Primary metal	1.17 (12)	1.58 (2)	1.80 (11)	—
Paper industry	0.81 (22)	0.89 (6)	1.92 (24)[a]	1.34 (5)
Printing and publishing	0.37 (7)[a]	0.47 (2)	1.53 (14)	—
Textile mill industry	0.62 (39)[a]	1.06 (16)	1.54 (46)[a]	1.82 (24)
Others				
Cooks, except private household	0.99 (7)	0.87 (13)	2.33 (64)[b]	2.67 (36)
Hairdressers and cosmetologists	1.06 (20)	3.00 (6)[a]	1.10 (13)	0.84 (8)
Kitchen workers except private household	0.60 (32)	1.59 (17)	1.85 (51)[b]	1.86 (16)

[a] p ≤ 0.05

[b] p ≤ 0.0.

by the Roswell Park Memorial Institute in Buffalo, N.Y.[150] Lifetime occupational histories of patients admitted during the period 1956 to 1965 were analyzed for specific forms of cancer and compared with those of patients diagnosed for nonneoplastic conditions. The epidemiologic limitations of the study population (hospital based and from a discrete geographic area) allow only an interpretation of a general cancer pattern in the context of other data concerning cancer and its relationship to occupation. However, since data on women workers are so few, the study provides new tentative information. The comparison group was made up of women whose lifetime employment consisted almost entirely of clerical occupations. The relative risk estimates for different cancers within each occupational group were computed according to classic case control methodology to indicate the degree of association between the occupation and cancer.

Operatives in the apparel industry showed a consistently higher relative risk for cancer of female organs than other occupations (Table 6). In addition to cancer of the breast, corpus uteri and cervix uteri, cancer of the buccal cavity had a relative risk of 5.71 (smoking adjusted, seven cases, probability value of 0.001) and lymphoma showed a relative risk of 2.3, although not statistically significant with only seven cases. No other occupational category in this study had a marked trend for cancers of several sites.

The apparel industry employs over one million women in the U.S., and their close contact with fabric exposes them to chemicals used for dyeing, finishing, mothproofing, flame retarding, and wrinkle resistance. Benzidine-based dyes, formaldehyde (possibly in association with hydrogen chloride to form *bis* (chloromethyl) ether (BCME), silicone sprays, trichloroethylene, perchloroethylene, chloroprene, styrene, asbestos, and tris-(2,3-dibromopropyl) phosphate (tris-BP) are all possible contaminants in the work environment of the apparel industry. Asbestos, benzidine, and BCME are confirmed human carcinogens.[186] In the past there have been many long-term workers, though in recent years the industry has been more unstable economically.

Hairdressers and cosmetologists showed the highest relative risk of cancer of the corpus uteri and were the only occupations with a high relative risk of cancer of the ovary: 3.0 (probability 0.01, ten cases). Cancer of these two sites is relatively rare, particularly when compared with breast and cervix uteri cancers. Graham and Graham[187] have concluded that the incidence of ovarian cancer has been increasing since the turn of the century, when it was uncommon in both western Europe and North America. In 1965, the New York State Annual Report of the Bureau of Cancer Control attributed 7% of all female cancer deaths to ovarian cancer (8.4/100,000), a marked increase over rates of 30 years before.

Cancer of the breast, except for those in the apparel industry, consistently showed a lower relative risk for women in the occupations studied. The observations for women exposed to a variety of chemicals may be related to their demographic characteristics, though it does not seem that such differences would be marked between them and the control group of secretarial women. In view of the findings of Petrakis[178] that during adult life the nonlactating breast glands of women secrete and reabsorb breast fluid, it seems possible that the breast epithelium could be affected by the accumulation of toxic substances in breast tissue, even though there is no supportive evidence in the data presented in the Roswell Park Study. With sensitive and accurate analysis techniques, small quantities of nicotine and its metabolite cotinine can be measured, and Petrakis et al.[179] have identified them in breast fluid aspirated from women 15 min after a single cigarette had been smoked. Nicotine was found in amounts considerably higher than in plasma, 50 to 200 ng/ml, compared to 10 to 20 ng/ml. Cotinine concentrations of 200 to 300 ng/ml were comparable to plasma levels. The plasma levels used for comparison were concentrations reported in the literature and were not from the same individuals from whom the breast fluid was taken. Petrakis considers these observations on nicotine, cotinine, and, in addition, barbiturates to be evidence that exogenous substances can be secreted into the nonlactating breast glands and may be concentrated by the "resting" breast. The concern is whether these substances and their metabolites cause adverse effects on breast epithelium. Animal studies by Dao[180] of quantitative determination of tissue concentrations of 3-methylcholanthrene showed that concentration in the fatty and breast tissues was considerably higher than intestine, lungs, and kidney following a single large dose to the rat. Dao further concluded that mammary glands do not synthesize benzopyrene hydroxylase in response to the presence of aromatic hydrocarbons concentrated there and that the mammary fat functions as a storage depot for unmetabolized hydrocarbons with slow clearance. The significance of chemical contamination of breast fluid in the etiology of malignancy remains an open question.

Mortality patterns among women working in the rubber industry have now been described by Monson and Nakano.[181] Standard mortality ratios (SMR) for lung, uterus, bladder, brain, and lymphatic cancer and myeloma were 100 or greater. The SMR for all causes of death was 78, to be expected for healthy working populations (Table 7). There were 21 deaths (vs. 10.8 expected) for those who had started work between 1920 and 1939. An excess of cancer of the uterus (not analyzed separately for cervix and fundus uteri) was seen particularly among women working in the industrial division with hoses, belts, tubing, molded rubber toys, and gloves. Asbestos, β-naphthylamine, uncured rubber, and rubber cement are among the toxic substances in

TABLE 7

Standard Mortality Ratio (and observed deaths) Women in Rubber Industry[181]

Cause of death	Standard mortality ratio	Observed deaths
Lung cancer	100	(15)
Breast cancer	82	(52)
Uterus cancer	107	(39)
Bladder cancer	189	(7)
Brain cancer	108	(7)
Lymphatic and myeloma	111	(14)
Leukemia	97	(9)
Total malignant neoplasms	85	(237)

that work environment. The possible association with lung, bladder, and brain cancer was suggested in the earlier study of male rubber workers in the same plants.[182]

In the report of a large epidemiologic study of women workers exposed to asbestos, Newhouse et al.[183] described the difficulties of tracing women for epidemiologic studies and the means within the British medical system for locating 77% of the known exposed group. The mortality of women workers in an asbestos factory appeared to follow a pattern comparable to that of the men, with a highly significant excess of cancers of the lung and pleura. Of the 716 women traced for more than 20 years, 1.5% died of mesothelial tumors, and 6 of the 11 cases occurred in women with less than 2 years employment in the factory. Newhouse suggested that further attention be accorded cancer of the ovary, in view of the four deaths registered and two others being possibly due to the same cause. Graham and Graham[177] have demonstrated that some mesotheliomas closely resemble ovarian carcinoma histologically, and in some instances they cannot be distinguished one from the other if the anatomical site of origin is unknown. They propose that abdominal cancers diagnosed in women with asbestosis may well have been ovarian tumors, particularly since the distribution of cancer type differed for men. In a study of 15 women with asbestosis who died, there were 4 lung cancers and 9 abdominal cancers; whereas for 15 men with asbestosis who died, 10 had lung cancer and only 1 had carcinoma peritonei.[184]

As in the epidemiologic study of Dresden workers by Jacob and Anspach,[185] Newhouse found a far higher ratio of observed to expected lung cancer for women than for men: 13 for women and 2.5 for men. Jacob and Anspach found ratios of 16 and 2.1 for women and men, respectively, although the ratio of male to female cancers was 9.9 to 1. Newhouse suggested, as an explanation for the difference, that the effect is more easily detected in a cohort of women because of their lower lung cancer rates in the general population. The question is still clearly open until more epidemiologic studies of women workers are done. The Dresden sample of 1124 women and 1512 men occupationally exposed to asbestos showed a sharp increase in lung cancer among women and men from 1958 to 1964, but, additionally, six cases of pleural mesotheliomas in women and none in men. Exposure data were not available.

The apparently higher relative risk for clothing workers reported in the Roswell Park Study had earlier been noted for a population in Leeds, England, where tumors of the urinary bladder were reviewed by Anthony and Thomas.[186] The relative risk for all weavers, finishers, dyers, and tailors with 20 years in the occupation ranged from 2.9 to 12.9. The relationship was also found for women, where the relative risk was 2 for weavers and 13.5 for tailors, the latter with a p value less than 0.001. For clothing workers overall, the relative risk was 1.8. Among medical workers examined in the Leeds study, nurses showed the highest relative risk of 2.1, though there were only 5 cases. No known bladder carcinogens could be identified in the work environment of the clothing industry, whereas benzidine used by nurses for bedside testing for occult blood was suggested as a possible cause for that group.

The identification of aromatic amines, particularly the naphthylamines and benzidine, as causes of occupational bladder cancer in British factory workers eventually led to a review of the use of many of the same compounds in chemical and biological laboratories. The possible extent of carcinogenic effects has been difficult to establish, as there has been little epidemiologic interest in the scattered and discrete small populations in hospitals, research, and academic institutions and even less interest in the conditions of exposure to toxic substances. Li et al.[187] examined cancer mortality among chemists of the American Chemical Society in the late 1960s and found a significantly higher proportion of deaths from cancer among male chemists when compared with other professional men. However, there were only 115 women, in addition to the 3522 men in the study population, and the results are far less definitive. There were 15 deaths from breast cancer when 7 were expected on the basis of data from the U.S. white female population. One explanation could have been the high proportion of unmarried women (40%) of high socio-economic status.[188] A surprising finding was the high suicide rate, 11% of the deaths which was 5 times that of the U.S. white female population. As this study was based on deaths in the period 1948 to 1967, the observations by George and Searle[189] that widespread use of carcinogenic aromatic amines in laboratories developed only after the 1940s should be borne in mind.

Although laboratory use of chemicals is likely to be on a smaller scale than is the case in the industrial setting, careless use and inadequate ventilation may well increase the risk of exposure to a comparable level. With no epidemiologic evidence available, the inherent danger of laboratory use of toxic substance must be considered. Veys[199] has provided a useful summary of the use of aromatic amines, particularly benzidine, dimethylbenzidine (*o*-tolidine), and dimethoxybenzidine (*o*-dianisidine), which are used either for spraying chromatograms, occult blood testing, or blood glucose determination. Testing for chlorine water content in swimming pools and for nitrites in water works are also common procedures. Inhalation, ingestion from contaminated hands and skin, or mucous membrane absorption are all possible routes of exposure under these work conditions. Although educational efforts have been directed at improving laboratory practices and substituting less toxic substances, the past work experience of cohorts of workers must be remembered when taking work histories for many years into the future. Warnings concerning the use of benzidine in 1965 led to substitutes for many routine uses of aromatic amines. Other carcinogens, e.g., polycyclic aromatic hydrocarbons, have been extensively used in research laboratories with likely contamination of the experimenter, technicians, and animal handlers. Emphasis on accident hazards of chemical reactions in the past resulted in a late awareness of the need for safe use of carcinogens and substances with human health effects.

Suspicion of the possible adverse effects of anesthetic gases on operating room personnel exposed to trace amounts originated from a study of female Russian anesthetists.[200] The reported association of inadequately ventilated exhaust systems and an excess of spontaneous abortion was sufficient to stimulate a large-scale, collaborative study by the American Society of Anesthesiologists (ASA) and the National Institute of Occupational Saftey and Health (NIOSH).[123] On the basis of the known structural similarities between some inhalation anesthetics and known human carcinogens, e.g., trichloroethylene with vinyl chloride: isoflurane, methoxyflurane, and enflurane with bis-(chloromethyl)-ether and chloromethyl methylether, the study was designed to include age-standardized cancer rates.[120] Comparisons were made between 1008 female physicians in the ASA and 566 female physicians in the American Academy of Pediatrics (AAP). The age-standardized cancer rates per 100 respondents were 3.0 ± 0.6 (± standard error) and 1.6 ± 0.5, respectively, a difference which was statistically significant. For 6407 members of the American Association of Nurse Anesthetists compared with 5400 members of the American Nursing Association, the age-standardized cancer rates per 100 respondents were 2.6 ± 0.2 and 1.8 ± 0.2, respectively, a difference which was also statistically significant. When the 11,843 members of the Association of Operating Room Nurses and the Association of Operating Room Technicians were compared with the 5400 members of the American Nurses Association, the difference in cancer rates was not statistically significant although the rate for the operating room personnel was 2.3 ± 0.2, i.e., considerably in excess of 1.8 ± 0.2. Overall, the incidence of lymphoma and leukemia showed an approximately three-fold excess in the exposed groups compared to the unexposed, which was statistically significant. The excess of cancers of the breast, cervix, fundus uteri, and thyroid did not appear to be as marked and further interpretation was limited by the number of cases reported and the study design. There were no differences in age-standardized cancer rates among the men in the ASA and in the AAP who responded to the questionnaire. Further studies of these professional groups are now in progress and most hospitals have installed gas-scavenging devices in operating rooms. Control of private dental offices has been more difficult and studies of the more mobile dental assistant population do not appear to be feasible.

Waste anesthetic gases are not the only environmental hazard present in the operating room. Hexachlorophene is under study in Sweden as a suspected human teratogen among hospital personnel.[193] Ethylene oxide is widely used as a sterilant and has been found to be an animal carcinogen.[193] Linde and Bruce[194] have also assessed the exposure of ten anesthetists to ionizing radiation in the operating room over a 6-week period and concluded that under unmonitored conditions, the 100 milligroetgen per week limit could be reached in addition to the chemical hazards of anesthetic gases. As in most work settings when a detailed analysis of the total hazardous environment is made, there is little likelihood that a single active agent is acting in isolation to cause an adverse health effect.

XV. FEMALE-INTENSIVE OCCUPATIONS

Laboratories and the jewelry and electronics industries are three examples of female-intensive environments where hazardous chemicals have been part of the accepted conditions of work. The lack of perception that women are in daily contact with physical and chemical agents has been one reason for the total lack of epidemiologic studies among women in these occupations.

A. Laboratories

The brief sections on laboratory safety in chemistry books and manuals discuss the mechanical safety hazards such as fire, explosion, corrosive agents, proper glassware storage and set up, and the inappropriate fittings for corks and stoppers for reagent bottles. The description of hazards in the chemical laboratory listed in the opening chapters of standard laboratory manuals has changed very little from the early 1930s to the 1970s.[195] Most are concerned with the issues of safety while presenting only the most cursory descriptions of health hazards. In contrast with radiation laboratory workers, chemists have not adopted the smallest possible dose as their criterion for establishing acceptable exposures to chemical substances. Considering these last two points, the laboratories using organic compounds, particularly, have usually been unhealthy places of employment. Chemistry laboratories are also notoriously poorly ventilated. The hood space is rarely adequate and the hoods are often improperly designed or installed. This is true today as well as in the 1950s and 1960s.

A technician in a hospital, biology, or chemistry laboratory devotes considerable time to processes involving organic compounds. Basic methods in frequent use are distillation, crystallization, extraction, and chromatography. During the 1950s and early 1960s, extractions were performed with ethyl and diethyl ether, although their use was limited industrially because of the great fire-hazard potential. Common water-immiscible solvents were petroleum ether, benzene, carbon tetrachloride, chloroform, ethylene dichloride, butanol, and ligroin. In crystallization, a highly effective means of purifying a solid substance, the most common solvents used were the following: water, ligroin, methanol, benzene, ethanol (95%), chloroform, acetic acid, carbon tetrachloride, acetone, carbon disulfide, ether, toluene, petroleum ether, and aniline.

An evaluation of a pesticide analytical laboratory was reported in 1968 by Applegate[196] and could represent the possible extreme conditions experienced by laboratory workers. In a pesticide analytical laboratory, large quantities of volatile solvents are used to extract pesticides from various types of biological samples. In the air-conditioned laboratory examined, all evaporations and concentrations of volatile solvents approached but did not reach the maximum levels allowable in 1968. Organic solvents used in the daily processing of samples allowed a build-up of vapors in the laboratory to the extent that a background reading for hydrocarbons was 340 to 380 ppm each morning before analytic procedures began.

The chemicals used over a 5-day period were chloroform, hexane, ethyl acetate, petroleum benzin, acetonitrile, and *N,N*-dimethylformamide. The threshold limit values in 1968 ranged from 10 ppm for *N,N*-dimethylformamide to 500 ppm for hexane. During the study period, the atmospheric hydrocarbon concentrations rose markedly by noon each of the five weekdays to reach 1200 to 1500 ppm by 3 p.m. each day. The demonstration of such high levels, despite ventilation, indicates the likely hazard present in less well-equipped laboratories.

A repetitive theme in chapters and papers on laboratory hazards, particularly in relation to chemical contamination, is the level of apathy and indifference toward safety and health.[197] Wood and Spencer[198] additionally comment that microbiology laboratories are also chemical laboratories where strong chemical carcinogens are in frequent use: naphthylamines for nitrate reduction tests, benzidine for detection of hydrogen peroxide and bacterial cytochromes, β-propiolactone as a sterilant, and isonicotinic acid hydrazide for the tuberculosis-sensitivity test. Benzidine has been extensively used in a variety of microbiological tests and has been particularly useful for screening large numbers of organisms. Laboratory exposure to aromatic amines has been associated with known cases of bladder cancer. Sodium selenite is commonly used in media for the isolation of salmonellae and is an animal teratogen.[199] In dehydrated media it becomes an airborne inhalation hazard.

B. Jewelry Industry

Today one half of the country's jewelry industry is located in Rhode Island and 30.6% of the manufacturing plants in the state are involved in the jewelry industry, employing 24,600 people. The industry is of long standing and has traditionally employed a high proportion of women. A 1976 project organized by Brown University students has resulted in a very detailed evaluation of processes and hazardous conditions in the industry and the following information comes from their observations and booklet.[200]

Small factories in stables, lofts, basements, and houses invariably of 19th century vintage are characteristic of the unorganized Rhode Island jewelry industry which is dependent on an unstable fashion market and labor-intensive, high-volume piece work. Trade secrets, nonstandardized processes, and sweat shop conditions all contribute to a particularly complex and hazardous chemical environment.

Several major processes are involved in the jewelry industry: metal casting, stamping and pressing, grinding, polishing, buffing, metal cleaning, electroplating, soldering, spray painting, lacquering, enameling, and gluing. About the framework of these main procedures is a variety of preparation and finishing jobs, such as set up and charge, stringing, racking, dipping, carding, and packaging. Women perform all of these operations to a varying degree, although they usually have the jobs that prepare and finish a "major" operation and transfer production pieces from one process to another. Most processes in jewelry manufacturing are usually carried out in the same shop, so that harmful working conditions can affect all those in the general vicinity of the hazard as well as those working with it directly. High heat in summer and poor ventilation in winter are the rule rather than the exception.

The most popular casting process for costume jewelry is rubber mold casting. White metal, an alloy usually composed of 32% tin, is cast into rubber molds at 300 to 400°F. Higher percentages of tin comprise the better quality white metals along with varying amounts of lead, copper, zinc, arsenic, mercury, cadmium, and beryllium. The rubber molds themselves are cut with soldering irons. When the natural rubber molds combust, benzene-soluble hydrocarbons such as benzo(a) pyrene and anthracenes are released. Before the molten white metal is poured, talc is used to dust the rubber mold. Asbestos- and silica-contaminated talcs are common in the Rhode Island industry. The liquid metal is transferred from open vat to mold with a ladle by the "pot tender". The metals are usually compounded in the jewelry plant. Lead is stored in-house in powder form; beryllium in small ingots of 2% Be-Cu alloy composition. Each formulation is likely to be unique so that little knowledge of its constituents is ever available.

Investment or lost-wax casting produces the most ornate or detailed jewelry, such as fine filigreed designs of school rings that require little finishing. Copper alloys and precious metals are generally cast at approximately 3000°F, though low-temperature white metal is occasionally cast by this method. The lost-wax molds are made from a pastry mixture of lime- or clay-base plaster (up to 30% silica) and very fine silica powder (up to 70% silica). "Shakeout" is the industry's term for the breaking of the plaster molds about the newly cast jewelry piece and is traditionally done by hand with the sand flying into the workers' breathing area. The Rhode Island Department of Health has measured levels of silica during shakeout at 32 times the threshold limit value. In die casting, molten metal is forced into a metal mold or die. Zinc-aluminum and copper alloys are commonly used, while white metal is used only occasionally. Muriatic acid (impure hydrochloric acid) is employed as an industrial cleaner for the metal dies.

After a jewelry piece is cast, it must be ground, polished, and buffed to finish the metal surface or prepare it for plating. These operations involve mechanical abrasion of the jewlery casting to grind off the rough edges and impart smoothness and a sheen to the metal surface. Much of the grinding, polishing, and buffing in the jewlery industry is done by hand. Different colored metal surfaces and the brightest lusters are obtained with very finely powdered buffing abrasives such as lime, unfused aluminum oxide, iron oxide, and chromium oxide. Airborne particles and dusts are generated in the work area by the high-powered wheels and in some instances, oils are added to the wheels causing mists.

After the cast jewelry has been ground, polished, and buffed, it is usually plated with a more attractive or durable alloy, unless it was originally cast with a precious metal. Before the plating can be done, the metal surface of the production piece must be free of all grease, oils, abrasives, and/or metal oxides. Three categories of cleaning materials are used for the essential preelectroplating process: organic solvents, acids, and alkalis.

In the 1950s and 1960s, by far the most common degreasing solutions were trichloroethylene and perchloroethylene. Methyl chloroform, trichloroethane, and ethylene dichloride were also used. Only very recently, with the rising suspicion of trichloroethylene and perchloroethylene as human carcinogens, have attempts been made to replace these solvents with other organic solvents thought to be less harmful.

The solvents are placed in large, tub-like degreasing machines and heated until they vaporize. Racks of jewelry are hung in the solvent vapors to be cleaned. The top layer of the degreasing tanks is supposed to be lined with cooling coils to condense the trichloroethylene vapors back into the tank. The pieces of jewelry that have been cleansed are also supposed to be moved to the cooling zone of the degreasing tank to remove the solvent on each article before it is carried to the electroplaters. Jewelry workers are often pressured to accelerate production so that metal pieces are removed from the cooling zone much too quickly. Quite frequently the tanks are poorly ventilated, the condensing coils malfunction, the amperage of the vaporizers is increased, and workers are not informed of the hazards of organic solvents. Sulfuric, hydrochloric, and nitric acids are most commonly used to clean and activate metal in addition to the alkalis, sodium and potassium hydroxide. Splashing usually occurs around degreasers so that acid and alkaline mists can be generated when the tank temperature rises. Oxides of nitrogen and arsine can be formed under these conditions. "Brighteners" tend to be trade secrets used during an early stage of plating, the "copper strike", and may include metallic cobalt, selenium, saccharin, thiourea, dextrin, and molasses. Hydrogen cyanide gas can form in the vicinity of tanks used for cyanide-copper, acid-gold, cyanide-gold, rhodium, and silver plating.

Other processes include soldering, annealing, gluing, lacquering, enameling, and plastic embedding so that lead, cadmium, and fluorine fumes, carbon monoxide, asbestos dust, epichlorohydrin and polyamine vapor, lacquer and enamel solvent aerosols, and methyl methacrylate vapors can be in the work environment of a jewelry maker. During the 1950s and 1960s, benzene was still being used as a solvent and thinner. Toluene and xylene are more likely to be used now.

Women have traditionally been employed "racking up", which involves hanging the individual pieces of jewelry on to metal racks for cleaning and plating. They are likely to be seated at a long work table with piles of metal racks beside them on the floor and hundreds of pieces of jewelry before them, rapidly filling a rack with 15 to 20 pieces of jewelry. The environment is one of intense concentration, speed, and fumes from degreasing and plating tanks which are usually in close proximity. Any effort to consider the biological effect of a single chemical agent would be virtually futile due to the nonspecialist nature of the industry. Most shops use many processes over a period of time.

C. Electronics Industry

Over the 100 years since the invention of the electric light bulb, women have been in the majority in the manufacture of electronic products. Exposure to beryllium in the fluorescent lamp industry caused illness and death in the 1940s and women who became pregnant were particularly at risk.[156] Today more than 75% of the workers making semiconductors and printed wiring circuit boards are women. Current inspection of plants by state and federal occupational safety and health agencies across the country frequently show ventilation inadequacy, with solvent exposures sufficient to cause dizziness, headaches, and euphoria in workers.[9]

TABLE 8

Chemicals used in Production of Printed Circuits[201]

Dusts and solvents	Resins, adhesives, sealants, rubbers, and plastics	Acids and alkalis
Laminates	Polysulphides	Acetic acid
Glass fibers	Expoxies based on bisphenol A reaction products	Chromic acid
Asbestos	Styrene monomer	Citric acid
Mica	Urethanes	Fluoroboric acid
Methylene chloride	Diisocyanates	Hydrochloric acid
Carbon tetrachloride	Chlorinated naphthalenes	Hydrofluoric acid
Trichloroethylene	Diphenylamines	Nitric acid
1,1,1-Trichloroethane	Naphthalamines	Sulphuric acid
Perchloroethylene	Polyvinyl chloride	Sodium cyanide
1,1,2-Trichlorotri-fluoro ethane	Polytetrafluoroethylene	Sodium hydroxide
White spirit		Ammonium hydroxide
Naphtha		
Acetone		
Ethyl methyl ketone		
Cyclohexanone		
Methyl alcohol		
Ethyl alcohol		
Isopropyl alcohol		

Ross[201] has provided an extensive listing of the hazardous agents associated with the production of printed circuits from the receiving and storage of raw materials through machining, precleaning, etching, cleaning, plating, soldering, coding, and marking. Dusts and solvents can act as allergens, skin sensitizers, and carcinogens. Acids and alkalis may be corrosive and irritating to skin. Resins, adhesives, sealants, rubber, and plastics may be skin sensitizers and carcinogens (Table 8).

Soldering and welding operations also result in the formation of toxic gases such as phosgene and, as in the jewelry industry, the soldering process may involve solders of diverse metal content, including cadmium and lead. Resin core solders can release formaldehyde and fluorides.

Polyesters heat cured with peroxides or epoxy resins cured with phenol cause skin and eye irritation. Toluene diisocyanate and similar compounds are used to form polyurethane. Polychlorinated biphenyls and chloronaphthalenes are used to protect parts from corrosion. Electroplating involves use of nickel and chromium solutions with resulting acid mists. Cyanide baths are used in zinc, cadmium, and gold plating.

Health hazard evaluations by NIOSH in the mid 1970s have repeatedly recommended installation of better ventilation systems, particularly in soldering, plating, degreasing operations, spraying, and washing of circuit boards. Today many electronics companies have installed closed systems and "clean rooms". The economic history of the industry has been considerably more progressive than in the jewelry industry, and we can fairly confidently rate the hazards of the electronic industry as the less severe, an opinion based in part on the relative size and age of buildings used in the two industries.

REFERENCES

1. **Butler, E. G.,** Women and the Trades: Pittsburgh 1907—8, Russell Sage Foundation, New York, 1911.
2. **Hamilton, A.,** *Exploring the Dangerous Trades,* Little, Brown, Boston, 1943.
3. **Zenz, C., Ed.,** *Occupational Medicine: Principles and Practical Applications,* Year Book Medical Publishing, Chicago, 1975.
4. Occupational Diseases: A Guide to their Recognition, U.S. Department of Health, Education and Welfare, Public Health Service, Center for Disease Control, National Institute of Occupational Safety and Health, Washington, D.C., 1977.
5. **Hamilton, A. and Hardy, H.,** *Industrial Toxicology,* 3rd ed., Publishing Science, Acton, Mass., 1974.
6. **Hunt, V. R.,** Reproduction and work. *Signs: J. Women Culture Soc.,* 1, 543, 1975.
7. **Hunt, V. R.,** How the occupational environment affects worker health in Women in the Workplace, Symp. Oakland, Calif. Am. Ind. Hyg. Assoc., 1973, Chap. 1.
8. **Stellman, J.,** *Women's Work, Women's Health,* Pantheon, New York, 1977.
9. **Hricko, A. and Brunt, M.,** Working for Your Life, Labor Occupational Health Program, University of California, Berkeley, 1976.
10. **Blum, A. and Ames, B.,** Flame retardent additives as possible cancer hazards, *Science,* 195, 17, 1977.
11. **Rom, W. N.,** Effects of lead on the female and reproduction, a review, *Mt. Sinai J. Med.,* 43, 542, 1976.
12. **Vermande-Van Eck, G. and Meigs, J. W.,** Changes in the ovary of the Rhesus monkey after chronic lead intoxication, *Fertil. Steril.,* 11, 223, 1960.
13. Criteria Document for Trichloroethylene, U.S. Department of Health, Education, and Welfare, National Institute of Occupational Safety and Health, 73—11025, Washington, D.C., 1971.
14. **Frant, R. and Westendorp, J.,** Medical control of exposure of industrial worker to trichloroethylene, *Arch. Ind. Hyg. Occup. Med.,* 1, 308, 1950.
15. **Bolanowski, W. and Golacka, J.,** Absorption and excretion of tetrachloroethylene in humans under experimental conditions, *Med. Pr.* 23, 109, 1972.
16. **Chase, H. P., Barnett, S. E. and Welch, N. N.,** Pesticides and U.S. Farm Labor Families, *Rocky Mount. Med. J.,* 70, 27, 1973.
17. **Welch, R. M., Levin, W. and Conney, A. H.,** Estrogenic action of DDT and its analogs, *Toxicol. Appl. Pharmacol.,* 14, 358, 1969.
18. **Bitman, J., Cecil, H. C., Harris, H. C. and Fries, G. F.,** Estrogenic activity of *o,p'*-DDT in the mammalian uterus and rat oviduct, *Science,* 162, 271, 1968.
19. **Duby, R. T., Travis, H. F. and Terrill C. E.,** Uterotropic activity of DDT in rats and mink and its influence on reproduction in the rat, *Toxicol. Appl. Pharacol.,* 18, 348, 1971.
20. **Bengtsson, G. and Ullberg, S.,** The autoradiographic distribution pattern after administration of diethylstilbestrol compared with that of natural estrogens, *Acta Endocrinol.,* 43, 561, 1963.
21. **Backstrom, J., Hansson, E. and Ullberg, S.,** Distribution of C^{14}-DDT and C^{14}-Dieldrin in pregnant mice determined by whole body autoradiography *Toxicol. Appl. Pharmacol.,* 7, 90, 1965
22. **Lutwak-Mann, C.,** Drugs and the blastocyst, in *Fetal Pharmacology,* Boreus, L., Ed., Raven Press, New York, 1973, 419.
23. **Briggs, M. H. and Briggs, M,.** *Biochemical Contraception. Prospects for Human Development,* Academic Press, London, 1976, 191.
24. **Dallenback-Hellweg, G.,** *Histopathology of the Endometrium,* 2nd ed., Springer-Verlag, New York, 1975, 44.
25. **Novak, E. R., Jones, G. S., and Jones, H. W.,** *Textbook of Gynecology,* 9th ed., Williams & Wilkins, Baltimore, 1975.
26. **Cecil, H. C., Harris, S. J., Bitman, J., and Reynolds, P.,** Estrogenic effects and liver microsomal enzyme activity of technical Methoxyclor and technical 1,1,1-trichloro-2,2, bis(P-Chlorophenylethane) in sheep, *J. Agric. Food Chem.,* 23, 401, 1975.
27. **Ware, W.,** Effect of DDT on reproduction in higher animals, *Residue Rev.,* 59, 119, 1975.
28. **Fabro, S.,** Passage of drugs and other chemicals into the uterine fluids and preimplantation blastocyst, in *Fetal Pharmacology,* Boreus, L., Ed., Raven Press, New York, 1973, 443.
29. **Guyton, A. C.,** *Function of the Human Body,* 4th ed., W. B. Saunders, Philadelphia, 1974, 452.
30. **Moya, F. and Smith, B. E.,** Uptake, distribution and placental transport of drugs and anesthetics, *Anesthesiology,* 26, 465, 1965.
31. **Metcalfe, J., Bartels, H., and Moll, W.,** Gas exchange in the pregnant uterus, *Physiol Rev.,* 47, 782, 1967.
32. **Longo, L. D.,** Carbon monoxide in the pregnant mother and fetus and its exchange across the placenta, *Ann. N.Y. Acad. Sci.,* 174, 313, 1970.

33. **Blanchard, R. L.**, Correlation of lead-210 and strontium-90 in human bones, *Nature (London)*, 211, 995, 1966.

34. **Baglan, R. J., Brill, A. B., and Schulert, A.**, Utility of placental tissue as an indicator of trace element exposure to adult and fetus, *Environ. Res.*, 8, 64, 1974.

35. **Scanlon, J. S.**, Umbilical cord blood lead concentration, *Am. J. Dis. Child.*, 121, 325, 1971.

36. **Harris, P. and Holley, M. R.**, Lead levels in cord blood, *Pediatrics*, 49, 606, 1972.

37. **Kubasik, N. P. and Volosin, M. T.**, Concentrations of lead in capillary blood of newborns, *Clin. Chem.*, 18, 1415, 1972.

38. **Rajegowda, B. K., Glass, L., and Evans, H. E.**, Lead concentrations in the newborn infant, *J. Pediatr.*, 80, 116, 1972.

39. **Haas, T., Wieck, A. G., Schaller, K. H., Mache, K., and Valentine, H.**, Die usuelle Bleisbelastung bei Neugeborenen und ihren Muttern, *Zentralbl. Bakteriol., Parasitenk., Infektionskr. Hyg., Abt. Orig., Reihe B:*, 155, 341, 1972.

40. **Gershanik, J. J., Brooks, G. G., and Little, J. A.**, Blood lead values in pregnant women and their offspring, *Am. J. Obst. Gynecol.*, 119, 508, 1974.

41. **Fahim, M. S., Fahim, Z., and Hall, D. G.**, Effects of subtoxic lead levels on pregnant women in the state of Missouri, *Res. Commun. Chem. Pathol. Pharmacol.*, 13, 309, 1976.

42. **Hytten, F. E. and Leitch, L.**, *The Physiology of Human Pregnancy*, 2nd ed., Blackwell Scientific, Oxford, 1971, 379.

43. **Skerfring, S. and Vostal, J.**, Symptoms and Signs of Intoxication, *Mercury in the Environment*, Friberg, L. and Vostal, J., Eds., CRC Press, Cleveland, 1972, 93.

44. Maximum allowable concentrations of mercury compounds, *Arch. Environ. Health*, 19, 891, 1969.

45. **Khera, K. S. and Tabacova, S. A.**, Effects of methylmercuric chloride on the progeny of mice and rats treated before or during gestation, *Food Cosmet. Toxicol.*, 11, 245, 1973.

46. **Nolan, G. A., Buelhler, E. V., Geil, R. G., and Goldenthal, E. J.**, Effects of trisodium nitriloacetate on cadmium and methylmercury toxicity and teratogenicity in rats, *Toxicol. Appl. Pharmacol.*, 23, 222, 1972.

47. **Monsour, M.**, Placental transfer of mercuric nitrate and methyl mercury in the rat, *Am. J. Obstet. Gynecol.*, 119, 557, 1974.

48. **Berlin, M. and Ullberg, S.**, Accumulation and retention of mercury in the mouse, *Arch Environ. Health*, 6, 589, 1963.

49. **Harris, B., Wilson, G. and Printz, H.**, Embryotoxicity of methyl mercury chloride in golden hamsters, *Teratology*, 6, 139, 1972.

50. **Spyker, J. M. and Smithberg, M.**, Effects of methylmercury on prenatal development in mice, *Teratology*, 5, 181, 1972.

51. **Garret, N. E., Garret, R. J. B. and Archdeacon, J. W.**, Placental transmission of mercury to the fetal rat, *Toxicol. Appl. Pharmacol.*, 22, 649, 1972.

52. **Null, H., Gartside, P. S. and Wei, E.**, Methylmercury accumulation in brains of pregnant, non-pregnant and fetal rats, *Life Sci.*, II, 12, 65, 1973.

53. **Scharpf, L. G., Hill, T. D., Wright, P. L., and Keplinger, M. L.**, Teratology studies in methylmercury hydroxide and nitrilotriacetate sodium in rats, *Nature (London)*, 241, 461, 1973.

54. **Yamaguchi, S. and Hiromitsu**, Trans-placental transport of mercurials in rats at the subclinical dose levels, *Environ. Physiol. Biochem.*, 4, 7, 1974.

55. **Greenwood, M. R., Clarkson, T. W., and Magos, L.**, Transfer of metallic mercury into the fetus, *Experentia*, 28, 145, 1972.

56. **Clarkson, T. W., Magos, L. and Greenwood, M. R.**, The transport of elemental mercury into fetal tissues, *Biol. Neonate*, 21, 239, 1972.

57. **Nordberg, F. and Skerfring, S.**, Metabolism, in *Mercury in the Environment*, Friberg, L. and Vostal, J., Eds., CRC Press, Cleveland, 1972, 37.

58. **Suzuki, T., Miyaina, T., and Katsunuma, H.**, Comparison of mercury contents in maternal blood, umbilical cord blood and placental tissues, *Bull. Environ. Contam. Toxicol.*, 5, 502, 1971.

59. **Hamilton, A. and Hardy, M.**, *Industrial Toxicology*, 3rd ed., Publishing Sciences, Acton Mass., 1974, 135.

60. **Wannag, A. and Skjaerasen, J.**, Mercury accumulation in placenta and fetal membranes. A study of dental workers and their babies, *Environ. Physiol. Biochem.*, 5, 348, 1975.

61. **Rahola, T., Hattula, T., Korolainen A., and Miettinen, J. K.**, Elimination of protein-bound and ionic mercury ^{203}Hg in man, *Scand. Clin. Lab. Invest.*, 27 (Suppl. 116), 77, 1971.

62. **Lauwerys, R. R. and Buchet, J. P.**, Occupational exposure to mercury vapors and biological action, *Arch. Environ. Health*, 27, 65, 1973.

63. **Casarett, L., J. and Doull, J., Eds.**, *Toxicology — The Basic Science of Poisons*, Macmillan, New York, 1975, 37.

64. Finnegan, J. K., Haag, H. B., and Larson, P. S., Tissue distribution and elimination of DDD and DDT following oral administration to dogs and rats, *Proc. Soc. Exp. Biol. Med.*, 72, 357, 1949.

65. Pillmore, R. E., Cottontail rabbit: feeding test, *U.S., Fish and Wildl. Serv. Cir.*, 167, 47, 1963.

66. Pillmore, R. and Finlay, R. B., Residues in game animals resulting from forest and range insecticide applications, *Trans. North Am. Wildl. Conf.*, 28, 409, 1963.

67. Backstrom, J., Hansson, E. and Ullberg, S., Distribution of ^{14}C-DDT and ^{14}C-dieldrin in pregnant mice determined by whole body autoradiography, *Toxicol. Appl. Pharmacol.*, 7, 90, 1965.

68. Denes, A., Problems of food chemistry concerning residues of chlorinated hydrocarbons, *Nahrung*, 6, 48, 1962.

69. Wasserman, M., Wasserman, D., Zellermayer, L., and Gom, M., Pesticides in people. Storage of DDT in people of Israel, *Pestic. Monit. J.*, 1, 15, 1967.

70. Rappolt, R. T., Mengle, D., Hale, W., et al., Kern County: Annual generic pesticide input: blood dyscrasias, p-p'-DDE and p,p'-DDT residues in human fat, placentas with related stillbirths and abnormalities, *Ind. Med. Surg.*, 37, 513, 1968.

71. Curley, A., Copeland, M. F., and Kimbrough, R. D., Chlorinated hydrocarbon insecticides in organs of stillborns and blood of newborn babies, *Arch. Environ. Health*, 19, 628, 1969.

72. Zavon, M. R., Tye, R., and Latorre, L., Chlorinated hydrocarbon insecticide content of the neonate, *Ann. N.Y. Acad. Sci.*, 160, 196, 1969.

73. O'Leary, J. A., Davies, J. E., Edmundson, W. F., and Feldman, M., Correlation of prematurity and DDE levels in fetal whole blood, *Am. J. Obstet. Gynecol.*, 106, 939, 1970.

74. Laben, R. C., Archer, T. E., Crosby, D. G., and Peoples, S. A., Lactational output of DDT fed prepartum to dairy cattle, *J. Dairy Sci.*, 48, 701, 1965.

75. Davies, J. E. and Edmundson, W. F., *The Epidemiology of DDT*, Futura, New York, 1972.

76. Polishuk, Z. W., Wasserman, D., Wasserman, M., Cucos, S. and Rom, M., Organochlorine ompounds in mother and fetus during labor, *Environ. Res.*, 13, 278, 1977.

77. Villeneuve, D. C., Willes, R. E. F., Lacroix, J. B., and Phillips, W. R. J., Placental transfer of ^{14}C-Parathion administered intravenously to sheep, *Toxicol. Appl. Pharmacol.*, 21, 542, 1972.

78. Juchau, M. R., Placental metabolism in relation to toxicology, in *CRC Critical Reviews in Toxicology*, CRC Press, Cleveland, 2, 125, 1973.

79. Welch, R. M., Harrison, Y. E., Gommi, B. W., Poppers, P. J., Finster, M., and Conney, A. H., Stimulatory effect of cigarette smoking on the hydroxylation of 3,4 benzypyrene and the N-demethylation of 3 methyl-4-monomethylaminoazobenzene by enzymes of the placenta, *Clin. Pharmacol. Ther.*, 10, 100, 1969.

80. Wang, I. Y., Rasmussen, R. E., Creasy, R., and Crocker, T. T., Metabolites of benzo (a) pyrene produced by placental microsomes from cigarette smokers and non-smokers, *Life Sci.*, 20, 1265, 1977.

81. Nebert, D. W., Winker, J., and Gelboin, H. V., Aryl hydrocarbon hydroxylase activity in human placenta from cigarette smoking and non-smoking women, *Cancer Res.*, 29, 1763, 1969.

82. Dawson, E. B., Gravy, W. D., Clark, R. R., and McGanity, W. J., Effect of trace metals on placental metabolism, *Am. J. Obstet. Gynecol.*, 103, 253, 1969.

83. Porritt, N., *The Menace and Geography of Ecclampsia*, Oxford University Press, 1934.

84. Parizek, J., The peculiar toxicity of cadmium during pregnancy, *J. Reprod. Fertil.*, 9, 111, 1965.

85. Amin-Zaki, L., Elhassani, S., and Majeed, M. A., Intra-uterine methylmercury poisoning in Iraq, *Pediatrics*, 54, 587, 1974.

86. Suzuki, T., Takemoto, T., Shishido, S., and Kani, K., Mercury in human amniotic fluid, *Scand. J. Work Environ. Health*, 3, 32, 1977.

87. Van Vunukis, H., Langone, J. J., and Milinsky, A., Nicotine and cotinine in the amniotic fluid of smokers in the second trimester of pregnancy, *Am. J. Obstet. Gynecol.*, 120, 64, 1974.

88. Hytten, F. E. and Leitch, I., *The Physiology of Human Pregnancy*, 2nd ed., Blackwell Scientific, Oxford, 1971, 329.

89. Wilson, J. G., Environmental Factors: Teratogenic drugs, in Prevention of Embryonic, Fetal and Perinatal Disease, Fogarty Int. Center Ser. Prev. Med. Vol 3, Brent, R. L. and Harris, M. I., Ed., National Institutes of Health, U.S. Department of Health, Education and Welfare, Washington, D.C., 76—853, 1976, 147

90. Wilson, J. G., *Environment and Birth Defects*, Academic Press, New York, 1973,

91. Wilson, J. G., Teratogenic interaction of chemical agents in the rat, *J. Pharmacol. Exp. Ther.*, 144, 429, 1964.

92. Brent, R. L., Environmental Factors: Miscellaneous in prevention of embryonic, fetal and perinatal disease, Fogarty Int. Ser. Prev. Med. Vol 3, Brent, R. L. and Harris, M. I., Eds., National Institutes of Health, U.S. Department of Health, Education and Welfare, Washington, D.C., 76—853, 1976, 211.

93. Shepard, T. H., *Catalog of Teratogenic Agents,* Johns Hopkins University Press, Baltimore, 1973.

94. Angle, C. R. and McIntire, M. S., Lead poisoning during pregnancy, *Am. J. Dis. Child.,* 108, 436, 1964.

95. Karlog, O. and Moller, K. O., Three cases of acute lead poisoning, *Acta Pharmacol. Toxicol.,* 15, 8, 1958.

96. Rom, W. N., Effects of lead on the female and reproduction, *Mt. Sinai J. Med.,* 43, 542, 1976.

97. Palmisano, P. A., Sneed, R. C., and Cassady, G., Untaxed whiskey and fetal lead poisoning, *J. Pediatrics,* 75, 869, 1968.

98. Scanlon, J., Human fetal hazards from environmental pollution with certain non-essential trace elements, *Clin. Pediatr.,* 11, 135, 1972.

99. Bell, W. B., Influence of lead on normal and abnormal cell growth, *Lancet,* 1, 267, 1924.

100. Hamilton, A. and Hardy, H., *Industrial Toxicology,* 3rd ed., Publishing Sciences, Acton, Mass., 1974, 120.

101. Masters, W. H. and Johnson, V. E., *Human Sexual Response,* Little, Brown, Boston, 1966.

102. Jones, K. L., Smith, D. W., Ulleland, C. N., and Streissguth, A. P., Pattern of malformation in offspring of chronic alcoholic mothers, *Lancet,* 1, 1267, 1973.

103. Takeuchi, Biological reactions and pathological changes in human beings and animals caused by organic mercury contamination, in *Int. Conf. Environ. Mercury Contam., 1970,* Hartung, R. and Dinman, B. D., Eds., Ann Arbor Science, Ann Arbor, Mich., 1972, 247.

104. Poland, A. and Kende, A., 2,3,4,8 — Tetrachlorodibenzo-p-dioxin: environmental contaminant and molecular probe, *Fed. Proc.,* 35, 2404, 1976.

105. Menges R. W., Selby, L. A., Marienfeld, C. J., Aue, W. A., and Green, D. L., A tobacco related epidemic of congenital limb deformities in swine, *Environ. Res.,* 3, 285, 1970.

106. Crowe, M. W. and Swerczek, T. W., Congenital arthrogryposis in offspring of sows fed tobacco (nicotiana tabacum), *Am. J. Vet. Res.,* 35, 1071, 1974.

107. Tanimura, T., Katsuya, T., and Nishimura, H., Embryotoxicity of acute exposure to methyl parathion in rats and mice, *Arch. Environ. Health,* 15, 609, 1967.

108. Fish, S. A., Organophosphorus-cholinesterase inhibitors and fetal development, *Am. J. Obstet. Gynecol.,* 96, 1148, 1966.

109. Kimbrough, R. D. and Gaines, T. B., Effect of organic phosphorus compounds and alkylating agents on the rat fetus, *Arch. Environ. Health,* 16, 805, 1968.

110. Bus, J. S. and Gibson, J. E., Bidren: Perinatal toxicity and effect on the development of brain acetylcholinesterase and choline acetyltransferase in mice, *Food Cosmet. Toxicol.,* 12, 312, 1974.

111. Budreau, C. H. and Singh, R. P., Tetratogenicity of embryo toxicity of Demeton and Fenthion in CF #1 mouse embryo, *Toxicol. Appl. Pharmacol.,* 24, 324, 1973.

112. Rice, J. M., Environmental Factors: Chemicals in Prevention of Embryonic, Fetal and Perinatal Disease, Fogarty Int. Ser., Vol 3, Brent, R. L. and Harris, M. I., Eds., National Institute of Health, U.S. Department of Health, Education and Welfare, Washington, D.C., 76—853, 1976, 163.

113. Report of the Secretary's Commission on Pesticides and their Relationship to Environmental Health, Parts 1 and 2, U.S. Department of Health, Education and Welfare, Washington, D.C., 1969.

114. Muller, G. L. and Graham, S., Intrauterine death of the fetus due to accidental carbon monoxide poisoning, *N. Engl. J. Med.,* 252, 1075, 1955.

115. Ginsberg, M. D. and Myers, R. E., Fetal brain damage following maternal carbon monoxide intoxication: an experimental study, *Acta Obstet. Gynecol. Scand.,* 53, 309, 1974.

116. Kline, J., Stein, Z. A., Susser, M. and Warburton, D., Smoking: a risk factor for spontaneous abortion, *N. Engl. J. Med.,* 297, 793, 1977.

117. Oakley, G. P., Birth defect surveillance in the search for and evaluation of possible human teratogens, *Birth Defects Original Articles Series,* 12, 1, 1976.

118. Summary of NIOSH Recommendations for Occupational Health Standards, U.S. Department of Health, Education and Welfare, Washington, D.C., October, 1977.

119. Strobino, B., Kline, J., and Stein, Z. A., Chemical and physical exposures on parents: effects on human reproduction and offspring, *Early Human Dev.,* 1, 371, 1977.

120. Corbett, T. H., Cornell, R. G., Endres, J. L., and Lieding, K., Birth defects among the children of nurse-anesthetists, *Anesthesiology,* 41, 341, 1974.

121. Pharoah, P. D. D., Alberman, E., and Doyle, P., Outcome of pregnancy among women in anesthetic practice, *Lancet,* 1, 34, 1977.

122. Knill-Jones, R. R., Rodrigues, L. V., Moir, D. D., and Spence, A. A., Anesthetic practice and pregnancy: controlled survey of women anesthetists in the U.K., *Lancet,* 1, 1325, 1972.

123. Report of an ad hoc committee on the effect of trace anesthetics on the health of operating room personnel, *Am. Soc. Anesthesiol.,* Occupational disease amoung operating room personnel. A national study, *Anesthesiology,* 41, 321, 1974.

124. **Green, H. G.,** Infants of alcoholic mothers, *Am. J. Obstet. Gyneol.,* 118, 713, 1974.

125. **Carson, M. and Reid, M.,** Warfarin and fetal abnormality, *Lancet,* 1, 1356, 1976.

126. **Rice, J. M.,** Environmental Factors: Chemical in Prevention of Embryonic Fetal and Perinatal Disease, Fogarty Int. Ser., Vol. 3, 76—853, Brent, R. L. and Harris, M. I., Eds., National Institute of Health, U.S. Department of Health, Education and Welfare, Washington, D.C., 1976, 163.

127. **Hornstein, L., Crowe, C., and Gruppo, R.,** Adrenal carcinoma in child with history of fetal alcohol syndrome, *Lancet,* 2, 1292, 1977.

128. **Mays, C. W., Taylor, G. N., and Fisher, D. R.,** Estimated toxicity of Ca-DTPA to the human fetus, *Health Phys.,* 30, 247, 1976.

129. **Bauman, D. E. and Davis, C. L.,** Biosynthesis of milk fat, in *Lactation,* Vol. 2, Larson, B. L. and Smith, V. R., Eds., Academic Press, New York, 1974.

130. **Laug, E. P., Prickett, C. S., and Kunze, F. M.,** Survey analysis of human milk and fat for DDT contents, *Fed. Proc.,* 9, 294, 1951.

131. **Quimby, G. E., Armstrong, J. F., and Durham, W. F.,** DDT in human milk, *Nature (London),* 207, 726, 1965.

132. **Egan H., Goulding, R., Roburn, J., and Tatton, J. O.,** Organochlorinated pesticide residues in human fat and human milk, *Br. Med. J.,* 2, 66, 1965.

133. **Wilson, D. J.,** DDT concentrations in human milk, *Am. J. Dis. Child.,* 125, 814, 1973.

134. **Kroger, M.,** Insecticide residues in human milk, *J. Pediatr.,* 80, 401, 1972.

135. **Curley, A. and Kimbrough, R.,** Chlorinated hydrocarbon insecticides in plasma and milk of pregnant and lactating women, *Arch. Environ. Health,* 18, 156, 1969.

136. **Savage, E. P., Tessari, J. D., Malberg, J. W., Wheeler, H. W., and Bagby, J. R.,** Organochlorine pesticide residues and PCBs in human milk, Colorado, 1971—1972, *Pestic. Monit. J.,* 7, 1, 1973.

137. **Davies, J. E., Edmundson, W. F., Maceo, A., Barquet, A., and Cassady, J.,** An epidemiologic application of the study of DDE in whole blood, *Am. J. Pub. Health,* 59, 435, 1969.

138. **Bakken, A. F. and Seip, M.,** Insecticides in human breast milk, *Acta Pediatr. Scand.,* 65, 535, 1976.

139. Federal Register, United States, 42: April 1, No. 63, P17187, 1977.

140. **Miller, R. W.,** Pollutants in breast milk, *J. Pediatr.,* 90, 510, 1977.

141. **Peters, H. A., Johnson, S. A. M., Cam, S., Oral, S., Muftu, Y., and Ergene, T.,** Hexachlorobenzene-induced porphyria: effect of chelation on the disease, porphyrin and metal metabolism, *Am. J. Med. Sci.,* 251, 314, 1966.

142. Convention concerning Protection against Hazards of Poisoning arising from Benzene, International Labour Office, 54, 246, 1971.

143. **Vozovaya, M. A., Malyarova, L. K., and Emkieva, R. M.,** Soderzhanie khloristogo metilena v biosredakh v period beremennosti i kormlenica u rabotnits zavoda rezino-tekhnicheskikh izdelif, *Gig. Tr. Prof. Zabol.,* 18, 42, 1974.

144. *Report on The Employment of Women and Children and the Berne Conventions of 1906,* League of Nations, Rep. 3, Int. Labour Conf., Washington, Harrison and Sons, London, 1919.

145. **Murthy, G. K. and Rhea, U.S.,** Cadmium, copper, iron, lead, manganese and zinc in evaporated milk, infant milk products and human milk, *J. Dairy Sci.,* 54, 1001, 1971.

146. Task Group on Metal Accumulation, Accumulation of toxic metals with special reference to their absorption, excretion and biological half-times, *Environ. Physiol. Biochem.,* 3, 65, 1974.

147. **Hammond, P. B. and Aronson, A. L.,** Lead poisoning in cattle and horses in the vicinity of a smelter, *Ann. N.Y. Acad. Sci.,* 111, 595, 1964.

148. **Donovan, P. P., Feeley, D. T., and Canavan, P. P.,** Lead contamination in mining area in western Ireland, *J. Sci. Food Agric.,* 20, 43, 1969.

149. **Goldblatt, D., Greenwood, M. R. and Clarkson, T. W.,** Chronic metallic mercury poisoning treated with N-acetylpenicillamine, *Neurology,* 21, 439, 1971.

150. **Decoufle, P., Stanislawczyk, K., Houten, L., Bross, I. D. J., and Viadana, E.,** A retrospective survey of cancer in relation to occupation, National Institutes of Health, U.S. Department of Health, Education and Welfare, Washington, D.C., US DHEW (NIOSH) 77—178, 1977.

151. **Stuik, E. J.,** Biological response of male and female volunteers to inorganic lead, *Int. Arch. Arbeitsmed.,* 33, 83, 1974.

152. **Roels, H. A., Lauwerys, R. R., Buchet, J. P., and Vrelust, M.-Th.,** Response of free erythrocyte porphyrin and urinary d-aminolevulinic acid in men and women moderately exposed to lead, *Int. Arch. Arbeitsmed.,* 34, 97, 1975.

153. **Wibowo, A. A., del Castilho, P. D., Herber, R. F. M., Verberk, M. M., Salle, H. J. A., and Aielhuis, R. L.,** Blood lead and serum iron levels in non-occupationally exposed males and females, *Int. Arch. Occup. Environ. Health,* 39, 113, 1977.

154. **Dickens, C.,** The Uncommercial Traveller — All the Year Around, *Vol. 1, New Series 1,* Chapman and Hall, London, 1861.

155. Seppalainen, A. M., Hernberg, S., Tola, S., and Kock, B., Subclinical neuropathy at "safe" levels of lead exposure, *Arch. Environ. Health*, 30, 180, 1975.

156. Hardy, H. L., Beryllium poisoning. Lessons on control of man-made disease, *N. Engl. J. Med.*, 273, 1188, 1965.

157. Hardy, H. L. and Stoeckle, J. D., Beryllium Disease, *J. Chron. Dis.*, 9, 152, 1959.

158. McCallum, R. I., Rannie, I., and Verity, C., Chronic pulmonary berylliosis in a female chemist, *Br. J. Ind. Med.*, 18, 133, 1961.

159. Beryllium Criteria Document for a Recommended Standard, Occupational Exposure to Beryllium, HSM 72—10268, National Institute for Occupational Safety and Health, U.S. Department of Health, Education and Welfare, Washington, D.C., 1972.

160. Jaffe, R. B., Schruefer, J. J., Bowes, W. A., Creasy, R. K., Sweet, R. L., and Lavos, R. K., High risk pregnancies: maternal medical disorders, in *Prevention of Embryonic, Fetal and Perinatal Disease*, Brent, R. L. and Harris, M. I., Eds., U.S. Department of Health, Education and Welfare, Washington, D.C., US DHEW (NIH) 76—853, 1976, 27.

161. Hamilton, A. and Hardy, H., *Industrial Toxicology*, 3rd ed., Publishing Science, Acton, Mass., 1974, 272.

162. Quibb, G. P., Axelrod, J., and Brodie, N. B., Species, strain and sex differences in metabolism of hexobarbitose, amidopyrine anti-pyrine and aniline, *Biochem. Pharmacol.*, 1, 152, 1958.

163. Kato, A., Nakajima, T., Fujiwara, Y., and Murayama, N., Kinetic studies on sex differences in susceptibility to chronic benzene intoxication with special reference to body fat content, *Br. J. Ind. Med.*, 32, 321, 1975.

164. Gutheran, E. and Fernedez, J., Control of industrial exposure to tetrachloroethylene by measuring alveolar concentrations, *Br. J. Ind. Med.*, 31, 159, 1974.

165. Dale, W. D. and Quimby, G. E., Chlorinated insecticides in the body fat of people in the U.S., *Science*, 142, 593, 1963.

166. Hoffman, W. S., Fishbein, W. I., and Andelman, M. B., Pesticide content of human fat tissue, *Arch. Environ. Health*, 9, 387, 1964.

167. Hoffman, W. S., Adler, H., and Fishbein, W. I., Relation of pesticide concentration in fat to pathological changes in tissues, *Arch. Environ. Health*, 15, 758, 1967.

168. Hayes, W. J., Review of the metabolism of chlorinated hydrocarbon insecticides, especially in mammals, *Ann. Rev. Pharmacol.*, 5, 27, 1965.

169. Edmundson, W. F., Davies, J. E., and Maceo, A., Drug and environmental effects on DDT residues in human blood, *South. Med. J.*, 63, 1440, 1970.

170. Robinson, J. and Hunter, C. G., Organochlorine insecticides concentrations in human blood and adipose tissues, *Arch. Environ. Health*, 13, 558, 1966.

171. Morgan, D. P. and Roan, C. C., Absorption, storage and metabolic conversion of ingested DDT and DDT metabolites in man, *Arch. Environ. Health*, 22, 301, 1971.

172. Skerlj, B., Brozek, J., and Hunt, E. E., Subcutaneous fat and age changes in body build and form in women, *Am. J. Physiol. Anthropol.*, 11, 577, 1953.

173. Polishuk, Z. W., Wassermann M., Wassermann, D., Groner, Y., Lazarovici, S., and Tomatis, L., Effects of pregnancy on storage of organochlorine insecticides, *Arch. Environ. Health*, 20, 215, 1970.

174. Peterson, J. E. and Robison, W. H., Metabolic products of p,p'-DDT in the rat, *Toxicol. Appl. Pharmacol.*, 6, 321, 1964.

175. Brown, J. R., Organochlorine pesticide residues in human depot fat, *Can. Med., J.*, 97, 367, 1967.

176. Lassiter, D. V., Occupational carcinogenesis, *Adv. Mod. Toxicol.*, 3, 63, 1977.

177. Graham, J. and Graham, R., Ovarian cancer and asbestos, *Environ. Res.*, 1, 115, 1967.

178. Petrakis, N. L., Genetic factors in the etiology of breast cancer, *Cancer*, 39, 2709, 1977.

179. Petrakis, N. L., Gruenke, L. D., Beelen, T. C., Castagnoli, N., and Craig, J. C., Nicotine in Breast Fluid of Non-lactating Women, *Science* 199, 303, 1978.

180. Dao, T. L., Studies on mechanisms of carcinogenesis in the mammary gland, *Prog. Exp. Tumor Res.*, 11, 235, 1969.

181. Monson, R. R. and Nakano, K. K., Mortality among rubber workers. II. Other employees, *Am. J. Epidemiol.*, 103, 297, 1976.

182. Monson, R. R. and Nakano, K. K., Mortality among rubber workers. I. White male union employees in Akron, Ohio, *Am. J. Epidemiol.*, 103, 284, 1976.

183. Newhouse, M. L., Berry, G., Wagner, J. C., and Turok, M. E., A study of the mortality of female asbestos workers, *Brit. J. Ind. Med.*, 29, 134, 1972.

184. Keal, E. E., Asbestosis an abdominal neoplasms, *Lancet*, 2, 1211, 1960.

185. Jacob, G. and Anspach, M., Pulmonary neoplasia among Dresden asbestos workers, *Ann. N.Y. Acad. Sci.*, 132, 536, 1965.

186. Anthony, H. M. and Thomas, G. M., Tumors of the uinary badder. An analysis of the occupations of 1,030 patients in Leeds, England, *J. Natl. Cancer Inst.*, 45, 879, 1970.

187. **Li, F. P., Fraumeni, J. F., Mantel, N., and Miller, R. W.,** Cancer mortality among chemists, *J. Natl. Cancer Inst.,* 43, 1159, 1969.

188. **Lilienfeld, A. M.,** The epidemiology of breast cancer, *Cancer Res.,* 23, 1503, 1963.

189. **George, W. H. S. and Seale, C. E.,** Chemical Carcinogens as Laboratory Hazards in Chemical Carcinogens, Searle, C. E., Ed., *Am. Chem. Soc., Monogr.* 173, Washington, 1976.

190. **Veys, C. A.,** Aromatic amines: the present status of the problem, *Ann. Occup. Hyg.,* 15, 11, 1972.

191. **Vaisman, A. I.,** Working conditions in surgery and their effect on the health of anesthesiologists, *Eksp. Khir. Anesteziol.,* 3, 44, 1967.

192. **Halling, H.,** Misstänkt samband mellan hexaklorofenexposition och missbildningsbörd, *Lakartidningen,* 74, 542, 1977.

193. **Halling, H.,** Suspected link between exposure to hexachlorophene and malformed infants, *Ann. N.Y. Acad. Sci.,* 1978, in press.

194. **Linde, H. W. and Bruce, D. L.,** Occupational exposure of anesthetists to halothane, nitrous oxide and radiation, *Anesthesiology,* 30, 363, 1969.

195. **Streitwieser, A. and Heathcock, C. H.,** *Introduction of Organic Chemistry,* Macmillan, New York, 1976.

196. **Applegate, H. G.,** Volatile solvents in pesticide analytical laboratories, *Arch. Environ. Health,* 17, 312, 1968.

197. **Fawcett, H. H.,** Exposures of personnel to laboratory hazards, *Am. Ind. Hyg. Assoc. J.,* 33, 559, 1972.

198. **Wood, J. M. and Spencer, R.,** Carcinogenic hazards in the microbiology laboratory, in *Safety in Microbiology,* Shaptan, D. A. and Board, R. G., Eds., Academic Press, London, 1972.

199. **Robertson, D. S. F.,** Selenium — a possible teratogen, *Lancet,* 1, 518, 1970.

200. **Quinn, M. M.,** Personal communication, 1978.

201. **Ross, W. McL.,** Environmental problems in the producton of printed circuits, *Ann. Occup. Hyg.,* 15, 141, 1972.

Chapter 5

THE BIOLOGICAL ENVIRONMENT

I. INTRODUCTION

There is an extensive literature on laboratory-acquired infections and the wide range of bacterial, viral, rickettsial, parasitic, and fungal organisms implicated in illness and death.[1] In some instances the case reports have identified disease in laboratory workers as a result of infection from agents previously only observed as pathogenic in animals or lower forms.[2] At the end of World War II a marked increase in infections among laboratory workers led to a survey directed to 4725 research, public health, hospital, and clinical laboratories; biological manufacturers; colleges; medical, agricultural, and veterinary schools; and experimental stations, of which 2143 responded. The usual limitations of incomplete ascertainment and selective reporting obtained, but it appeared from the laboratories reporting infections for a 20-year period that research institutions had working conditions which resulted in the highest risk for infection. Table 1 shows the estimated incidence for different types of laboratories as well as different occupations. A monitoring of published accounts was maintained by the same authors until 1963 and they identified the predominant infections reported over a period of 33 years (1930 to 1963) in approximate order of the number of reported cases (Table 2).

The sources of infection appeared to stem predominantly from working directly with the agent, exposure to an aerosolized source, and accidents which together accounted for 50 to 80% of the infections. Infected animals or ectoparasites, working with clinical specimens, handling of discarded glassware, and autopsy contact contributed the remainder.

The death rate is an indicator of the severity of laboratory infections, for which a combined case fatality rate of 4.0% was estimated in 1969.[3] By comparison, the case fatality rate for motor vehicle accidents was 2.7%. Effective vaccines, toxoids, or drug therapy were available for 37 of the 133 causative agents of clinical infection recognized at that time. Only 8 of the 78 viral diseases (58% of the total) had effective vaccines. Most of the microorganisms can be identified in the feces or urine of inoculated animals. The laboratory worker therefore may be exposed to infectious microorganisms at a far higher dose level than is likely to occur outside the laboratory and the route of exposure may be atypical for the organism, e.g., inhalation of an organism naturally transmitted by an arthropod.

The American Public Health Association has in the past monitored laboratory infections and has published industrial hygiene recommendations.[4] A common complaint of industrial hygienists has been the problem associated with the social climate of research laboratories where many of the requirements for safe operation of a laboratory are incompatible with the philosophy of risk developed by an academic research biologist. In addition, viruses are being used as biochemical tools by scientists who have not experienced training in microbiology or bacteriology. The evident enforcement of the Occupational Safety and Health Act of 1970 has stimulated reassessment of traditional laboratory practices. Common sources of exposure to infectious material include accidental oral aspiration through a pipette, accidental inoculation by a needle and syringe, animal bites and scratches, spray from syringes, centrifuge accidents, cuts

TABLE 1

Estimated Incidence of Laboratory-acquired Infections in Various
Types of Laboratories and Among Various Types of Personnel in
the U.S.: 1930—1959[2]

	No. of Infections/year/ thousand employed
Type of laboratory	
Research institutes	4.1
Public health laboratories	0.7
Hospital laboratories	0.8
Biological manufacturers	0.5
Agricultural and veterinary schools and experimental stations	0.5
Colleges and medical schools	0.3
Clinical laboratories	0.2
Types of personnel	
Trained scientific	1.9
Animal caretakers, janitors, dishwashers	0.4
Students (not in research)	0.2
Others (occupation not shown)	1.0

from contaminated glassware and instruments, and spills of pathological cultures on bench tops and floor.

The high probability that exposure to infectious agents will occur has led to a recommendation that serum samples be collected from all employees upon commencing work with viral pathogens and yearly thereafter with storage until 1 year after termination of employment.[5] A change of philosophy can be recognized in a recent epidemiologic report on tick-borne encephalitis in which flaviviruses were implicated. Neutralization tests were not performed because of the potential hazards to laboratory personnel.[6]

Research laboratory contact with arboviruses has been more intensively controlled than for most other infectious agents, in part because of their virulence and also because of the marked increase in their use since 1950. The American Committee on Arthropod-borne Viruses, Subcommittee on Laboratory Infections surveyed laboratories in the U.S. in the mid-1960s. Among 91 laboratories, 428 overt laboratory-acquired infections due to arboviruses, were reported. There had been 16 fatalities. Over 50% of the laboratories employed 5 to 14 employees, 29% had less than 5, and 13% employed more than 15. The distribution of infections in terms of specific arboviruses did not show a consistent pattern because some outbreaks of infection occurred in a single laboratory providing several cases, some viruses were very seldom used, and some were in frequent use for a variety of research and clinical purposes.[7]

In several instances an arbovirus was first found to be capable of producing disease in people as a result of laboratory infection. Some viruses not known to cause human disease through natural exposure conditions have produced infections in laboratory workers. Acquisition of laboratory infections is not always similar to transmission of the disease when it occurs naturally, that is transmission by an arthropod may not be necessary for infection. Dried virus preparations are ideal for aerosol transmission and contaminated dust from animal cages can also be readily inhaled. Laboratory-adapted strains of some arboviruses, although they may have passed through animals many times, may still be pathogenic for human beings. Their virulence is usually assumed

TABLE 2

Predominant Laboratory-acquired Infections World-wide Reports: 1930—1963[1]

Bacterial	Viral	Rickettsial	Fungal	Parasitic
Brucellosis	Hepatitis	Q Fever	Coccidioidomycosis	Toxoplasmosis
Tuberculosis	Psittacosis	Typhus	Histoplasmosis	Trypanosomiasis
Tularemia	Encephalitis	Spotted fever	Ring worm	Amebiasis
Typhoid	LCM	Scrub typhus	Blastomycosis	Malaria
Streptococcal infections	Yellow fever	Rickettsial	Sporotrichosis	Ascariasis
Shigellosis	Newcastle	Pox	Dermatomycosis	Strongyloidiasis
Anthrax	Rift valley			Coccidiosis
Erysipeloid	LGV		Moniliasis	Leishmaniasis
Relapsing fever	Coxsackie		Nocardiosis	Giardiasis
Staphylococcal infections	Poliomyelitis			
Diphtheria	B virus			
Rat bite fever	Kyasanur forest			
Plague	Adenovirus			
Salmonellosis	Vesicular stomatitis			
Treponema pallidum	Bunyamivera			
Vibrio fever	Colorado tick fever			
Tetanus	Trachoma			
PPLO	Ovine dermatitis			
	Bat salivary gland			
	19 other viruses			

TABLE 3

Proved or Probable Sources of Laboratory-acquired Arbovirus Infections[7]

Probable source	Percent of total
Experimentally infected animals	21.7
Not indicated	19.6
Aerosol source, centrifuge, pipette blowing	17.3
Agent handled	16.4
Accidents	10.0
Preparation of vaccines, antigens	8.2
Experimentally infected chick embryo	2.1
Discarded glassware	2.1
Autopsy	1.9
Clinical specimens	0.7

to have been moderated by such procedures but reduction in infectivity apparently can be inadequate.[8]

Before 1950, laboratory-acquired infections were primarily attributable to bacterial infections, with viral infections making up only about 20% of the total. Since that time over 80% of the currently classified arboviruses have been recognized for the first time, and among the viral infections acquired in laboratories arboviruses have been implicated in more than half. The source of infection is often obscure but most probably results primarily from aerosol production and inhalation of the virus (Table 3). Recommendations have been made to maintain a regular testing program for all laboratory staff for antibodies to the viruses being used so that the effectiveness of safety procedures can be evaluated and unexpected infections prevented. The World Health Organization and the Center for Disease Control of the U.S. Department of Health, Education and Welfare have been collecting, pooling, and accumulating blood serums of convalescents from specific arbovirus infections for immunization and treatment procedures.

Epidemiologic studies of the occupations which involve exposure to human blood and blood products have identified a high risk of subclinical and clinical viral hepatitis. The World Health Organization has reported a prevalence of clinical hepatitis among medical and ancillary hospital staff three to six times higher than workers in other occupations.[9] Serologic sampling for hepatitis B surface antigen and antibody by radioimmunoassay has in recent years allowed more reliable evaluation of the importance of subclinical infection. Prior contact with type B hepatitis virus can be established serologically for individuals so that estimates of relative hepatitis B risk for hospital personnel according to occupational category and work practices is now possible.

When discrete occupational groups have been examined, asymptomatic but serological positive individuals were identifiable. Overt illness may occur in about 15% of a hospital-employed population with serologic evidence of hepatitis B infection and it appears that subclinical infection predominates for such populations.[10] Pattison et al. in a study of hospital workers observed no difference in the proportion of men and women who were seropositive. For those with prior history of hepatitis, 34% were seropositive compared with 13% of those who had not had a clinical history of hepatitis. Exposure to blood products and blood was the most important factor in increasing hepatitis B infection risk, in contrast to direct patient contact which did not provide an increased risk. Duration of employment and possibly age were also associated with an increase in the percent of seropositive individuals, particularly for those employed more than 10 years, 30% of 67 examined. The lowest socioeconomic group based on the Hollingshead Index had a considerably higher percent of seropositive individuals, 32% vs. 16% in Categories 1 through 4.

Pattison et al. took socioeconomic status into account for each occupational category or work area and showed that (excluding physicians) excess risk was greatest for operating room personnel followed by laboratory workers. The comparison was with personnel of all hospital wards except surgery. Technicians and practical nurses were at highest risk and physicians, registered nurses, and nursing aids were not at increased risk.[10] In the period of the late sixties and early seventies there appeared to be a change in the epidemiology of hepatitis B associated with illicit drug use, which could possibly explain the unusually high infection rate in those employed less than 3 years in the hospital Pattison et al. examined between 1972 and 1974.[11] Exposure to antigen-positive blood and hepatitis B virus was a more probable event during that period.[12] The general observation of licensed practical nurses and technicians is that there is a high frequency of routine blood exposure, often with no precautions taken. Hospital characteristics in terms of socioeconomic status of patients served and strictness of work supervision undoubtedly affect the experience of the health care personnel who work in a particular hospital. There appears to be an inevitable risk associated with hospital employment which will not be markedly diminished until better occupational health programs are instituted and there is routine immunization when it becomes available.

Plasma fractionation procedures involve work practices which result in more extensive exposure of employees to human blood than is found in hospitals. Taylor et al. showed high antibody titers in 55 to 92% of workers associated with different phases of plasma fractionation.[13] Clinical hepatitis was more prevalent among those working in the plasma fractionation area, particularly where there was plasma dumping into large vats. Those without evidence of hepatitis but with plasma fractionation work experience had 83% with high antibody titers, compared to 55% for those with only some experience in that activity and 18% for control subjects with no plasma fractionation contact.

The sources of entry have usually been identified as parenteral (associated with minor cuts and puncture wounds), intranasal, and conjunctival. Dry plasma, aerosolization of plasma and liquid powder during centrifugation, and manual scraping of fibrinogen from centrifuges have been identified as sources of hepatitis virus in contaminated environments. Taylor et al. were of the opinion that administration of immune serum globulin had no significant prophylactic effect for exposures of this occupational nature and supported that view with the recommendations of a Public Health Service Advisory Committee on Immunization Practices.[14] General hygiene and safety measures along with periodic monitoring of employees for seroepidemiological evidence of subclinical hepatitis prevalence was recommended. Cohen et al. surveyed 14 U.S. plasma fractionation facilities and described in detail the work practices and hazards.[15] Strong protection and hazard awareness programs were present in some plants but in others there was considerable indifference to many problems, e.g., disposition of contaminated clothing and glassware. They concluded that poorly designed procedural methods of fractionation and poor work practices provided a high-risk work environment, comparable in severity to surgical, dental, and laboratory workers whose experience with hepatitis infection has also been documented.[16-18]

Hemodialysis centers also cover a range from well-controlled efficient units to overcrowded, understaffed, and poorly equipped centers.[19] Szmuness et al. did a point-prevalence study of hepatitis B infection in 15 U.S. hemodialysis centers and detected hepatitis B antigen in 2.4% of the medical staff and specific antibody to HB Ag (HB

Ab) in 31.3%. They concluded that all personnel of dialysis centers are heavily exposed to infection from the beginning of their employment but were not able to identify a particular transmission route with any more definition than had already been described — accidental inoculation and contamination of the conjunctiva and other mucosa. Unexpected sources of infection have come to light when careful analysis of work practices has been done. An outbreak of hepatitis in a hospital-based clinical laboratory was traced to the introduction of a computerized system for specimen collection and data dispersal.[20] Contamination of the computer cards and handling by laboratory personnel with minor cuts was implicated in the sudden increase in hepatitis in one laboratory on the basis of the importance of percutaneous exposure reported in several studies.

Although the best documented episodes of infectious disease outbreaks of occupational origin come from laboratories, there are also other high-risk occupations. Newcastle disease virus is widely distributed in fowls and has led to infection in poultry workers. The clinical disease has been well described in laboratory workers in whom symptoms of conjunctivitis and more rarely central nervous system involvement have occurred. In poultry and kitchen workers conjunctivitis has been common. Nelson et al. described an outbreak of conjunctivitis in 39 women and 1 man among 90 workers who were employed on a chicken eviscerating line. No secondary cases occurred among family contacts and it was noted that no time was lost from work. The company records showed recurring episodes at about 3-month intervals. Isolation of Newcastle disease virus was successful in four of ten cases attempted.[21]

Certain occupations appear not to have been identified as high-risk populations appropriate for epidemiologic studies. Laundry workers particularly receive contaminated clothing from many sources but have not been examined for infectious disease prevalence as an occupational group. Occupations involving contact with young children carry the high risk for childhood diseases for the individual who has not developed immunity. Abattoir workers, meat packers, and pet shop workers must all accept the risk of infection as part of their jobs. Some infective organisms may provide difficulties in diagnosis and treatment. For example, *Mycobacterium balnei* has been associated with pustular lumps on the arms and fingers resembling tuberculosis verrucosa cutis in two women who cleaned out fish aquariums as pet shop workers. Adequate chemotherapy is necessary for 12 to 18 months and for 24 months when extensive infection occurs.[22]

II. MATERNAL INFECTION AND EFFECTS ON THE FETUS

There is a variety of occupational settings where exposure to infective agents can result in adverse effects on a pregnant woman and the fetus — hospitals, laboratories, laundries, food processing, animal handling, and biological manufacturing.

The presence of infectious newborns in a nursery presents a particular hazard to pregnant nurses. Table 4 shows the known infectious viruses which may be present in the newborn due to intrauterine infection. Rubella virus can be isolated from throat swabs of the newborn for several months after birth and shedding of virus may continue for a year. Infection of the mother in the first trimester usually results in placental infection. About 22% of babies born following first trimester rubella infection and about 10% following second trimester infection have severe congenital abnormalities observed as deafness, congenital heart disease, microcephaly, hepatosplenomegaly, and mental retardation.[23] About 10% of women of childbearing age in the U.S. are at risk for rubella infection, though the availability of immunization against rubella should provide a preventive measure for all health personnel. However, the report of

TABLE 4

Effects of Maternal Viral, Bacterial, Protozoal, and Rickettsial Infection[23]

	Abortions	Developmental defects	Congenital infections	Stillborn	Prematurity	Postnatal	Infant morality
Coxsackie	X	X	X	X		X	X
Cytomegalovirus		X	X			X	
Herpes simplex		X	X			X	X
Rubella		X	X	X	X	X	
Varicella zoster	X	X	X	X	X	X	X
Venezuelan equine encephalitis	X	X	X				
Toxoplasmosis		X	X				
Echo virus		X	X				
Hepatitis	X		X	X			X
Influenza	?	?		?	?		
Mumps	X						
Rubeola	X		X	X	X	X	
Vaccinia	X		X	X	X		X
Variola	X		X				X
Western equine en-cephalitis			X				
Brucellosis	X						
Listeriosis	X		X	X	X	?	X
Plague	X			X			
Syphilis		X	X	X			
Q Fever			X				

an outbreak among physicians and nurses in February 1978 in a large Los Angeles hospital indicates that such a practice is not routine. The suspected index patient was an obstetrical resident. His rash was diagnosed retrospectively when two more residents and two nurses developed rubella symptoms and two of them were serologically confirmed to have rubella. About 200 pregnant patients were exposed to these health professionals within their first 16 weeks of pregnancy. Follow-up and counseling of patients have been necessary for evaluation by rubella antibody tests. The California Department of Health is now recommending that health care personnel in the state, both male and female, likely to be in contact with pregnant women be screened for antibodies to rubella in addition rubella vaccine is to be given to all susceptible persons, taking due caution with women of childbearing age who may become pregnant within the following 3 months. The high turnover rate among hospital personnel demands that such a program be continuous in its implementation.[24] In New York State the screening of female hospital employees is required by state law. However, this approach does not cover male health-care personnel who can infect both patients and their co-workers. Other recent hospital outbreaks have been reported in Colorado and in Great Britain, which may indicate a general lack of concern for the role of infectious disease as a highly predictable environmental hazard for workers and patients. Maternal rubella infection and congenital abnormalities in the child is one of the best understood relationships for which adequate prevention is readily available. It is therefore all the more difficult to understand the lack of responsible prevention programs in the occupational setting.

The high risk for hepatitis infection among laboratory and clinical personnel in hospitals and other health-related institutions is of considerable importance for the large population of childbearing age in those occupations.[25] Occupational health programs have been notoriously poor throughout hospitals of all sizes in the U.S. which, coupled with the professional attitudes which prevails particularly among those in clinical occupations, has resulted in little or no precautionary philosophy of protection against hepatitis infection and its effects.[26]

Hepatitis-associated antigen can cross the placenta and has been identified in cord blood. Congenital hepatitis results in stillbirth or abortion of the fetus.[27] Keys et al. have summarized the known effects on the newborn as jaundice, hepatosplenomegaly, and hemolytic anemia with a liver function test indicating an obstructive type of jaundice. Although about 80% of infants survive for at least 1 year, 50% of these show a chronic persistent liver disease. Chronic maternal infection can result in births in successive pregnancies to infants with hepatitis.[28] There appear to be no epidemiologic studies of hospital personnel in terms of hepatitis infection and pregnancy outcome to indicate the extent of an effect in their children.

Many of the microorganisms listed in Table 4 are likely to be encountered by the pregnant woman only in an occupational setting such as a laboratory, hospital, laundry, or abattoir. In contrast, *Coxiella burnetii,,* the rickettsial agent of Q fever, is common and widespread in wild and domestic animals as a latent infection. *C. burnetii* can be isolated from the placentae and milk of domestic animals and appears to be associated with a sudden rise in antibody titer during pregnancy.[29] Asymptomatic recrudescence of infection during pregnancy also occurs in women and case reports have been published for a woman who had laboratory-acquired Q fever early in pregnancy and for others who were infected 3 or 4 years before conception. *C. burnetii* was isolated from placentae and milk a month after delivery. Four of these women experienced normal pregnancies and deliveries, and their babies had no history of Q fever or other abnormalities. *C. burnetii* was isolated in the curettage material of one of the five whose pregnancy was terminated in the third month. High levels of *C. burnetii* specific IgM antibodies have been detected in cord blood indicating *in utero* infection. In some parts of the world there is a high silent endemicity, e.g., Mediterranean countries and areas of the U.S., and Fiset et al. have shown immunologic evidence of *in utero* infection in the general population of the United Arab Republic. However it is far more difficult to study the children longitudinally and so far there is no information concerning late effects for the developing child. The use of sheep as experimental animals has led to transmission of Q fever to laboratory personnel probably by a natural infection route.[30]

For some infective agents the adverse effect on the fetus leading to fetal loss is probably the result of systemic effects of maternal illness rather than direct placental or fetal infection. Bubonic plague historically was known to cause spontaneous abortion in most cases with some evidence for occasional true intrauterine infection. Mann and Moskowitz have reported the successful pregnancy of a woman who developed plague in the fifth month of pregnancy and was treated with streptomycin.[31]

Brucellosis infection provides more uncertainty. The disease can be both acute and chronic in human beings and the etiologic agents *Brucella abortus, B. suis,* and *B. melitensis* are associated with infectious abortion in their respective hosts (cattle swine, and sheep/goats). Porreco and Haverkamp described a case study similar to the previously discussed case of plague, again with a successful outcome of pregnancy following tetracycline therapy.[32] The illness began at the end of the eighth month of pregnancy and after hospitalization and recovery at home delivery was at 41 weeks gestation. The placenta was normal macroscopically and microscopically and endometrial and placental cultures were negative. Brucellosis is an uncommon disease in the U.S. because of milk pasteurization. The high-risk occupations are slaughterhouse workers, veterinarians and their assistants, farmers, and laboratory personnel. The brucellae are known to lodge in the human female generative tract resulting in tubo-ovarian and pelvic abscesses, chronic salpingitis, cervicitis, and menstrual disturbances. Chronic brucellosis is also associated with major symptoms of depression, nervousness, headache, lassitude, and emotional instability. There is some disagreement on the extent to which the brucellae induce human abortion. There is enough evidence to indicate that abortion does result but how frequently is far from certain. Human chorioamniotic tissues and the fetus can be infected but probably abortion overall is rare, possibly because of the lack of placental erythritol, a carbohydrate which is the preferred nutrient for brucellae species growth. Erythritol is found in the placentae of sows, ewes, goats, and cows, where brucellosis runs an acute course with abortion resulting.[33]

The possibility of postnatal infectivity of the infant infected utero with rubella or cytomegalovirus led Haldane et al. to make a questionnaire survey of nurses in an attempt to identify transmissible birth defects of virologic origin in their children. As an exploratory study with considerable epidemiologic limitations it nevertheless provides very useful data on the nursing experience and its possible reproductive effect. From 1997 responses to 3670 questionnaires they identified 1582 nurses who had a total of 4196 pregnancies. Those who worked during pregnancy were divided into three groups — one group had cared for infants in hospitals, the second group cared for infants in the home (other than their own infants), and the third group cared for adults. Group 4 did not carry on professional activity during pregnancy. Pregnancy outcome was categorized into premature births, stillbirths, abortions, and congenitally defective infants. The percentage of congenitally defective children was 11.1% for the children of nurses who worked with infants in hospitals and in the home and 8.5% for the children of nurses who cared only for adults or did not work professionally during pregnancy. More detailed breakdown of Groups 1 and 2 to identify nurses who cared for children with congenital defects showed that for Group 1 (hospital nursing) 14 of 77 (18.2%) of their children had congenital defects. For Group 2 (home nursing) there were 8 of 31 (25.8%) of the children who had congenital defects. When premature births, stillbirths, and abortions were added to the congenitally defective children for these two categories there were 32 of 77 (28.5%) adverse pregnancies experienced by nurses in Group 1 and 15 of 31 (48.4%) adverse pregnancies experienced by nurses in Group 2. Infective illness during pregnancy was reported with twice the frequency in Groups 1 and 2 when compared with Groups 3 and 4. For those who experienced infectious disease and in addition cared for infants with congenital defects when pregnant, there were 16 of 88 (18.2%) children with congenital defects born to them compared with 28 of 332 (8.4%) children born to those who had no infective illness and had not cared for infants with congenital defects. Despite the acknowledged limitations of a retrospective mail survey study, Haldane et al. recommended that consideration be given to reassignment of pregnant nurses to working with noninfective patients and virologic screening of potentially high-risk infective infants to minimize risk to those caring for them.

"Further investigations of a similar nature are required, both in nurses and in other female occupation groups, as a possible basis for preventive measures to one type of pregnancy hazard."(1969)[34]

III. BIOLOGICALLY ACTIVE AGENTS

There is no federal standard to control levels of antibiotics in the air environment of the workplace. Large-scale production of antibiotics began in the late 1940s and synthetic penicillin exposure has now been experienced by workers for many years. Schmunes et al. have examined 169 subjects exposed to penicillin and ampicillin during manufacture.[35] The ampicillin dust level in workroom air ranged from less than 0.1 to 263 mg³. Highest levels were found in the blending, capsule filling, and milling operations (3.7 to 262 mg/m³). At the packaging line levels had decreased to 0.005 to 0.789 mg/m³. Symptoms experienced by 67% of the workers were localized rash, rhinorrhea and sneezing, generalized pruritis without rash; itching eyes; hives; swollen eyes, face, and lips; wheezing; chronic diarrhea; black hairy tongue; and generalized rash. There was a statistically different incidence of symptoms for the three groups designated by severity of ampicillin dust level. Hemagglutinating antipenicillin antibodies were present in the sera of 73 of the 169 workers tested and the presence or absence of antibodies was associated with presence or absence of symptomatology. The conclusion was that the correlation of chronic symptomatology with titer of antibody was indicative of an immune reaction. Respiratory symptoms were first observed in 1947 in penicillin workers in the U.S. from breathing cultures contaminated with *Aspergillis niger* and since then there have been repeated reports of sensitization to penicillin acquired through direct contact or inhalation of the powder. Ampicillin has been found to cause allergic eczematous contact dermatitis especially among medical personnel, but the additional irritation stemming from dust levels higher than the federal standard for inert nuisance dust (15mg/m³) could explain local dermatitis, rhinorrhea and sneezing, pruritis, and itching eyes on a nonallergic basis in those exposed to antibiotics during manufacture.[36]

Modification of the bacteria of the intestine and other organs has also been reported following occupational exposue to streptomycin, tetracycline, and penicillin and the occurrence of black hairy tongue provides evidence that there can be disturbance of the natural flora.

The question can be raised concerning women working in these antibiotic dust environments and the reliability of intrauterine devices, which may be dependent for their efficacy on the irritant response of the endometrium. Therapeutic doses of antibiotics are suspected in the infrequent failure of these devices.

REFERENCES

1. **Pike, R. M., Sulkin, S. E., and Schulze, M. L.**, Continuing importance of laboratory acquired infections, *Am. J. Public Health,* 55, 190, 1965.
2. **Sulkin, S. E. and Pike, R. M.**, Laboratory acquired infections, *JAMA,* 147, 1740, 1951.
3. **Phillips, G. B.**, Control of microbiological hazards in the laboratory, *Am. Ind. Hyg. Assoc. J.,* 30, 170, 1969.
4. **Inhorn, S. L.**, Ed., *Quality Assurance Practices for Public Health Laboratories,* American Public Health Association, Washington, D.C., 1978.
5. **Stark, A.**, Policy and procedural guidelines for the health and safety of workers in virus laboratories, *Am. Ind. Hyg. Assoc. J.,* 36, 234, 1975.
6. **Bannister, S. M., Cruse, R. P., Rothner, A. D., and Halpin, T.**, Imported tick-borne encephalitis — Ohio, *Morbidity Mortality Weekly Rep.,* 27, 164, 1978.
7. **Hanson, R. P., Sulkin, S. E., Buescher, E. L., Hammon, W. McD., McKinney, R.W., and Work, T. H.**, Arbovirus infections of laboratory workers, *Science,* 158, 1283, 1967.
8. **Sulkin, S. E. and Pike, R. M.**, *The Prevention of Laboratory Infections. Diagnostic Procedures for Viral and Rickettsial Diseases,* 3rd ed., American Public Health Association, New York, 1964.
9. Viral Hepatitis, Tech. Rep. Ser. No. 512, World Health Organization, Geneva, 1973.
10. **Pattison, C. P., Maynard, J. E., Berquist, K. R., and Webster, H. M.**, Epidemiology of hepatitis B in hospital personnel, *Am. J. Epidemiol.,* 101, 59, 1975.
11. **Garibaldi, R. A., Hanson, B., and Gregg, M. B.**, Impact of illicit drug-associated hepatitis morbidity reports in the U.S., *J. Infect. Dis.,* 126, 288, 1972.
12. **Devenyi, P. and Jourdain, P.**, Viral hepatitis in health care personnel working with drug abusers, *J. Occup. Med.,* 15, 779, 1973.
13. **Taylor, J. S., Schmunes, E., and Holmes, A. W.**, Hepatitis B in plasma fractionation workers, *JAMA,* 230, 850, 1974.
14. U.S. Department of Health, Education and Welfare, Center for Disease Control, Immune serum globulin protection against viral hepatitis, recommendation of the Public Health Service Advisory Committee on Immunization Practices, *Morbidity Mortality Weekly Rep.,* 21, 194, 1972.
15. **Cohen, S. R., Butler, G. J., Schmunes, E., and Holmes, A. W.**, Hepatitis among plasma fractionation workers, *J. Occup. Med.,* 18, 685, 1976.
16. **Koff, R. S. and Issebacher, K. J.**, Changing concepts in the epidemiology of viral hepatitis, *N. Engl. J. Med.,* 278, 1371, 1968.
17. **Byrne, E. B.**, Viral hepatitis: an occupational hazard of medical personnel: experience of the Yale-New Haven hospital 1952 to 1965, *JAMA,* 195, 362, 1966.
18. **Levin, M. L., Maddrey, W. C., Wands, J. R., and Mendeloff, A. I.**, Hepatitis B. transmission by dentists, *JAMA,* 228, 1139, 1974.
19. **Szmuness, W., Prince, A. M., Grady, G. F., Mann, M. K., Levine, R. W., Friedman, E. A., Jacobs, M. J., Josephson, A., Ribot, S., Shapiro, F. L., Steinzel, K. H., Suki, W. N., and Vyas, G.**, Hepatitis B infection, *JAMA,* 227, 901, 1974.
20. **Pattison, C. P., Boyer, K. M., Maynard, J. E., and Kelly, P. C.**, Epidemic hepatitis in a clinical laboratory, *JAMA,* 230, 854, 1974.
21. **Nelson, C. B., Pomeroy, B. S., Schrall, K., Park, W. E., and Lindeman, R. J.**, An outbreak of conjunctivitis due to Newcastle Disease virus occurring in poultry workers, *Am. J. Public Health,* 42, 672, 1952.
22. **Van Dyke, J.**, Chemotherapy for aquarium granuloma, *JAMA,* 233, 1380, 1975.
23. **Sever, J. L., Fucillo, D. A., and Bowes, W. A.**, Environmental Factors. Infection and Immunization in *Prevention of Embryonic, Fetal and Perinatal Disease,* NIH 76-853, National Institutes of Health, U.S. Department of Health, Education and Welfare, Washington. D.C.. 1976, 199.
24. U. S. Department of Health, Education and Welfare, Exposure of patients to rubella by medical personnel, *California, Morbidity Mortality Weekly Rep.,* 27, 123, 1978.
25. **Williams, S. V., Huff, J. C., Feinglass, E. J., Gregg, M. B., Hatch, M. H., and Matsen, J. M.**, Epidemic viral hepatitis type B in hospital personnel, *Am. J. Med.,* 57. 904, 1974.

26. Hospital Occupational Health Services Study, (NIOSH) 75-101, National Institute of Occupational Safety and Health, U.S. Department of Health, Education and Welfare, Washington, D.C., 1976.

27. Keys, T. F., Sever, J. L., Hewitt, W. L., and Gitnick, G. L., Hepatitis associated antigen in selected mothers and newborn infants, *J. Pediatr.*, 80, 650, 1972.

28. Alterman, K., Neonatal hepatitis and its relation to viral hepatitis of mother, *Am. J. Dis. Child.*, 105, 395, 1963.

29. Fiset, P., Wissenian, C. L., and El Batawi, Y., Immunologic evidence of human fetal infection with Coxiella burnetii, *Am. J. Epidemiol.*, 101, 65, 1975.

30. Curet, L. B. and Paust, J. C., Transmission of Q fever from experimental sheep to laboratory personnel, *Am. J. Obstet. Gynecol.*, 114, 566, 1972.

31. Mann, J. M. and Moskowitz, R., Plague and pregnancy, *JAMA*, 237, 1854, 1977.

32. Porreco, R. P. and Haverkamp, H. D. Brucellosis in pregnancy, *Obstet. Gynecol.*, 44, 597, 1974.

33. Carpenter, C. M. and Boak, R., Isolations of *Brucella abortus* from a human fetus, *JAMA*, 96, 1212, 1931.

34. Haldane, E. V., van Rooyen, G. E., Embil, J. A., Tupper, W. C., Gordon, P.C., and Wanklin, J. M., A search for transmissible birth defects of virologic origin in members of the nursing profession, *Am. J. Obstet. Gynecol.*, 105, 1032, 1969.

35. Schmunes, E., Taylor, J. S., Petz, L. D., Garratty, G., and Fudenberg, H. H., Immunologic reactions in penicillin factory workers, *Ann. Allergy*, 36, 313, 1976.

36. Hjorth, N. and Wilkinson, D. S., Contact dermatitis. V. Occupational dermatitis from ampicillin, *B. J. Dermatol.*, 81, 80, 1969.

Chapter 6

INFLUENCE OF ENVIRONMENTAL AGENTS ON MALE REPRODUCTIVE FAILURE

Jeanne M. Manson and Ruth Simons

I. INTRODUCTION

The incidence of reproductive failure in the human population is relatively high with estimates that 7% of all newborns (200,000 of 3 million live births) in the U.S. have birth defects each year. More than 560,000 lives a year are claimed by infant death, spontaneous abortion, stillbirth, and miscarriage as a result of defective fetal development. The cause of 65 to 70% of developmental defects in the human population is unknown.[1]

The high percentage of reproductive failure in the human population necessitates examining the role played by occupational and environmental exposures on the process of reproduction in men and women. Epidemiologic and laboratory animal studies have demonstrated that reproductive function is highly sensitive to toxic agents in the environment. Common industrial agents including vinyl chloride, lead, hydrocarbons, and pesticides have been identified as human reproductive toxicants.[2]

Reproductive studies have tended to focus almost exclusively on associations between maternal exposure to toxic agents during pregnancy and subsequent birth defects in the newborn. Reproductive effects resulting from exposure of parents at other stages of their lives have not been systematically examined. Paternal exposure in particular has been infrequently examined in relation to reproductive events. In this chapter agents capable of causing toxicity to the male reproductive system will be discussed. The effects caused by these agents include male infertility as well as adverse pregnancy outcome via mutation of sperm.

Two potential exposure routes exist that may account for an association between paternal exposure and reproductive outcome: (1) paternal exposure results in maternal exposure, and the agent operates through the mother, or (2) exposure causes damage to sperm cells which results in infertility or abnormal development of the embryo.[2] If mutated sperm fertilize an ovum, the most likely outcome is spontaneous abortion insofar as all of the cells in the resulting embryo will have chromosomal anomalies. Other less likely outcomes include the occurrence of stillbirths, birth defects, and childhood diseases.

Environmental agents that damage male germ cells, leading to infertility and mutation, are not likely to be recognized by current epidemiologic studies unless they are of overwhelming magnitude. Nevertheless, current epidemiologic studies have identified a number of environmental agents that adversely affect male reproduction. Lead and dibromochloropropane (DBCP) have been associated with decreased sperm counts and sperm abnormalities in exposed workers, leading to infertility.[3,4] Occupational exposure of male workers to vinyl chloride, anesthetic gases, chloroprene, and hydrocarbons has been associated with adverse pregnancy outcome in the unexposed wives.[2] Thus, there is a need to study the mechanisms responsible for male infertility and whether groups of chemical and physical agents are likely to influence sperm production, motility, capacitation, and reproductive tract function.

II. SURVEY OF THE LITERATURE

Tables 1 through 4 summarize findings in the literature on agents causing male reproductive toxicity. In general, agents have been examined for their effects on fertility, testicular histology, endocrinology, and testicular biochemistry. Information on the mechanism of action of these agents on the male reproductive system is scarce and is inferred mostly from mechanism studies in other tissues. Most of the agents listed in the tables cause reversible effects on male reproductive function; sterility and pathologic effects on the testis are rarely permanent with physical and chemical insult.

Disturbances of testicular function may manifest themselves by one or several of the following signs: loss of libido, impotence, sterility, abnormal seminal secretions (azoospermia, teratospermia, oligospermia), and presence of anatomical lesions in spermatogenic tissues. These manifestations are brought about by agents acting directly on the testis or accessory organs, or indirectly on the neuroendocrine system.

The paucity of observations in Tables 1 and 3 for human populations is not a result of negative studies but rather reflects the absence of studies. The similarity in response of humans and laboratory animals to some of the more extensively studied agents is apparent. The purpose of this summary is to underline the important deficiencies of information in the area of human reproductive effects. Unpredicted fertility deficits have recently been identified by workers themselves exposed to DBCP and it appears from the summary presented in the tables that other comparable conditions are likely to be found.[8]

III. CELLULAR AND HORMONAL ASPECTS OF TESTICULAR FUNCTION

Mitotic activity in the seminiferous tubules starts at about 10 years of age and active spermatogenesis starts some 3 years later.[81] The seminiferous tubules are lined by a highly complex and stratified epithelium consisting of two populations of cells: non-proliferating Sertoli cells and proliferating germ cells. The latter undergo continuous migration as they differentiate from spermatogonia at the periphery of the tubules to mature sperm at the luminal free surface. (Figure 1). The Sertoli cells are tall, columnar elements extending from the base of the seminiferous epithelium to the tubule lumen. Because germ cells develop in the microenvironment provided by Sertoli cells, control of germ cell differentiation is mediated by Sertoli cells. Antifertility agents, hypophysectomy, and steroid hormones may exert effects primarily on the Sertoli cells which are transmitted to germ cells.

Leydig or interstitial cells are scattered between seminiferous tubules and are found in clusters. At the age of 9 to 10 years, Leydig cells multiply and androgen secretion increases. Leydig cells are the primary source of testosterone, which controls the functional activity of accessory sex organs and development of secondary sexual characteristics.[83]

The function of the testis is controlled by at least two pituitary hormones, luteinizing hormone (LH) and follicle-stimulating hormone (FSH). The testis controls the output of these two pituitary hormones by negative feedback, as the concentrations of both hormones in the pituitary and blood are elevated after castration (Figure 2). LH stimulates Leydig cells in the testis to synthesize steroid hormones, principally testosterone. When testosterone levels in the blood are low, the pituitary releases LH, which stimulates Leydig cells in the testis to make more testosterone. Thus, an inverse relationship exists between levels of testosterone and LH, and LH release by the pituitary is controlled by levels of circulating testosterone.[84] (Figure 2).

The control mechanisms regulating FSH levels are unclear. FSH is generally recognized as being important in the initiation of spermatogenesis at puberty and maintenance of optimal testicular function in the adult. The Sertoli cell is believed to be the primary target for FSH within the testis, with Leydig cells mediating the effect.[85,86] There is evidence in rodent species for the existence of a factor termed "inhibin" produced by the germinal cells of the testis that selectively inhibits secretion of FSH from the pituitary. The role of inhibin is to control the rate of sperm production via feedback control of FSH levels (Figure 2). When germinal cells are damaged, inhibin levels are lowered and FSH levels are elevated. A surge of FSH from the pituitary results in stimulation of spermatogonial cell division to repopulate the seminiferous tubules.[84]

Treatment of males with agents that destroy germinal cells, such as cadmium, alkylating agents, diamines, and antimitotic agents, results in a selective increase in plasma FSH levels, while plasma LH and testosterone levels remain normal.[84] The inverse correlation between sperm concentration in semen and FSH levels in serum or urine holds well in cases of azoospermia but is variable in cases of oligospermia. Thus, FSH elevation without corresponding increase in LH or testosterone levels can be diagnostic of specific damage to the germinal epithelium with normal function and morphology of Sertoli and Leydig cells.[87,88]

Sperm production is affected by many factors such as general health, age, frequency of ejaculation, season of the year, temperature, photoperiod, nutrition, stress, and toxic substances.[81] The process of spermatogenesis can be divided into three principal phases: spermatocytogenesis, meiosis, and spermiogenesis. In spermatocytogenesis, spermatogonia proliferate by mitosis to give rise to new stem cells to replace those removed from the population by differentiation into spermatocytes (Figure 3). There are two types of spermatogonial stem cells: those which serve as an emergency source of new stem cells (reserve) and those which proceed to differentiate into spermatocytes (renewing). Reserve stem cells remain quiescent unless the supply of renewing stem cells is depleted through formation of B_1 spermatogonia which differentiate into primary spermatocytes. Type A spermatogonia may degenerate during mitotic divisions so that the total number of spermatozoa produced is less than the number of Type A spermatogonia present at the beginning of spermatogenesis.[81] In Sprague-Dawley rats, there is a total cell loss of 22% between late spermatogonial and advanced spermatid stages. In man, a cell loss of 35% from early spermatocyte to the spermatid stage has been reported.[89] The testis selects against many more potential gametes than the number allowed to complete spermatogenesis during these early stages. Evidence suggests that a considerable amount of selection in the testis is against spermatogonia with abnormal chromosomes. Studies have shown that the incidence of polyploid spermatogonia is very high in mice but that polyploid primary spermatocytes are seldomly observed.[89] Degenerating spermatogonia are phagocytized by Sertoli cells.

Spermatocytes undergo two maturational, meiotic divisions to reduce chromosomal number and produce a cluster of spermatids. As meiosis progresses, primary spermatocytes become larger and migrate from the basement membrane of the Sertoli cell toward the luminal surface projecting into the seminiferous tubule. Sertoli cells are divided into two compartments based on composition of germ cells; the basal compartment contains spermatogonia and early spermatocytes, while the adluminal compartment contains late spermatocytes and spermatids.[82] The significance of this compartmentalization is that early germ cells are protected from many toxic agents in the blood stream by the blood-testis barrier that is operative in the basal compartment (see next section). More mature germ cells that have completed mitosis and meiosis move into the adluminal compartment.

TABLE 1

Male Reproductive Effects: Environmental Agents, Human Studies

Agent	Exposure Conditions	Species	Type of Study	Effects	Ref.
Anesthetic gases	Occupational	Male workers	Reproductive history	Increased incidence congenital anomalies offspring	5, 6
Chloroprene	Occupational	Male workers	Semen analysis; reproductive history	Decrease motility and number of sperm; threefold excess miscarriages in wives	7
Dibromochloro-propane	Occupational	Male workers	Semen analysis: reproductive history	Decreased sperm count; infertility	8
High altitude	14,000 ft	Male	Semen analysis	Decreased sperm count and motility; increased number abnormal sperm	9
Hydrocarbons	Occupational	Male workers	Reproductive history	Twofold increased incidence childhood cancer with occupational hydrocarbon exposure of father	10
Kepone	Environmental	Male	Reproductive history	Decreased fertility males	11
Lead	Occupational	Male workers	Semen analysis	Decreased sperm count and motility; increase abnormally-shaped semen	3
Microwaves	Occupational	Male workers	Semen analysis; reproductive history	Decreased libido; decreased sperm count and mobility, increase abnormally-shaped sperm	12
Carbon Disulfide	Occupational	Male workers	Semen analysis, reproductive history	Impotence, loss of libido	13
Irradiation	Occupational	Male workers	Gonadotropic hormone and semen analysis	Depression gonadotropic hormone levels; alterations in spermatogenesis	14, 15

Oral contraceptives	Occupational manufacture	Male workers	Reproductive history, physical exam, blood analysis	Gynecomastia, decreased libido, infertility	16
Vinyl chloride	Occupational	Male workers	Reproductive questionnaire	Adverse pregnancy outcome wives; excess fetal loss	17
Cigarette smoking	Environmental	Male	Semen analysis	Increase in abnormally shaped sperm	18
Elevated temperature	Occupational, environmental $30 \rightarrow 37°C$	Male	Semen analysis, histology	Inhibition spermatogenesis, testicular pathology	13

TABLE 2

Male Reproductive Effects Environmental Agents — Animal Studies

Agent	Exposure conditions	Species	Type of study	Effects	Ref.
		Heavy Metals			
Cadmium chloride	4 to 8 mg/kg s.c., i.m., i.v. single dose	Dog; rats, mice, rabbits, guinea pigs, hamsters, opossums, goats, and monkeys cited	Histology, semen analysis	Damage to testicular blood vessels; disruption of blood-testis barrier; destruction seminiferous tubules; reduced fertility	19
Methyl mercuric chloride	10 mg to 1 g/liter for 30 min in water	Steelhead trout	Percentage eggs fertilized by treated sperm	Reduced viability of sperm at 1 ppm and greater	20
Methyl mercury hydroxide and mercuric chloride	1 mg/kg i.p. single dose	Mice	Serial mating	Inhibition early stages spermatogenesis; reduced fertility	21
Nickel sulfate	25 mg/kg/day oral, 120 days	Rat	Histology	Damage to testicular parenchyma; decreased fertility	22
Lead-cadmium interaction	25 μg each	Rat	Histology	Absence of spermatogenesis; synergistic effect simultaneous exposure lead-cadmium	23

Food additives and contaminants

Compound	Dose	Species	Method	Effect	Ref.
Aflatoxin B1	5 mg/kg/ i.p. single exposure	Mice	Dominant lethal	Reduced Fertility	24
Dibutyl phthalate	2000 mg/kg/ day oral, 4 days	Rat	Histology	Morphologic damage and reduction weight testes	25
Diethyl adipate	Single i.p. dose	Mice	Dominant lethal	Reduced percentage pregnancies; increased numbers early fetal deaths	26
Glutamic acid	25 mg/kg/day 1 month oral	Rabbits	Histology/general toxicology	Inhibition of spermatogenesis; reduced fertility; atrophy of testes	27
P-Hydroxy-aceto-phenone (PHA) and P-hydroxy-butyrophenone (PHB)	0.06% in diet 314 to 465 days	Rats	Histology	Atrophy adrenals and testes; interference spermatogenesis	28
Nitrofuran compounds	10 mg/100g oral, 7 days	Rat, guinea pig	Histology	Atrophy testes; degeneration seminiferous tubules	29, 30
Pesticides					
DDT	200 mg/kg/day 14 days oral	Juvenile rats	Histology, dominant lethal	Reduced weight testes; alterations spermatogenesis; small litters	31
DBCP (dibromo-chloropropane)	100 mg/kg single dose	Rat	General toxicology	Reduced weight testes; alterations spermatogenesis	32, 33

TABLE 2 (continued)

Male Reproductive Effects Environmental Agents — Animal Studies

Agent	Exposure conditions	Species	Type of study	Effects	Ref.
Carbaryl	7, 14, 70 mg/kg/day up to 12 months	Rat	Endocrine, semen analysis	Reduced motility sperm; alterations spermatogenesis	34
DDVP (Dichlorvos)	20 mg/kg/day 2 days oral	Juvenile rats	Histology, dominant lethal	Reduction spermatogenic cells and leydig cells; reduced fertility	35
Malathion	40 mg/kg/day 19 days, oral	Juvenile rats	Histology	Reduction spermatogenic cells and Leydig cells	35
Niridazole (antibilharzial drug)	50 mg/kg/day 5 days oral	Guinea pigs	Histology	Inhibition spermatogenesis; damage to seminiferous tubules	36
Kepone	200 ppm diet 42 days	Japanese quail	Histology	Fluid-filled and atrophic testes; disruption germinal epithelium; alterations spermatogenesis	37
HMPA (hexamethyl-phosphor-amide)	100 to 500 mg/kg	Rats, mice, rabbits	Dominant lethal	Infertility	38
Physical agents					
High oxygen tension	Various	Various	Review	Gonadal injury; testicular atrophy, disorganization germinal cells; arrest spermatogenesis	39
Irradiation	200 to 1000 R	Mice	Histology/general toxicology, dominant lethal	Reduction testes wt, alterations spermatogenesis, embryonic lethality	40, 41
Elevated CO_2	1.8/1.0 mixture air/CO_2, 6 hr	Mice	Semen analysis, serial mating	Abnormally shaped sperm; low conception rate	42

Agent	Dose/Exposure	Species	Test	Effects	Ref.
Elevated temperature	Various	Rats	Histology, hormone profile	Atrophy and pathology testis, prostate and seminal vesicles; Lowered testosterone levels; seminiferous tubule pathology; abnormal sperm	43
Other agents					
Carbon tetrachloride	0.3 ml/100 g i.p. of 50% solution	Rat	Histology	Atrophy and necrosis testes	44
Carbon disulfide	Inhalation	Rat	Histology	Alterations spermatogenesis	45
Cyclosiloxanes	Various sub-chronic dermal, oral	Rabbits	Histology	Testicular pathology; depression spermatogenesis	46, 47
Ethylene oxide	1000 ppm, 4 hr	Rat	Dominant lethal	Increase postimplantation fetal death, decreased fertility	48
Chloroprene	Various	Mice, rats, drosophila	Dominant-lethal, semen analysis, cytogenetics, recessive-lethal	Testicular atrophy; abnormal semen profile; reduced fertility; increased embryonic mortality; chromosome anomalies	7
Hair dyes	Oral to adult males	Drosophila	Recessive-lethal	Mutagenic primarily to spermatids and spermatocytes	49
Nitrous oxide	Inhalation 20%, 35 days	Rats	Histology	Damage to seminiferous tubules; suppression spermatogenesis	50
Tris (flame retardant)	2.27 g/kg once a week for 3 months, dermal	Rabbits	Histology	Testicular atrophy, degeneration spermatozoa	51

TABLE 3

Male Reproductive Effects Drugs (Human Studies)

Agent	Exposure conditions	Species	Type of study	Effects	Ref.
Alcohol	Chronic alcoholism	Human	Autopsy	Testicular atrophy, azoospermia; testicular pathology;	13, 52
Amebicide	Therapeutic 1 to 2 g/day	Human	Clinical	Inhibit sperm motility; abnormal morphology; immature cells in ejaculate	53
Anticonvulsants	Therapeutic	Human	Survey of children of epileptics	Increased level developmental disabilities in children	54, 55
Antineoplastic agents	Therapeutic	Human	Clinical, epidemiologic	Reduced fertility	56
Clomiphene	200 mg/day 2 to 12 months	Human	Semen analysis	Reduction sperm numbers	57
Diamines	Therapeutic	Human	Testicular biopsy	Reduction spermatids, abnormal morphology spermatids, azoospermia	58
Diethylstilbesterol	Transplacental exposure male offspring	Human	Clinical	Epididymal cysts, hypotrophic testes, capsular induration testes, sperm abnormalities	59
Iodine	Therapeutic doses	Adolescent males	Clinical	Atrophy of testes	13
Testosterone enanthate	Male contraception	Human	Clinical	Sterility	60

TABLE 4

Male Reproductive Effects Drugs — Animal Studies

Agent	Exposure conditions	Species	Type of study	Effects	Ref.
Antibiotics					
Adriamycin	0.125, 0.250, and 0.5 mg/kg i.v. single dose	Rabbits, dogs	Histology	Alterations spermatogenesis	61
Urologic antibiotics	Various	Rat	Histologic and enzymatic analysis	Alterations spermatogenesis	62
Alkylating agents					
Alkylating agents	Various	Rat	Cytogenetic, fertility	Chromosomal anomalies in different stages of spermatogenesis; infertility	63, 64
CNU-ethanol	0.36 to 81.45 mg/kg i.p. single dose	Mice	Cytogenetic	Chromatid aberrations in spermatogonia	65
Ethyl methane sulfonate	25 mM feeding 24 hr	Drosophila	Recessive lethal	Dose-response alkylation and sex-linked recessive lethals	66
Nitrogen mustards	Various	Drosophila	Recessive lethal	Differential cell stage response to each chemical	67
Trenimon	0.125 to 0.250 mg/kg i.p. single dose	Mice, hamsters	Dominant lethal	Damage to spermatozoa and spermatids; chromosome anomalies in embryos	68, 69

TABLE 4 (continued)

Male Reproductive Effects Drugs — Animal Studies

Agent	Exposure conditions	Species	Type of study	Effects	Ref.
			Other drugs		
alpha-Chlorohydrin	15 mg/rat, 8 days	Rats	Serial mating	Reversible sterility	13
Amphotericin B	2 mg/kg/day 10 days i.v.	Rabbit	Histology	Alterations spermatogenesis	70, 71
Clomiphene	34 to 100 μg/day 22 to 55 days orally	Rats	Histology	Atrophy testes, tubular and interstitial elements damaged	72
Cyproterone	0.3 to 10 mg/day s.c., 12 days	Juvenile rats	Hormonal assay; histology	Atrophy seminal vesicles, increased gonadotropin levels	73
Diamines	500 mg/kg single dose, oral	Mice, rats, dogs, monkeys	Dominant lethal, histology	Decreased fertility; embryolethality; sperm abnormalities	74
Dinitropyrroles	100 mg/kg oral	Rats	Histology	Interference meiosis	75
Ethionine	0.5% diet	Rat	Histology	Testicular damage; arrest spermatogenesis	76, 77
Fluoroacetamide	5 to 20 mg/kg diet, 1 to 28 days	Rat	Histology	Alterations spermatogenesis	78
Iodine	Various, review	Rabbits, rats, mice, guinea pigs	Histology, serial mating	Testicular degeneration; sterility	13
Methadone	0.067 mg/mℓ in drinking water 24 hr	Rat	Dominant-lethal	Increased neonatal death rate; growth retardation	79, 80

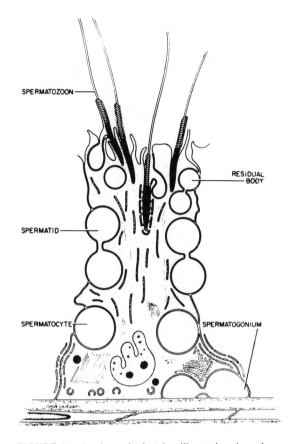

FIGURE 1. A schematic drawing illustrating the columnar shape of the Sertoli cell extending from the base of the seminiferous tubule to the lumen and the germinal cell population. (Adapted from Dym, M., Raj, H. G., and Chemes, H. E., in *The Testes in Normal and Infertile Men,* Troen, T. and Nankin, H. R., Eds., Raven Press, New York, 1977, 97.)

The process of spermiogenesis consists of three developmental processes: acrosome formation, nuclear condensation, and tail formation. Spermatids lose most of their cytoplasm and undergo remarkable transformation into spermatozoa without cell division. During spermiogenesis, cytoplasm containing Golgi bodies, vesicles, degenerating mitochondria, lipid droplets, and ribosomes is extruded from the germinal cell and phagocytized by Sertoli cells.[81]

Sperm undergo maturation and achieve motility while transported through the epididymis from the testis to the ejaculatory duct. The epididymal environment is needed for sperm to become capable of fertilizing an ovum. Sperm retain their fertilizing ability in the epididymus for 20 to 35 days in most laboratory species, but they lose their ability to produce viable embryos before losing their ability to penetrate the egg.[81]

The duration of each of these spermatogenic stages in laboratory animals and humans is given in Table 5. At any point in time spermatogenic cells exist in each of these stages. If a given agent specifically damages cells in the premeiotic stages in man, then abnormal sperm will not appear in the ejaculate until 11 to 15 weeks after exposure. Up to 11 weeks after exposure, normal sperm will be present in the ejaculate. This time interval will remain constant only in cases of acute exposure; chronic expo-

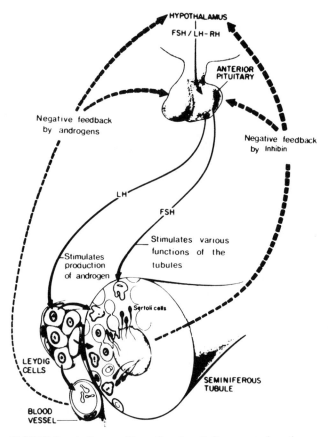

FIGURE 2.   A diagram illustrating the pituitary controls acting on the testis and the negative feedback by androgens and inhibin on LH and FSH production, respectively. (Adapted from Setchell, B. P., Davies, R. V., and Main, S. J., in *The Testis*, Vol. 4, Johnson, A. D. and Gomes, W. R., Eds., Academic Press, New York, 1977, 190.)

sure will ultimately result in constant production of abnormal sperm in the ejaculate, or infertility.

IV. BLOOD-TESTIS BARRIER

Evidence exists for the presence of a permeability barrier in the testis. The distinctive composition of testicular fluid relative to blood plasma and the exclusion of radiolabeled compounds from seminiferous tubules suggest compartmentalization of the testis. The blood-testis barrier lies between the lumen of interstitial capillaries and the lumen of seminiferous tubules. The barrier is largely attributed to tight junctions between Sertoli cells (Figure 1). As seen with the electron microscope, tracer substances that reach the seminiferous epithelium tend to remain in the basal region of Sertoli cells, rarely penetrating beyond the zone occupied by spermatogonia.[91]

Studies on the transfer of a few drugs from the blood into testicular fluids have been performed. The mutagen, alpha-chlorohydrin, and metabolites readily enter testicular fluid from the blood. Equilibration occurs between rete testis fluid and blood levels within 45 min in rats.[92] The rate of transfer of barbiturates from blood into rete testis fluid of rats suggests that the rate of penetration obeys simple diffusion kinetics and depends on lipid solubility rather than pKa value or molecular weight.[93] The rates

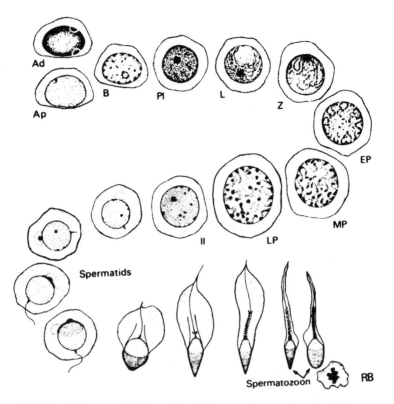

FIGURE 3. Diagrammatic illustration of the steps in spermatogenesis in man. Spermatogonia are at the top left and spermatozoa at the bottom right. Labels: Ad, dark type A spermatogonia; Ap, pale type A spermatogonia; B, type B spermatogonia; Pl, preleptotene primary spermatocytes; L, leptotene spermatocytes; Z, zygotene spermatocytes; EP, early pachytene spermatocyte; MP, midpachytene spermatocyte; LP, late pachytene spermatocyte; II, secondary spermatocytes. Spermatids are shown at various steps of spermiogenesis. A spermatozoon is illustrated from the lateral and frontal position (RB, residual body). (From Hafez, E. S. E., in *Techniques of Human Andrology*, Hafez, E. S. E., Ed., Elsevier, Amsterdam, 1977, 39. With permission.)

of penetration of these drugs into testicular fluid could be predicted from partition coefficients. Additional evidence has shown that the blood-testis barrier expresses a wide range of permeability toward families of compounds as dissimilar as ions, proteins, steroids, and various pharmacologic agents.[94]

The blood-testis barrier in rats is established between the 16th and 19th days of postnatal life in close temporal association with the appearance of junctional complexes between Sertoli cells.[95] Considering the importance of the germ line to species survival and the vulnerability of this proliferating cell population to mutagenic agents, it seems appropriate that developing germ cells be sequestered within a compartment delimited by a permeability barrier. This barrier may shield meiotic cells from some environmental toxins that enter the circulation. It is likely that the blood-testis barrier is the cause of numerous false-negative results obtained in dominant-lethal testing of agents with known mutagenic activity.[96,97]

V. SEMINAL FLUID

The average fertile human ejaculate contains about 3 mℓ of semen consisting of 50

TABLE 5

Time Span Between Damage of Specific Cell Types and Onset Infertile Ejaculates[2]

Specific spermatogenic stage affected	Initial appearance of infertile ejaculates (weeks after treatment)				
	Rat	Mouse	Rabbit	Guinea pig	Man
Premeiotic stages				5—8	11-15
Spermatogonia		6—7	8—10		
Stem cells + type A	10				
Type A + intermediate	9				
Type B + resting	8				
Spermatocytes	6—7	4—5	6—7		
Spermiogenic stage			3—5	2—4	5—10
Spermatids and testicular sperm	3—5	2—3			
Epididymal phase	1—2	1	1—2	1	1—4

From Gomes, W. R., in *The Testis*, Vol. 3, Johnson, A. D., and Gomes, W. R., eds., Academic Press, New York, 1975, 485.

to 120 million sperm cells per milliliter suspended in seminal plasma. Approximately 60% of the volume of the seminal plasma is contributed by seminal vesicle secretion, 30% by the prostate gland, and the remainder from the urethral and bulbourethral glands, ampullae, epididymis, and testes.[98] The measurement of components in seminal fluid specific to the secretions of each of these organs can aid the clinician or researcher in evaluating the status of the male reproductive tract. This section will review the biochemical markers in seminal fluid, following the path of the spermatozoa from the testis outward.

Sperm cells, with accumulated rete testis fluid, pass into the caput epididymis, which absorbs most of the rete testis fluid and secretes components such as carnitine. Epididymal function can be ascertained by measurement of carnitine levels in seminal plasma. Carnitine may play a significant role in sperm maturation.[98,99]

Mature sperm cells move from the epididymis into the vas deferens and then to the ampulla. Upon ejaculation, sperm are mixed with secretions from the seminal vesicle and prostate, which provide the bulk of seminal fluid volume. In humans, the seminal vesicle secretes fructose, while in the rat the prostate and coagulating gland are the sources of fructose in the seminal fluid. Table 6 contains information on the chemical indicators of secretory activity of the accessory glands and their normal values in human seminal fluid.

VI. EXCRETION OF DRUGS INTO SEMINAL FLUID

Lutwak-Mann et al. have suggested that drugs excreted in semen may adversely affect fertility or cause mutation of sperm, leading to congenital malformations.[100] These investigators found thalidomide and/or metabolites in rabbit semen after administration of ^{14}C-thalidomide to male rabbits. Thalidomide added to semen in vitro bound to rabbit spermatozoa. Progeny of thalidomide-pretreated male rabbits exhibited poor neonatal survival, low birth weights, and an elevated incidence of birth defects. Similar

TABLE 6

Normal Values of Key Seminal Plasma Constituents

Component	Range	Mean	Secretory organ
Acid phosphatase ($IU \times 10^{-2}/ml$)	88—979	408	Prostate
Carnitine ($\mu mol/ml$)		0.319	Epididymis
Citric acid (mg/ml)	1.8—8.4	5.1	Prostate
Fructose (mg/ml)	0.7—5.0	3.0	Seminal vesicle
Glycerolphosphorylcholine ($\mu mol/ml$)		0.85	Epididymis
Prostaglandins			
A—B group ($\mu g/ml$)		50	Seminal vesicle
19—OHA—B group ($\mu g/ml$)		200	Seminal vesicle
Proteins (mg/ml)	21—66		Seminal vesicle
Zinc	25—424	197	Prostate

From Polakoski, K. L. and Zaneveld, L. J., in *Techniques of Human Andrology,* Hafez, E.S.E., Ed., Elsevier, Amsterdam, 1977, 265.

findings were obtained with methadone; male rats given methadone generated offspring with low birth weights and diminished neonatal survival.[101,102] Methadone is
excreted at high levels in the semen of man, with a semen/blood ratio of 0.82 to 4.72,
and is transmitted from male to female rabbits during coitus.[103,104] Likewise, the concentration of diphenylhydantoin was measured in plasma and semen of rabbits and
man.[105] In rabbits, a single i.v. injection resulted in a semen/plasma ratio of 0.2 for 8
hr. In epileptic human subjects maintained on oral diphenylhydantoin, the mean drug
concentration in semen was 2.31 $\mu g/ml$ while that in plasma was 13.8 $\mu g/ml$, giving
a ratio of 0.17. Antibiotic levels have been measured in human semen with the aim of
improving the treatment of venereal disease and chronic prostatitis.[106,107] Thus, drugs
in semen may directly influence the motility and viability of spermatozoa. Numerous
chemicals have been shown to alter sperm activity in vitro.[108] Little information is
available on the concentrations these chemicals might achieve in semen.

The significance of drug excretion into semen is not generally appreciated. In addition to the potential for spermatotoxic effects, drugs in semen can cause toxic reactions
in women. Cases of vaginitis have been reported in women whose sexual partners were
on vinblastine therapy.[109] Various drugs excreted into the semen of rats have caused
pharmacologic responses in female rats after coitus.[110] There is abundant evidence that
a variety of foreign substances can be rapidly absorbed through the vaginal
mucosa.[111,112] Thus, drugs transmitted via the semen during coitus are likely to enter
the systemic circulation of the female. This may constitute a significant route of exposure for the female as well as the embryo.

VII. SPERM ANALYSIS

At present, assessment of the fertility of men resides primarily in interpretation of
the ejaculate; pregnancy of the wife is the only other test of this potential, which is
subject to confounding factors such as female infertility, frequency of sexual contact,
and use of birth control. Considerable differences in opinion exist as to what constitutes a normal ejaculate which relate to variations in methods of collecting semen as
well as the source of the donor population. A number of studies have been performed
on the sperm count in ejaculates of fertile and infertile men with the goal of establish-

ing a range of sperm counts that would be predictive of the potential to conceive. In 1951, MacLead and Gold compared single sperm counts from 1000 men whose wives had just registered at a prenatal clinic with single counts from 1000 men whose wives had recently registered at an infertility clinic (Table 7). They concluded from this study that subfertility began when sperm counts were less than 20 million per milliliter of ejaculate.[113]

Findings from several recent studies have indicated that the level of 20 million sperm per milliliter of ejaculate is too high for accurate assessment of fertility.[114,115] These studies emphasize that low sperm count per se does not preclude pregnancy. No appreciable increase in fertility potential was obtained in men with sperm counts above 20 million sperm per milliliter but men with counts of 2 to 5 million per milliliter were capable of impregnating their wives.[114] Over 19% of men in one study whose wives conceived had sperm counts of 20 million per milliliter or less.[115] These findings have led some investigators to set the division between fertility and infertility at sperm counts of 10 million per milliliter or 50 million per ejaculate. This figure is supported not only by conception rates but also by plasma hormone levels. Significant elevations in plasma FSH levels, indicative of germinal epithelium damage, occurred in men with sperm counts less than 10.1 million per milliliter and total sperm counts below 25.1 million per ejaculate.[115]

In addition to sperm count, sperm motility, and volume of the ejaculate have been found to be unstable parameters and not highly predictive of fertility.[114-116] By contrast, sperm morphology has been found to be the most stable semen parameter and highly reliable in the prediction of the fertile state. Sperm concentration and morphology are believed to be the best indicators because they were shown to be stable in a study where sequential analysis of semen was conducted over a six-month period.

Extensive studies have been performed on the induction of abnormal sperm morphology by physical and chemical agents in laboratory animals.[116-118] Sperm morphology in mice can easily be determined microscopically from stained smears of epididymal sperm.[118] The relevancy of sperm morphology for assay of spermatotoxic agents has become evident from three lines of evidence:

1. Sperm shape is genotypically determined by autosomal and sex-linked genes. The shape of the sperm head is so highly heritable that strains of inbred mice can be distinguished by sperm morphology alone.
2. A low level of abnormally shaped sperm normally occurs in control animals that is dependent on genotype; this fraction is increased in a dose-dependent fashion following exposure of mice to mutagenic agents and is not increased by exposure to nonmutagenic compounds. Twenty-five diverse chemical agents representing a range of mutagenic, carcinogenic, and teratogenic potential have been studied for this effect.[117]
3. Induced elevations in sperm abnormalities are transmitted to subsequent generations following Mendelian rules.[118]

The majority of chemicals chosen produced sperm abnormalities 4 weeks after exposure with maximum levels 40 times above background. Induced sperm abnormalities in mice can be scored under two conditions. Mature sperm from treated adult animals can be analyzed, as well as sperm of F_1 male progeny of treated F_0 males. The former monitors sperm prior to fertilization, while the latter assays mutations passed on to the offspring.[118]

Methods developed for assessing sperm shape abnormalities in mice have been applied to humans.[118] Sperm morphology in human males shows a high degree of individual constancy with considerable interindividual variation. In order to detect small

TABLE 7

Distribution of Sperm Counts

Sperm counts (million/ml)	Fertile (%)	Infertile (%)
< 10.1	2	9
10.1—20.0	3	5
20.1—40.0	12	13
40.1—60.0	12	11
60.1—80.0	14	13
80.1—100.0	13	9
> 100	44	38
Source of patients	Prenatal clinic	Infertility clinic

From macleod, J. and Gold, R. Z., *J. Urol.*, *66, 436, 1951.*

changes in sperm morphology following exposure, a baseline of semen quality should be established for each male. Changes detected in repeated measures could serve as indicators of potential mutagenic risk for each individual. Sperm morphology appears to be unaffected by frequency of ejaculation, in contrast to sperm number and motility. Studies of repeated semen analysis of the same individual have been reported in a few cases. In a study of six repeated measurements of 100 males, high variations in volume, number, and motility were found, while sperm morphology was identified as the most predictive and stable parameter for fertility.[114] The constancy of sperm morphology with time has been most clearly shown in a study where an individual with poor sperm morphology was followed for 11 years; the overall percentage of abnormal sperm and the relative types of abnormalities remained relatively constant.[119]

A few environmental agents have been studied for their effects on human sperm morphology. Lancranjan et al. found that the percentage of abnormal sperm in ejaculates from men working in a lead storage battery plant was directly proportional to blood lead values.[3] Significant levels of teratospermia were found in men with blood leads of 30 to 80 μg%. A study of spermatotoxic effects of cigarette smoking found that the percentage of abnormal sperm was directly related to the number of cigarettes smoked daily.[18] Significant differences were also found between semen of men who had smoked for more than 10 years and those who had smoked for shorter periods.

Although many studies have attempted to correlate semen quality with fertility, the extent to which abnormally shaped sperm participate in fertilization is unclear. In the mouse, the fraction of sperm with abnormal head shape remained unchanged in transit from the testis, through the epididymis and vas deferens, and into the uterus. The fraction of abnormally shaped sperm around the egg was greatly reduced, however.[120] Another study demonstrated that while midpiece and flagellar abnormalities inhibited progression of human sperm in vivo and in vitro, headshape abnormalities did not present a handicap to migration.[121] This suggests that sperm with abnormalities in headshape, but with normal motility and intact acrosomes, can still fertilize. Another significant issue is that abnormally shaped sperm may have mutations in genes specific for determining headshape which are expressed only during the latter stages of spermatogenesis. Mutation of other genes whose activities are essential for embryogenesis may not be picked up by screening for headshape abnormalities in sperm. Despite these uncertainties, the presence of high levels of abnormally shaped sperm is clearly indicative of mutagenic damage to sperm and potentially indicative of the possibility of adverse pregnancy outcome.

It is well established that normally shaped sperm containing defective genomes are capable of fertilizing an egg. Chromosome anomalies such as Down's syndrome, translocations, and mosaicisms have been transmitted paternally and have been associated with failure of conception, spontaneous abortion, and abnormal progeny.[122] In a review of this topic, Salisbury et al. state that spermatozoa bearing gross genome imbalances are capable of fertilizing eggs and that the evidence for fertility of heteroploid gametes is "massive and unequivocal".[89] Spermatozoa take part in fertilization in numbers proportionate to those reaching the egg, regardless of whether they bear a normal haploid genome or a grossly imbalanced genome. In fact, spermatozoa lacking any genetic competence can penetrate the egg and initiate cell division and parthenogenic development. Resulting embryos die in preimplantation stages of development. Thus, it appears that genetic makeup of sperm does not limit their fertility and that, regardless of genetic composition, each sperm has an equal opportunity to fertilize an egg. Selective pressures do exist, however, against sperm with grossly abnormal genomes during spermatogenesis as well as in the female reproductive tract. If mutated sperm do fertilize an egg, the final selective pressure is embryonic death. In the reproductive process, embryonic death can be viewed as the final check for elimination of genetic abnormalities. Those embryos inheriting mutated genes that do not impair survival can escape the selective pressure of embryonic death, complete development, and display structural and functional deficits at birth.

VIII. SUMMARY AND CONCLUSIONS

Little attention has been directed toward elucidating the sensitivity of the pregnant woman and embryo to reproductive toxicants in the work-place, and even less toward comparable indexes in the male. The information presented in this chapter indicates that male reproductive toxicity is a significant human health effect that requires considerably more attention than it has received. Efforts to protect the validity of the next generation from environmental agents must include examination of insult to both the male and female reproductive systems. Test methods do exist which are capable of yielding information on reproductive toxicants and their mode of action. Research priorities need to be established for wide-scale application of these test methods in human and laboratory animal studies.

A number of environmental agents and drugs are capable of causing male reproductive failure in laboratory animals and humans. Agents such as heavy metals, pesticides, solvents, food additives and contaminants, alkylating agents, antibiotics, and synthetic steroids have been shown to cause male sterility as well as adverse pregnancy outcome resulting from mutation of sperm. Comparison of laboratory animal and human data underlines the necessity for more intensive research efforts in this area. Reproductive outcome is rarely examined in relation to occupational and environmental exposure either in human clinical or laboratory animal studies.

Various mechanisms operating in normal and abnormal male reproductive function have been discussed. The main cellular constituents of the testis, Sertoli, Leydig, and germ cells, have been described, as well as the hormonal interaction of these cells with the pituitary in normal and infertile states. Elevations in FSH levels can be prognostic of specific damage to the germinal epithelium. The process of spermatogenesis occurs in distinct stages which are differentially sensitive to spermatotoxic agents. A blood-testis barrier, consisting of tight junctions between the basal compartment of Sertoli cells, exists which protects premeiotic germ cells from some toxic agents that enter the bloodstream.

Analysis of specific biochemical markers in seminal fluid can be diagnostic of the function of accessory glands in the male reproductive tract. Evidence exists for the excretion of some drugs in seminal fluid. Drugs in semen may influence motility and viability of sperm, as well as cause allergic and pharmacologic reactions in women exposed during intercourse. This may constitute a significant route of exposure for the female as well as the embryo.

Studies have been performed on the number of sperm in the ejaculate with the goal of establishing a range of sperm counts predictive of the potential to conceive. Levels of sperm below 10 to 20 million per milliliter of ejaculate are considered to be indicative of subfertility. The most stable and predictive semen parameter in prediction of fertility potential is sperm morphology. Sperm shape is highly heritable and species specific; mutagenic agents cause dose-dependent elevations in the percentage of abnormal sperm in the semen. Sperm abnormalities induced by mutagens can be passed on to subsequent generations. The extent to which morphologically and chromosomally abnormal sperm participate in fertilization has been discussed. Existing evidence suggests that these sperm are capable of fertilizing the egg, although selective factors operate to prevent them from reaching the egg. If mutated sperm do fertilize an egg, the most likely outcome is early embryonic death. Other, less frequent, outcomes include structural and functional deficits in the offspring.

REFERENCES

1. Anon., National Foundation/March of Dimes: Facts, National Foundation, New York, 1975.
2. Strobino, B. R., Kline, J., and Stein, Z., Chemical and physical exposure of parents: effects on human reproduction and offspring, *Early Human Dev.*, 1(4), 371, 1978.
3. Lancranjan, I., Reproductive ability of workmen occupationally exposed to lead, *Arch. Environ. Health*, 30, 396, 1975.
4. Department of Labor, OSHA, Occupational exposure to 1,2-dibromo-3-chloropropane (DBCP), *Fed. Reg.*, Part VIII, 45537, 1977.
5. American Society of Anesthesiologists, *Ad Hoc* Committee, Occupational disease among operating room personnel, *Anesthesiology*, 41(4), 321, 1974.
6. Tomlin, P. J., Teratogenic effects of waste anesthetic gases, *Br. Med. J.*, 108, 1046, 1978.
7. Infante, P. F., Wagoner, J. K., and Young, R. J., Chloroprene: Observations of Carcinogenesis and Mutagenesis, paper presented at a Workshop on Methodology for Assessing Reproductive Hazards in the Workplace, National Institute for Occupational Safety and Health, Society for Occupational and Environmental Health, Washington, D.C., in press.
8. Whorton, D., Krauss, R. M., Marshall, S., and Milby, T. H., Infertility in male pesticide workers, *Lancet*, 2(8051), 1259, 1977.
9. Donayre, J., Guerra-Garcia, R., Moncloa, F., and Sobrevilla, L. A., Endocrine studies at high altitude. IV. Changes in the semen of men, *J. Reprod. Fertil.*, 16, 55, 1968.
10. Fabia, J. and Thuy, T. D., Occupation of father at time of birth of children dying of malignant diseases, *Br. J. Prev. Soc. Med.*, 28, 98, 1974.
11. Infante, P. F., Occupational Hazards: Do They Extend Beyond Plant Boundaries? paper presented at the Air Pollution Control Association Specialty Conference on Toxic Substances in the Air Environment, Cambridge, Mass., November 7 to 9, 1976.
12. Lancranjan, I., Marcanescu, M., Rafaila, E., Klepsch, I., and Popescu, H. I., Gonadic function in workmen with long-term exposure to microwaves, *Health Phys.*, 29, 381, 1975.
13. Hueper, W. C., Testes and occupation, *Urol. Cutaneous Rev.*, 46(3), 140, 1942.
14. Popescu, H. I., Klepsch, I., and Lancranjan, I., Elimination of pituitary gonadotropic hormones in men with protracted irradiation during occupational exposure, *Health Phy.*, 29, 385, 1975.

15. Lushbaugh, C. C. and Casarett, G. W., The effects of gonadal irradiation in clinical radiation therapy. A review, *Cancer (Philadelphia)*, 37, 1111, 1976.

16. Harrington, J. M., Stein, G. F., Rivera, R. O., and Morales, A. V., The occupational hazards of formulating oral contraceptives — a survey of plant employees, *Arch. Environ. Health*, 12, 37, 1978.

17. Infante, P. F., Wagoner, J. K., McMichael, A. J., Waxweiler, R. J., and Falk, H., Genetic risks of vinyl chloride, *Lancet*, p. 734, 1976.

18. Viczian, M., Ergebnisse von Spermauntersuchungen bei Zigarettenrauchern, *Z. Haut. Geschlechtskr.*, 44, 183, 1969.

19. Donnelly, P. A. and Monty, D. E., Toxicologic effects of cadmium chloride on the canine testes following various routes of administration, *Toxicol. Lett.*, 1, 53, 1977.

20. McIntyre, J. D., Toxicity of methyl mercury for steelhead trout sperm, *Bull. Environ. Contam. Toxicol.*, 9(2), 98, 1973.

21. Lee, I. P. and Dixon, R. L., Effects of mercury on spermatogenesis studied by velocity sedimentation, cell separation and serial mating, *J. Pharmacol. Exp. Ther.*, 194(1), 171, 1975.

22. Waltscheva, V., Slateva, M., and Michailov, I. V., Testicular changes due to long-term administration of nickel sulfate, *Pathol. Exp.*, 6(8), 116, 1972.

23. Der, R., Fahim, Z., Yousef, M., and Fahim, M., Environmental interaction of lead and cadmium on reproduction and metabolism of male rats, *Res. Commun. Chem. Pathol. Pharmacol.*, 14(4), 689, 1976.

24. Leonard, A., Dernudt, G., and Linden, G., Mutagenicity tests with aflatoxins in the mouse, *Mutat. Res.*, 22, 137, 1974.

25. Cater, B. R., Cook, M. W., Gangolli, S. D., and Grasso, P., Studies on dibutyl phthalate-induced testicular atrophy in the rat: effects on zinc metabolism, *Toxicol. Appl. Pharmacol.*, 41, 609, 1977.

26. Singh, A. R., Lawrence, W. H., and Autian, J., Dominant lethal mutations and antifertility effects of di-2-ethylhexyl adipate and diethyl adipate in male mice, *Toxicol. Appl. Pharmacol.*, 32, 566, 1975.

27. Trigrul, S., Teratogenic effects of glutamic acid, *Arch. Int. Pharmacodyn. Ther.*, 153(2), 323, 1965.

28. Lacassagne, A., Buu-Hoi, N., Hurst, L., and Giao, N., Complete inhibition by *p*-hydroxyacetophenone of rat liver carcinogenesis by butter yellow, *C. R. Acad. Sci.*, 258(23), 5763, 1964.

29. Miyaji, T., Miyamoto, M., and Ueda, Y., Inhibition of spermatogenesis and atrophy of the testis caused by nitrofuran compounds, *Acta. Pathol. Jpn.*, 14(3), 261, 1964.

30. Albert, P. S., Salerno, R. S., Kapoor, S. N., and Davis, J. E., The nitrofurans as sperm-immobilizing agents, their tissue toxicity, and their clinical application in vasectomy, *Fertil. Steril.*, 26(6), 485, 1975.

31. Drause, W., Hamm, K., and Weissmuller, J., The effect of DDT on spermatogenesis of the juvenile rat, *Bull. Environ. Contam. Toxicol.*, 14(2), 171, 1975.

32. Torkelson, T. R., Toxicologic investigations of 1,2-dibromo-3-chloropropane, *Toxicol. Appl. Pharmacol.*, 3, 545, 1961.

33. Reznik, J. A., and Sprincan, G. K., Experimental data on the gonadotoxic effect of nemagon, *Gig. Sanit.*, 6, 101, 1975.

34. Shtenberg, A. I. and Rybakova, M. N., Effect of carbaryl on the neuroendocrine system of rats, *Food Cosmet. Toxicol.*, 6(4), 462, 1968.

35. Krause, W., Hamm, K., and Weissmuller, J., Damage to spermatogenesis in juvenile rats treated with DDVP and malathion, *Bull. Environ. Contam. Toxicol.*, 15(4), 458, 1976.

36. Etribi, A., Ibrahim, A., El-Haggar, S., Arvad, H., and Metaivi, B., Effect of Ambilhar (niridazole) on spermatogenesis in guinea pigs, *J. Reprod. Fertil.*, 48, 439, 1976.

37. Eroschenko, V. P., Alterations in the testes of the Japanese quail during and after the ingestion of the insecticide kepone, *Toxicol. Appl. Pharmacol.*, 43, 535, 1978.

38. Jackson, H. and Craig, A. W., Antifertility action and metabolism of hexamethylphosphoramide, *Nature (London)*, 212, 86, 1966.

39. Balentine, J. D., Pathologic effects of exposure to high oxygen tensions, *N. Engl. J. Med.*, 275(19), 1038, 1966.

40. Cattanach, B. M., Murray, I., and Tracey, J. M., Translocation yield from the immature mouse testis and the nature of spermatogonial stem cell heterogeneity, *Mutat. Res.*, 44, 105, 1977.

41. Ehling, U. H., Comparison of radiation and chemically-induced dominant lethal mutations in male mice, *Mutat. Res.*, 11, 35, 1971.

42. Mukherjee, D. P. and Singh, S. P., Effect of increased carbon dioxide in inspired air on the morphology of spermatozoa and fertility of mice, *J. Reprod. Fertil.*, 13, 165, 1967.

43. Van Thiel, D. H., Gavaller, J., and Lester, R., Alcohol is a direct testicular toxin, *Clin. Res.*, 23, 396, 1975.

44. Kalla, N. R. and Bansal, M. P., Effect of carbon tetrachloride on gonadal physiology in male rats, *Acta Anat.*, 91, 380, 1975.

45. Artamonova, V. G. and Klishova, Z. N., Pathogenesis of chronic carbon bisulphide poisoning, *Gig. Tr. Prof. Zabol.*, 10, 22, 1972.

46. Palazzola, R., McHard, J., Hobbs, E., Faucher, O., and Calandra, J., Investigation of the toxicological properties of a phenylmethylcyclosiloxane, *Toxicol. Appl. Pharmacol.*, 21, 15, 1972.

47. Nicander, L., Changes produced in the male genital organs of rabbits and dogs by 2,6,-*cis*-diphenyl-hexamethyl-cyclotetrasiloxane, *Acta Pharmacol. Toxicol.*, 36, 40, 1975.

48. Embree, J. W., Lyon, J. P., and Hine, C. H., The mutagenic potential of ethylene oxide using the dominant-lethal assay in rats, *Toxicol. Appl. Pharmacol.*, 40, 261, 1977.

49. Blijleven, W., Mutagenicity of four hair dyes in Drosophila melanogaster, *Mutat. Res.*, 48(2), 181, 1977.

50. Kripke, B., Kelman, A., Shah, N., Balogh, K., and Handler, A., Testicular reaction to prolonged exposure to nitrous oxide, *Anaesthesiology*, 44(2), 105, 1976.

51. Osterberg, R. E., Bierbower, G. W., and Hekir, R. M., Renal and testicular damage following dermal application of the flame retardant, Tris (2,3-dibromopropyl) phosphate, *J. Toxicol. Environ. Health*, 3, 979, 1977.

52. Turner, T. B., Mezey, E., and Kimball, A. W., Measurement of alcohol-related effects in man: chronic effects in relation to levels of alcohol consumption. *Johns Hopkins Med. J.*, 141, 235, 1977.

53. Macleod, J., The effects of antispermatogenic compounds in relation to human male infertility, *Fertil. Steril.*, 1, 347, 1950.

54. Shapiro, S., Slone, D., Hartz, S. C., Rosenberg, L., Siskind, V., Monson, R. R., Mitchell, A. A., and Heinonen, O. P., Anticonvulsants and parental epilepsy in the development of birth defects, *Lancet*, 1, 272, 1976.

55. Meyer, J. G., The teratological effects of anticonvulsants and the effects on pregnancy and birth, *Eur. Neurol.*, 10, 179, 1973.

56. Sieber, S. M. and Adamson, R. H., Toxicity of antineoplastic agents in man, chromosomal aberrations, antifertility effects, congenital malformations and carcinogenic potential, *Adv. Cancer Res.*, 22, 57, 1972.

57. Heller, C. G., Rowle, M. J., and Heller, G. V., Clomiphene citrate: a correlation of its effect on sperm concentration and morphology, total gonadotropins, ICSH, estrogen and testosterone excretion, and testicular cytology in normal men, *J. Clin. Endocrinol. Metab.*, 29, 638, 1969.

58. Heller, C. G., Flageolle, B. Y., and Matson, L. J., Histopathology of the human testes as affected by bis(dichloroacetyl) diamines, *Exp. Mol. Pathol. Suppl.*, 2, 107, 1973.

59. Gill, W. B., Schumacher, G. F., and Bibbo, M., Pathological semen and anatomical abnormalities of the genital tract in human male subjects exposed to DES in utero, *J. Urol.*, 117, 477, 1977.

60. Steinberger, E. and Smith, K. D., Effect of chronic administration of testosterone enanthate on sperm production and plasma testosterone, follicle-stimulating hormone , and luteinizing hormone levels: a preliminary evaluation of a possible male contraceptive, *Fertil. Steril.*, 28(12), 1320, 1977.

61. Bertazzoli, C., Chiele, T., Ferni, G., Ricevuti, G., and Solcia, E., Chronic toxicity of adriamycin: a new antineoplastic antibiotic, *Toxicol. Appl. Pharmacol.*, 21, 287, 1972.

62. Timmermans, L., Influence of antibiotics on spermatogenesis, *J. Urol.*, 112, 348, 1974.

63. Jackson, H., Fox, B., and Craig, A., The effect of alkylating agents on male rat fertility, *Br. J. Pharmacol.*, 14, 149, 1959.

64. Auerbach, C., Mutagenic effects of alkylating agents, *Ann. N.Y. Acad. Sci.*, 68(3), 731, 1958.

65. Tates, A. D. and Natarajan, A. T., A correlative study of the genetic damage induced by chemical mutagens in bone marrow and spermatogonia of mice. I. CNU-ethanol, *Mutat. Res.*, 37, 267, 1976.

66. Aaron, C. S. and Lee, W. R., Molecular dosimetry of the mutagen ethyl methanesulfonate in Drosophila melanogaster spermatozoa: linear relation of DNA alkylation per sperm cell (dose) to sex-linked recessive lethals, *Mutat. Res.*, 49, 27, 1978.

67. Fahmy, O. G. and Fahmy, M. J., Cytogenetic analysis of the action of carcinogens and tumor inhibitors in Drosophila melanogaster. VI. The mutagenic cell stage response of the male germ line to nitrogen mustards, *Genet. Res.*, 1, 173, 1960.

68. Rochrborn, G., Mutagenic action of trenimon in the male mouse, *Humangenetik*, 1, 576, 1965.

69. Binkert, F. and Schmid, W., Pre-implantation embryos of Chinese hamster. II. Incidence and type of karyotype anomalies after treatment of the paternal post-meiotic germ cells with an alkylating mutagen, *Mutat. Res.*, 46, 77, 1977.

70. Ericsson, R. J. and Youngdale, G. A., Male antifertility compounds: structure and activity relationships of U-5897, U-15, 646 and related substances, *J. Reprod. Fertil.*, 21, 263, 1970.

71. Swierstra, E. E., Whitefield, J. W., and Fook, R. H., Action of amphotericin B(fungizone) on spermatogenesis in the rabbit, *J. Reprod. Fertil.*, 7, 13, 1964.

72. Kabra, S. P. and Prasad, M. R., Effect of clomiphene on fertility in male rats, *J. Reprod. Fertil.*, 14, 39, 1967.

73. Neumann, F., von Berswordt-Wallrabe, R., Elger, W., and Steinbeck, H., Activities of antiandrogens. Experiments in prepuberal and puberal animals and in fetuses, in *Testosterone*, Tamm, J., Ed., Hafner, New York, 1968, 134.

74. Coulston, F., Beyler, A., and Drobeck, H., The biologic actions of a new series of bis(cichloroacetyl)-diamines, *Toxicol. Appl. Pharmacol.*, 2, 715, 1960.

75. King, T., Berliner, V., and Blye, R., Pharmacology of 2,4-dinitropyrroles — a new class of antispermatogenic compounds, *Biochem. Pharmacol.*, 12 (Suppl. 69), 218, 1963.

76. Kaufman, N., Klavins, J., and Kinney, T., Testicular damage following ethionine administration, *Am. J. Pathol.*, 32, 105, 1956.

77. Goldberg, G., Pfau, A., and Ungar, H., Testicular lesions following ingestion of DL-ethionine studied by quantitative cytologic method, *Am. J. Pathol.*, 35(2), 383, 1959.

78. Steinberger, E. and Sud, B. N., Specific effect of fluoroacetamide on spermiogenesis, *Biol. Reprod.*, 2, 369, 1970.

79. Smith, D. J. and Joffe, J. M., Increased neonatal mortality in offspring of male rats treated with methadone or morphine before mating, *Nature (London)*, 253, 202, 1975.

80. Joffe, J. M., Peterson, J. M., Smith, D. J., and Soyka, L. F. Sublethal effects on offspring of male rats treated with methadone before mating, *Res. Commun. Chem. Pathol. Pharmacol.*, 13, 611, 1976.

81. Hafez, E. S. E., Physio - anatomical parameters of andrology, in *Techniques of Human Andrology*, Hafez, E. S. E., Ed., Elsevier, Amsterdam, 1977, 39.

82. Dym, M., Raj, H. G., and Chemes, H. E., Response of the testes to selective withdrawal of LH and FSH usng antigonadotropic sera, in *The Testis in Normal and Infertile Men*, Troen, T. and Nankin, H. R., Eds., Raven Pjess, New York, 1977, 97.

83. Connell, C. J. and Connell, G. M., The interstitial tissue of the testis, in *The Testis*, Vol. 4, Johnson, A. D. and Gomes, W. R., Eds., Academic Press, New York, 1977, 333.

84. Setchell, B. P., Davies, R. V., and Main, S. J., Inhibin, in *The Testis*, Vol. 4, Johnson, A. D. and Gomes, W. R., Eds., Academic Press, New York, 1977, 190.

85. Dufau, M. L. and Means, A., Eds., *Hormone Binding and Target Cell Activation in Testis*, Plenum Press, New York, 1974.

86. Means, A. R., Mechanism of action of follicle-stimulating hormone (FSH), in *The Testis*, Vol. 4, Johnson, A. D. and Gomes, W. R., Eds., Academic Press, New York, 1977, 163.

87. Franchimont, P., Chari, S., Hazee-Hagelstein, M. T., Debruche, M. L., and Duraiswami, S., Evidence for the existence of inhibin' in *The Testis in Normal and Infertile Men*, Troen, P. and Nankin, H. R., Eds., Raven Press, New York, 1977, 253.

88. Braunstein, G. D. and Swerdloff, R. S., Effects of aqueous extracts of bull and rat testicles on serum FSH and LH in the acutely castrate male rat, in *The Testis in Normal and Infertile Men*, Troen, P. and Nankin, H. R., Eds., Raven Press, New York, 1977, 281.

89. Salisbury, G. W., Hart, R. G., and Lodge, J. R., The spermatozoan genome and fertility, *Am. J. Obstet. Gynecol.*, 128(3), 342, 1977.

90. Gomes, W. R., Chemicals affecting testicular function, in *The Testis*, Vol. 3, Johnson, A. D. and Gomes, W. R., Eds., Academic Press, New York, 1975, 485.

91. Fawcett, D. W., Leak, L. V., and Heidger, P. M., Electron microscopic observations on the structural components of the blood-testis barrier, *J. Reprod. Fertil.*, Suppl. 10, 105, 1970

92. Edwards, E. M., Jones, A.R., and Waites, G. M., The entry of a-chorohydrin into body fluids of male rats and its effect upon the incorporation of glycerol into lipids, *J. Reprod. Fertil*, 43, 225, 1975.

93. Okumura, K., Lee, I., and Dixon, R., Permeability of selected drugs and chemicals across the blood-testis barrier of the rat, *J. Pharmacol. Exp. Ther.*, 194, 89, 1975.

94. Waites, G. M., Fluid secretion, in *The Testis*, Vol. 4, Johnson, A. D. and Gomes, W. R., Eds., Academic Press, New York, 1977, 91.

95. Vitale, R., Fawcett, D. W., and Dym, M., The normal development of the blood-testis barrier and the effects of clomiphene and estrogen treatment, *Anat. Rec.*, 176, 333, 1973.

96. Dixon, R. L. and Lee, I. P., Possible role of the blood-testicular barrier in dominant lethal testing, *Environ. Health Perspect.*, 6, 59, 1973.

97. Neaves, W. V., The blood-testis barrier, in *The Testis*, Vol. 4, Johnson, A. D. and Gomes, W. R., Eds., Academic Press, New York, 1977, 126.

98. Lewin, L. M., Biochemical markers in human seminal plasma as a means of evaluating the functioning of the male reproductive tract, in *The Testis in Normal and Infertile Men*, Troen, P. and Nankin, H. R., Eds., Raven Press, New York, 1977, 505.

99. Polakoski, K. L. and Zaneveld, L. J., Biochemical examination of the human ejaculate, in *Techniques of Human Andrology*, Hafez, E. S. E., Ed., Elsevier, Amsterdam, 1977, 265.

100. Lutwak-Mann, C., Schmid, K., and Keberle, H., Thalidomide in rabbit semen, *Nature (London)*, 214, 1018, 1967.
101. Smith, D. J. and Joffe, J. M., Increased neonatal mortality in offspring of male rats treated with methadone or morphine before mating, *Nature (London)*, 253, 202, 1975.
102. Joffe, J. M., Peterson, J. M., Smith, D. J., and Soyka, L. F., Sublethal effects on offspring of male rats treated with methodone before mating, *Res. Commun. Chem. Pathol. Pharmacol.*, 13, 611, 1976.
103. Gerber, N. and Lynn, R. K., Excretion of methodone in semen from methodone addicts; comparison with blood levels, *Life Sci.*, 19, 787, 1976.
104. Swanson, B. N. and Gerber, N., Excretion of methadone into semen of rabbits, *Proc. West. Pharmacol. Soc.*, 20, 477, 1977.
105. Swanson, B. N., Leger, R. M., Gordon, W. P., Lynn, R. K., and Gerber, N., Excretion of phenytoin into semen of rabbits and man, *Drug Metab. Dispos.*, 6(1), 70, 1978.
106. Hessl, J. M. and Stamey, T. A., The passage of tetracyclines across epithelial membranes with special reference to prostatic epithelium, *J. Urol.*, 106, 253, 1971.
107. Malmborg, A., Dornbusch, K., Eliasson, R., and Lindholmder, C., Excretion of antibiotics into semen, *Proc. 9th Int. Congr. Chemother.*, 4, 53, 1976.
108. Peterson, R. N. and Freund, M., The inhibition of the motility of human spermatozoa by various pharmacologic agents, *Biol. Reprod.*, 13, 552, 1975.
109. Paladine, W. J., Cunningham, T. J., Donavan, M. A., and Dumper, C. W., Possible sensitivity to vinblastine in prostatic or seminal fluid,. *N. Engl. J. Med.*, 292, 52, 1975.
110. Ericsson, R. J. and Baker, V. F., Transport of oestrogens in semen to the female rat during mating and its effects on fertility, *J. Reprod. Fertil.*, 12, 381, 1966.
111. Macht, D. I., On the absorption of drugs and poisons through the vagina, *J. Pharmacol. Exp. Ther.*, 10, 509, 1918.
112. Hartman, C. G., The permeability of the vaginal mucosa, *Ann. N.Y. Acad. Sci.*, 83, 318, 1959.
113. MacLeod, J. and Gold, R. Z., The male factor in fertility and infertility. II. Spermatozoon counts in 1000 cases of known fertility and in 1000 cases of infertile marriage, *J. Urol.*, 66, 436, 1951.
114. Sherins, R. J., Brightwell, D., and Sternthal, P. M., Longetudinal analysis of semen of fertile and infertile men, in *The Testis in Normal and Infertile Men*, Troen, P. and Nankin, H. R., Eds., Raven Press, New York, 1977, 473.
115. Smith, K. D. and Steinberger, E., What is oligospermia? in *The Testis in Normal and Infertile Men*, Troen, P. and Nankin, H. R., Eds., Raven Press, New York, 1977, 489.
116. Wyrobek, A., Sperm shape abnormalities in the mouse as an indicator of mutagenic damage, in *The Testis in Normal and Infertile Men*, Troen, P. and Nankin, H. R., Eds., Raven Press, New York, 1977, 519.
117. Wyrobek, A. J. and Bruce, W. R., Chemical induction of sperm abnormalities in mice, *Proc. Natl. Acad. Sci. U.S.A.*, 72(11), 4425, 1975.
118. Wyrobek, A. J. and Bruce, W. R., The induction of sperm — shape abnormalities in mice and humans, in press.
119. MacLeod, J., The significance of deviations in sperm morphology, in *The Human Testis*, Rosenberg, E. and Paulsen, C. A., Eds., Plenum Press, New York, 1970, 481.
120. Krzanowska, H., The passage of abnormal spermatozoa through the uterotubal junction of the mouse, *J. Reprod. Fertil.*, 38, 81, 1974.
121. Clavert, A., Brun, B., and Bollecker, G., Teratospermie et Migration des Spermatozoides *in vitro* et *in vivo*, *C.R. Seances Soc. Biol. Paris*, 169, 1281, 1975.
122. Hembree, W. C., Fang, J. F., and Jagrillo, G., Meiotic abnormalities in male reproductive function, in *The Testis in Normal and Infertile Men*, Troen, P. and Nankin, H. R., Eds., Raven Press, New York, 1977, 25.

Chapter 7

LEGAL CONSIDERATIONS BEARING ON THE HEALTH AND EMPLOYMENT OF WOMEN WORKERS

Kathleen Lucas-Wallace

I. INTRODUCTION

In the earlier part of this century, women workers living in western countries were singled out as needing "special" laws to protect them from low wages and long hours. Since that time, protecting the health of working women has continued to be a focal point in controversies involving the working conditions and job opportunities afforded women. Regardless of the desires and capabilities of working women, legislators and employers have repeatedly sought to protect women's health and their working environment. The three most frequently cited exceptions to this historical trend are (1) the "Eastern" communist countries in which women are presumed to be equally capable of working at most jobs, (2) the Scandinavian countries which have made national commitments to the full integration of women into the workforce, and (3) all nations during wartime.

Some of the protections in the U.S. come in the form of Social Security, Worker's Compensation, the Occupational Safety and Health Act,[1] Title VII of the Civil Rights Act of 1964 (as amended),[2] Executive Order 11246 (as amended),[3] the Fair Labor Standards Act,[4] the Equal Pay Act,[5] the Age Discrimination in Employment Act,[6] the Toxic Substances Control Act,[7] and the Employee Retirement Income Security Act.[8] Virtually every aspect of working is touched by one of the many statutory provisions. In the U. S. today, most employment contracts carry an addendum of legislature protections and governmental regulations designed to protect workers and to equalize employment opportunities.

In the U.S., one of the first pieces of legislation enacted to protect the health of women workers was aimed at the textile industry. The statute was upheld as a proper health measure by Massachusetts Supreme Court in 1876.[9] Later, in 1908, the U.S. Supreme Court followed the same reasoning and upheld a maximum hours law for certain women workers.[10] Then in 1923, the Supreme Court struck down a minimum wage law which applied only to women, holding it to be a "violation of their constitutional right to freedom of contract."[11] In effect, the Court was saying women workers are entitled to "special" legislative treament for they must be protected from working long hours, but they are not entitled to be the only workers receiving a minimum wage. To this day, the Court has never clearly defined the statutory and constitutional protections afforded women. At best, the Court's reasoning in sex-related cases has been confusing and circuitous.

This disparity between the treatment of men and women was partially resolved when the Court recognized the constitutionality of protective labor laws for men as well as women.[12] However, it was not until the adoption of the Equal Pay Act of 1963 and Title VII of the Civil Rights Act of 1964 were distinctions among workers based on sex statutorily outlawed as prohibited discrimination. Under Title VII, state protective laws which distinguished between the sexes were declared illegal. Taken together, the federal statutes outlawed distinctions based on sex when sex was not a bona fide occupational qualification for the job. No longer could states or employers legally make arbitrary distinctions between men and women with respect to employment practices.

Through these acts, women were given their first legal weapons to rid their workplaces of discriminatory treatment. As a result, more cases charging sex discrimination against women workers have been ruled on by the Supreme Court since 1970 than at any other time in its history.

However, the issue of special protective policies for women workers was recently resurrected when employers laid off or fired women from jobs involving exposure to hazardous chemicals which are suspected caacinogens, teratogens, and mutagens. These private policies were never embodied in legislation. A growing controversy has arisen over their legality. The question is whether the exclusionary policies can be justified in light of equal employment laws and the Occupational Safety and Health Act (OSHAct).

Before examining the equal employment questions, let us look at other statutory provisions which affect the health of workers and which form the background for the recent exclusionary policies.

II. WORKER'S COMPENSATION

At this time in the U.S., Worker's Compensation is a state-regulated system by which employees who have suffered injuries arising in the course of employment are compensated for their loss of earning power and for certain medical expenses. Because each state has its own statute and judicial precedent, the acts differ in the type of injuries covered and in the maximum and minimum amounts of money awardable to any one worker. To clear up any questions about the act, Worker's Compensation covers women workers to the same extent as it covers men.

Federal regulation of Worker's Compensation is not a dead issue. In 1972 the National Commission on State Worker's Compensation Laws issued a report recommending that federal legislation be passed if in 3 years the states failed to bring their laws into compliance with the Commission's recommendations. Some federal legislation covering a limited number of occupations was passed when the Longshoremen's and Harbor Worker's Compensation Act was amended in 1972. However, no comprehensive action has yet been taken by Congress.

The philosophy behind Worker's Compensation is that accidents will happen in many workplaces even in the absence of fault. Such injuries may leave workers so disabled that they are unable to continue working. In order for workers and their families to avoid becoming destitute as well as to avoid protracted litigation on the question of fault, states have enacted laws which short-circuit the judicial process by providing for an efficient and timely hearing on the employee's right to receive compensation. The primary role of the government is to settle disputed claims. Otherwise, the compensation program is a private matter between workers, employers, and insurance carriers.

In some ways, Worker's Compensation resembles social insurance programs. For in the U.S., the compensation programs are funded solely by employer contributions. The system is based upon employer liability in the sense that employers bear the full burden of the Worker's Compensation programs. By contrast, in Germany the workers themselves purchase the right to receive compensation in the event of disablement. History elucidates the reasons for the difference.

Historically, the German guilds were the workers' protective organizations. They provided all types of benefit programs for their members, including disability plans. This is in contrast to the U.S. where liability had been contingent upon successful suits under the adversary system. Over the years, the German benefit programs continued to be supported by workers, while in the U.S. employers who were viewed as potentially liable under a negligence theory were appointed by legislators to bear the financial burden of the program.

In other ways, Worker's Compensation in the U.S. resembles tort law. One person is injured and another person pays a portion of the injured party's loss, but Worker's Compensation is very different from tort liability.

First, tort law is based upon negligence or fault. Theoretically, under state compensation statutes neither negligence nor fault is an issue which affects the amount of or the right to receive such compensation. As to the right to receive compensation, the critical factor is the worker's relationship to the accident and not the negligence of either party.

Second, the goal of tort liability is to make the plaintiff whole. Unlike tort law, compensation plans seek to provide regular support to workers and their families. The support is generally less than the injured workers' wages. Most laws limit the benefits to one half or two thirds of the employee's average weekly wage, unless that sum exceeds the maximum amount awardable under the act. Some statutes also have a minimum award which sometimes benefits low-paid workers.

The compensation is for cash wage loss and the majority of medical expenses. Statutes cover only injuries resulting in disabilities which prevent workers from continuing to labor at their present job or to earn income at the preaccident rate. Pain and suffering are not compensable. Further, awards are not based on need. The sum awarded reflects the worker's actual loss of support. Although many awards include a factor for the workers's family responsibilities, the extent of compensation is often quite limited.

These plans differ from other countries in notable ways. For example, in Britain and New Zealand benefits are related to the number of dependents, and temporary sickness and accident claimants are awarded a uniform sum. In Britain, once the award is determined for a permanent disability, it continues even if the worker holds another job. This scheme was adopted because they view the injury as diminishing the worker's health, strength, and pleasures in life. As compared to the American practice of reconsidering the award when the worker is again in an earning position, the British model takes on the characteristics of a pension rather than a wage-loss system.

An important aspect of Worker's Compensation is that it was not a natural outgrowth of Anglo-American common law. Rather, it represents the adoption of a social policy to ease the plight of injured workers. In the late 19th and early 20th centuries, the number of injuries was increasing. Simultaneously, employee recoveries in tort were rapidly decreasing when and if the litigation was ever concluded. Injured workers and their families were often penniless. Legislators recognized a need for reform so they designed compensation programs to decrease the costs of lawsuits and to increase the benefits for workers. In effect, employers' litigation expenses were reallocated to benefit employees. Over the years, legislators have expanded the coverge of the acts, but the system has remained largely unchanged through the passage of time.

In exchange for income insurance, compensation programs require that workers and their families relinquish their right to sue employers for injuries covered by the acts. However, not all injuries and not all occupations are covered by the state laws. First, the occupation must be described or listed in the act itself. If not, the employee is left to common law rights and remedies. Some acts limit coverage to hazardous jobs. Others provide for much broader coverage. An enormous body of case law exists on questions of coverage, e.g., whether a launderer in a hotel is considered to be working in a laundry for purposes of the act.

Secondly, the worker must be an employee and not an independent contractor.

Thirdly, the injury must have arisen out of the employment. In general, there are three types of risks: (1) risks directly related to the employment, (2) risks personal to the claimant, and (3) so-called neutral risks which are risks having no particular relationship to either the employment or the employee.

Those directly related to employment are uniformly compensable. Those related to personal risks are uniformly noncompensable. Those related to the neutral risks are the most controversial and the most litigated.

A majority of state courts have held that employment need not be the primary cause of the injury. It must only contribute to the harm. Under the first category of risks, the connection with employment is very clear and the risks result in the most common types of injury. Machinery malfunctioning, explosions, falling from high places, and occupational diseases which disable the worker are examples of the types of risks compensable under most plans.

The second category of risks which are personal to the claimant are those the employee would have suffered whether or not she was an employee. Natural death, non-occupational diseases, or heart failure are examples of personal risks which may not arise from employment. Litigation over this category is initiated when a worker's personal propensity for weakness is aggravated by her employment. For example, if a woman with a weak heart is faced with an employment emergency in which she must shut down the product line and in the process she suffers heart damage, should she be compensated? In general, the law does not inquire into the degree of causation. The only question asked is whether her employment contributed to the injury. If the answer is yes, compensation may be awarded.

The third category of risks are the most difficult to resolve because causation is not easily established by the worker. Traditionally, the employee bears the burden of proving an affirmative connection between the injury and her employment. For example, if a woman is working in a factory and she is hit by a piece of tin from someone's roof, should she be compensated for her loss? In the majority of states she could not recover because she could not prove a causal connection between the risks of her employment and her injury. A modern trend is developing which recognizes that the loss must fall on either the employee or the insurance fund. Under this theory, the worker is allowed to recover because "but for" the employment, the injury would not have occurred at that particular time and in that particular manner. The connection is made through the fact that the worker was performing her job at the time she suffered the injury.

In all compensation cases, the worker must have been disabled. Impotence alone has not been held compensable because there was no showing of its effect on the employee's earning capacity.[13] Many scholars believe the same resoning would be applied to a woman's claim for interference with her childbearing capacity. Therefore, under the weight of prior case law, damage to the reproductive capacity of male or female workers would not, by itself, be compensable under most Worker's Compensation laws.

Because an offspring is not an employee as defined by the acts, it would not have standing to claim compensation. The worker's offspring, like the uncovered employee, would be left to tort rights and remedies which require proof of employer negligence.

Although employers were recently required by Congress to treat pregnancy as a disability, the condition is not an employment disability within the meaning of Worker's Compensation. A substantial number of related issues have been addressed by the courts. These cases are discussed in the next section on equal employment opportunity.

III. POLICIES EXCLUDING CERTAIN CATEGORIES OF WORKERS

A. The Occupation Safety and Health Act (OSHAct) and The Toxic Substances Control Act

An international debate has emerged over the significance and the legal consequences of scientific evidence which indicates a relationship between exposure to certain substances and the capacity of workers to produce healthy offspring. The debate originally focused on women workers alone. Women were considered more significant because they are the childbearing sex.

However, similar effects on male reproductive capacity have gained recent recognition in the highly publicized cases of dibromochloropropane (DBCP) and kepone. In both instances, male workers were suffering from substantially reduced sperm counts, and some were sterile after 6 months of working with the chemical.

Further studies are being conducted to determine the reversibility of the injuries and the effect on the offspring of affected workers. These later studies move slowly because of the need to quantify parental exposure and observe the offspring during their procreative periods.

In the area of employment, the lag time between suspicions that a particular chemical might adversely affect workers or their offspring and confirmation of such injury by researchers and scientists has been troublesome. Lawyers who seek precise factual bases have been reluctant to enter the arena. Little litigation has been initiated because little hard data have been available on most agents. Lawyers have felt that the lack of widely accepted scientific data would present difficult evidentiary problems in proving a causal relationship between a chemical and the individual's injury.

Within the employer-employee sphere, the level of exposure to hazardous chemicals or toxins has not been a traditional subject of collective bargaining. Unions have bargained over high wages for hazardous jobs, but they have rarely negotiated on the extent of exposure. In many cases, unions have expected or depended upon governmental curtailment of excessive exposure.

The passage of the Occupational Safety and Health Act of 1970 (OSHAct) appeared to strengthen the government's enforcement posture. The broad enforcement powers of the OSHAct included, *inter alia:* (1) the establishment of the National Institute of Occupational Safety and Health (NIOSH) within the Department of Health, Education, and Welfare to conduct research on chemicals present in workplaces; (2) the delegation of authority to the Occupational Safety and Health Administration (OSHA) within the Department of Labor to issue standards which would bind all employers to specific levels of employee exposure and intake; and (3) the authority of the Secretary of Labor and OSHA to sue employers who violate the OSHAct or the standards issued pursuant to the Act.

Implementation of the legislative scheme has not been easy for OSHA. With the vast number of substances which some estimate to be over 20,000, individual standard setting would take decades. With the dearth of data on many chemicals and the lack of agreement among scientists on the safe levels of others, OSHA has struggled to reach a resolution on a few, widely used substances.

Administrator Eula Bingham's approach is to classify similar substances together. In an effort to issue one set of standards for several substances, she is undertaking to divide the chemical universe based upon common characteristics. If successful, this approach will reach many more workplaces than the single substance/single standard approach which OSHA has taken in the past.

To say that employers generally oppose OSHA is not an exaggeration. Reducing air levels or exposure levels will cost employers money. In some circumstances, such as with X-ray technicians, the cost of reducing the risk of radiation can be relatively inexpensive. With others, the cost of reducing exposure could be substantial. Employers generally have decried a new standard when the cost of reducing the hazard is predicted to be an ongoing expense. Employers are given no tax incentive to develop new technologies for reducing the risk. Therefore, the government has been acting alone in its efforts to compel the regulation of exposure through its limited litigation.

The inevitable antipathy between OSHA and employers has grown out of this lop-sided relationship. If the goal is to provide a safe and healthful workplace for all employees, employers need more incentive to incur the costs of research and development. Passage of the OSHAct alone has not been enough to ensure safe and healthful workplaces.

In 1976, Congress passed the Toxic Substances Control Act to encourage the development of adequate data on the effect of chemical substances and mixtures on health and the environment. The Act's policy is to regulate such chemicals "in such a manner as not to impede unduly or create unnecessary economic barriers to technological innovation." The Act specifically states that the development of the data "should be the responsibility of those who manufacture and those who process such chemical substances and mixtures...."[14] The Act authorizes the administrator to regulate such substances if there is presently an unreasonable risk of injury to health or the environment.

The scope of the Act is not limited to the use of toxins in the workplace. However, due to the presence of such substances in workplaces, the general regulation of chemicals under the authority of the Act will necessarily include regulation of chemical hazards in the working environment.

The Act does provide some reimbursement to those who conduct research and development pursuant to the administrative rules. The reimbursement provision is very limited in that claims submitted by the parties for their costs will be considered in light of the effect of the research on their competitive position. In effect, the Act's formula gives the administrator broad discretion in the award of costs and provides employers with little incentive to conduct their own research.

The Toxic Substances Control Act could complement the OSHAct. It certainly represents an important step toward providing manufacturers and processors with an economic incentive to conduct research and development on toxic agents.

In the past, when the Occupational Safety and Health Review Commission (OSHRC), OSHA's appellate body, was asked to consider whether the employers' costs to implement OSHA's standards exceeded the benefits, the Commission consistently held that the cost defense carries a very high burden of proof. Employers unsuccessfully argued before the commission that they had no funds to abate the hazard,[15] that compliance costs were greater than the costs of compensating injured employees,[16] that the implementation of the standard was too expensive[17] or impractical,[18] or that compliance costs would be borne by customers.[19]

A dramatic shift recently oocurred when the courts were faced with the argument that a justifiable cost-benefit analysis is a prerequisite to OSHA's promulgation of standards. In several important cases, two U.S. courts of appeal struck down OSHA's enforcement efforts when OSHA was unable to show a cost-benefit analysis and one court found one of the standards "affordable" to the regulated industry. Specifically, the Fifth Circuit after staying the enforcement of the benzene standard wrote:

OSHA must "assess the expected benefits in light of the burdens to be imposed by the standard. Although the agency does not have to conduct an elaborate cost benefit analysis . . . , it does have to determine whether the benefits expected from the standard bear a reasonable relationship to the costs imposed by the standard . . . The only way to tell whether the relationship between the benefits and costs of the benzene standard is reasonable is to estimate the extent of the expected benefits and costs . . . However, OSHA disclaimed any obligation to balance these costs against expected benefits . . .OSHA merely assumed that benefits from the reduction 'may be appreciable.' It based this assumption on a finding that benzene was unsafe at any level and its conclusion that exposures to lower levels of toxic materials would be safer than exposure to higher levels . . .[OSHA] contends . . .the standard promises appreciable benefits at a cost which industry can absorb. This justification is deficient in one crucial way; substantial evidence does not support OSHA's conclusion that benefits are likely to be appreciable. Without an estimate of benefits supported by substantial evidence, OSHA is unable to justify a finding that the benefits to be realized from the standard bear a reasonable relationship to its one-half billion dollar price tag.''[20]

The U. S. Supreme Court has granted certiorari in the benzene case. Hopefully, when the Court decides the case, it will set forth some guidelines on the cost-benefit question.

The basic issue which scholars and observers are now debating is the extent of authority delegated to the Secretary of Labor by the Act. Because the Act is relatively new and because chemical hazards which are now being documented may be costly to reduce or eliminate, the area is a hotbed of controversy.

New questions of informed consent, employer negligence, and unexpected tort liability have caused employers to adopt new policies to protect themselves from expensive lawsuits. These prophylactic policies have often drawn lines between male and female workers.

The distinctions which have been drawn in these policies appear to perpetuate the stereotype that women workers are more susceptible regardles of the scientific data or lack thereof on the particular substance. Some employers have excluded all women from jobs involving exposure to substances known or suspected of causing damage to the woman's reproductive capacity or to her offspring. In a few cases, women have been voluntarily sterilized and even then they have had to fight to keep their jobs.

Other employers have defined the excluded category as all women of childbearing age (usually 18 to 45 years), women of childbearing capacity, all pregnant women, or pregnant women at a particular time during their pregnancy. In the past year, pregnant women in the airline industry have sued to keep their jobs.[21] These cases involve the additional question of passenger safety.[22] Therefore, they are not rulings of general application. Nonetheless, these cases reflect the growing tension between the employment of women, the hazards of their workplaces, and the commitment of women to stay at their jobs.

Some employers in other industries, whose policies are soon to be tested in court, have excluded women workers from hazardous jobs based upon the possibility of reproductive injury while, at the same time, they have continued to employ men in jobs which expose them to hazardous substances in excess of the OSHA standard. Thus, on the one hand they are singling out women based upon protective health measures while, on the other hand, they are subjecting men to health risks in violation of an OSHA standard. This doube-edged position raises serious questions of discrimination against both sexes. From one point of view, women are denied employment; from another point of view, men are denied protection.

Many women view these so-called "health policies" as ways to keep women from gaining higher paying positions. On a more psychological level, working women adamantly reject the stereotypic view that they need more protection than men.

One breakthrough is now occuring within the union ranks. More and more unions are forming health and safety committees. They are becoming responsive to the laying off and firing processes being effectuated by employers as a result of the policy to exclude women. For example, the International Chemical Workers Union and the United Auto Workers have issued policies requiring employer justification for the adoption of an exclusionary policy and demanding negotiations on safety and health issues under certain circumstances. Local 1-5 of the Oil, Chemical, and Atomic Workers Union worked with the employer to confirm the cause of workers' sterility in the DBCP case.

Thus, we can perceive the dawning of a new era in occupational health. Workers and their representatives are beginning to ask more questions and make more demands regarding employee health policies. Like most other employment matters, there are many aspects to the complicated problems. Not the least of the factors are the workers' growing realizations that their inability to procreate healthy offspring, if they are capable of procreation at all, is related to the chemicals present in their workplaces.

The exclusion of women from workplaces has highlighted the problems, but men working with the same agents are beginning to fear the silent penalties that they, too, may be unknowingly paying. Men worry that their offspring may be found to have suffered carcinogenic or mutagenic effects as a result of their exposure. They are learning that even if they do not suffer from the damage themselves, the carcinogenic and mutagenic effects may not appear until after the next generation is born.

Recently there was a case in New Mexico in which a laboratory worker sued the Unversity of California and the Los Alamos Scientific Laboratory under the state's occupational disability and disease law. For 30 years the plaintiff had shaped uranium 235 and 238 into special-order devices. He had a number of ailments, including severe headaches and liver, hearing, and cancer of the eye problems. According to the testifying psychiatrist, he had a disabling anxiety neurosis caused by his occupational environment. His neurotic fear was that radiation would kill him. The court found that the neurosis was a disease and that the plaintiff was disabled by the disease. The judge ruled in favor of the worker and awarded the maximum benefit under the state's disability statute.[23]

This case is precedent setting. The facts demonstrate the increasing awareness of workers who are routinely exposed to hazardous substances. Women have been excluded from some jobs and men are often not adequately protected. The unavoidable legal question is who is suffering the discriminatory treatment — men who are not protected or women who have lost their jobs?

On the governmental level, OSHA is meeting with the agencies enforcing employment nondiscrimination laws[24] in an effort to determine a uniform policy. In the spring of 1977, OSHA held hearings on the proposed lead standard and requested testimony on "...groups with increased susceptibility to lead in the working population, such as women of childbearing age...."[25]

The four most controversial aspects which were addressed are (1) whether the standard and monitoring requirements should be set at a level and in a manner which protect all workers, including pregnant and potentially pregnant workers; (2) whether OSHA has the authority to require job reassignment and rate-retention without loss of seniority for all workers whose lead blood levels exceed that which is safe for them or their offspring; (3) whether the OSHAct should be read together with the Title VII of the Civil Rights Act of 1964; and (4) whether the OSHAct General Duty Clause,[26] independent of the issuance of an OSHA standard, requires employers to reduce the amount of toxins in the air or the amount of exposure to a level which protects male and female workers and perhaps the workers' progeny.

Those asserting OSHA jurisdiction argue that the stated purpose of the Act is "to assure so far as possible every working man and woman in the nation safe and healthful working conditions."[27] The Act further provides for the development of standards based upon "medical criteria which assure insofar as practical that no employee will suffer diminished health, functional capacity, or life expectancy as the result of his work experience."[28]

They maintain that the Act requires the Secretary of Labor to promulgate through rule making procedures, "any national consensus standard and any established federal standard unless [it is determined] that the promulgation of such a standard would not result in improved safety or health for specifically designated employees."[29] If a conflict in standards occurs, the Secretary may promulgate a single standard which "assures the greatest protection of the safety or health of the affected employees."[30] Although Section 655(a), cited immediately above, does not directly regulate the promulgation of standards for toxic materials or harmful physical agents,[31] it suggests that, at least in certain circumstances, it may be appropriate to establish a single "lowest common denominator" standard which assures "the greatest protection" for affected employees.

In dealing with toxins, the most pertinent section of the Act reads: "In promulgating standards dealing with toxic materials or harmful physical agents, under this subsection... [the Secretary] shall set the standard which most adequately assures, to the extent feasible, on the basis of the best available evidence, that no employee will suffer material impairment of health or functional capacity even if such employee has regular exposure to the hazard dealt with by such standard for the period of his working life."[32]

The major disagreement is over the meaning of the term "feasible." The Review Commission and the courts have construed the term to include technological feasibility as well as economic considerations which have a very high burden of proof.[33] No clear test has been adopted by either OSHA or the courts, but hopefully when the Supreme Court rules on the challenge to the benzene standard, it will give some guidance on the relative weight of cost arguments. Whether the court will find the cost of compliance more expensive than health considerations is a matter of conjecture. What can be said with some certainty is that cost will continue to be a hotly disputed factor.

Supporters of a comprehensive lower standard for air or exposure levels argue that the Act's General Duty Clause mandates full protection for all employees. The clause reads in pertinent part: "(a) Each employer shall — (1) furnish to each of his employees employment and a place of employment which is free from recognized hazards that are causing or likely to cause death or serious physical harm to his employees...."[34]

There is disagreement on the meaning and significance of the clause. Based upon the legislative history, courts have generally ruled that the duty is imposed only when the condition is a "recognized hazard," as "...matter for objective determination ... regardless of whether ... the particular employer is aware of it."[35]

As applied to the exclusion of one sex based on the presence of toxins in the workplace, if a court found: (1) that such exposure was a recognized hazard or that the particular employer had actual knowledge of the hazard, (2) that the excluded class of women was protected by the Act, and (3) that it was "feasible" for the employer to provide a safe and healthful workplace for the women, then the court would find the employer to be in violation of the General Duty Clause.

There are evidentiary problems in establishing the elements. Most cases would turn on the employer's knowledge of the hazards or on the feasibility of protecting employees. Arguing that OSHA has not yet issued a standard establishing a threshold level value (TLV) or that OSHA has issued one which protects only adults, the employer would try to deny that the hazard is one which is "recognized". However, the employer might suffer repercussions from asserting the OSHA defense in a later suit brought under EEO laws. For in an employment discrimination suit, the employer would want to prove that the exclusion of women is based upon a widely recognized danger to potentially pregnant women in order to justify discriminatory treatment. OSHA dealt with these questions when they issued the final regulations on lead. These regulations are very controversial and are the subject of several studies around the country.

Litigation was inevitable because all the parties feel they have a great deal to gain and a great deal to lose. Their positions are so clear because employers have not been financially motivated to assume the responsibility themselves. They are acting from a defensive position because Congress has not encouraged them to take the offensive. Meanwhile, employees who are now paying the penalties are losing their health or, if they are female, their jobs. OSHA will be determining its role in the conflict. Hopefully, Congressional interest will result in a tax incentive for employers in order to better balance the interests of the parties.

B. The Equal Employment Opportunity Aspect

Women workers have been excluded from jobs involving exposure to substances suspected or known to cause injury to their reproductive capacity or to their offspring. Employers have defended their actions on grounds of prospective tort liability, the alleged economic or technological infeasibility of eliminating the risk, and the humanitarian concern for the health of future generations. Women workers view the exclusions as prohibited discriminatory policies and as violations of the right to a safe and healthful workplace.

Some policies or their implementation will be found illegal; others may survive a challenge. The important point is that no general statement is applicable to all circumstances. Each company's policy must be viewed in light of the chemical creating the risk and its known effects. Each policy's implementation and the degree to which it adversely affects a category of workers must be compared to other policies adopted and applied by the company. In addition, the general compliance posture of the company can often determine its success or failure in a challenge against a single policy.

No one factor is the key to determining the validity of a particular policy. A number of factors will influence the result. It is the combination of factors which determines whether the policy or its implementation constitutes a violation of equal employment law.

First, one must ask who is excluded and why have they been excluded? Second, how has the policy been implemented?

When defining classes of excluded employees, employers do so based on distinctions such as sex, age, status, reproductive capacity, and toxic blood levels. Each distinction must be justified by the employer. The proffered justifications must be based upon accurate assumptions regarding each characteristic, and each characteristic must be related to job performance.

For example, if an employer excludes all women from jobs involving exposure to DBCP and assigns men to those jobs, the employer must show through comparative evidence that female workers are treated differently from male workers because women, and not men, are susceptible to the risk. Further, the employer must demonstrate the absence of "acceptable alternative policies or practices which would accomplish the business purpose advanced, or accomplish it equally well with a lesser differential ... impact."[36]

Courts would require proof that women could not be adequately protected and that men are free from similar risks. The company must introduce adequately researched and documented evidence. Mere speculation would not be sufficient to defeat an employment discrimination charge.

Therefore, a court would be looking to the type of job, the extent of exposure, the nature of the substance, its effect on both sexes, the scientific data supporting the exclusion, and the alternatives available to lessen the impact on the excluded sex. When considering the alternatives, most courts would scrutinize the protective measures available, the possibilities for temporary or permanent reassignments, and the degree of risk imposed on all employees. Thus, in the DBCP example above, scientific research indicates that men working with the substance for over 6 months may suffer sterility and perhaps carcinogenic effects. Therefore, the exclusion of only women would not be justified by the employer. Consequently, an employment discrimination charge would be upheld.

The Equal Employment Opportunity Commission (EEOC) has issued two decisions on forced resignations of pregnant X-ray technicians. In both cases, employers defended their actions on grounds of possible radiation risks to the unborn children. The Commission found the required resignations to be prohibited employment practices. Holding that less discriminatory alternatives were available and that such alternatives did not interfere with the safe and efficient operation of the businesses, the Commission required one employer to reassign the employee and the other to grant a temporary leave. The Commission reached its decisions by comparing the employers' treatment of similarly situated male and female employees.[37] Thus, when evaluating the necessity for an exclusion, decision makers compare prior practices and weigh the comparative risks and protective measures in addition to weighing the benefit and hardship to the employer and the employee.

Comparing the practices a company has followed in implementing the challenged policy and prior policies, a court would determine whether an employer had treated an excluded class of workers in the same way as other excluded classes. This principle of employment discrimination has become known as the disparate treatment theory. The theory allows a court to infer sex discrimination when similar classes of workers are treated in a disparate manner and the employer has no sex-neutral explanation for such treatment.

For example, if an employer fired all women who worked with a hazardous substance based on evidence that women could not be safely exposed to the chemical but reassigned all men whose blood levels exceeded that which is safe, an employer could be found to be treating similarly situated women and men differently becuse all workers for whom exposure is unsafe had not been treated in a similar manner. Such differential treatment would tend to prove that the company had violated equal employment laws. Therefore, adopting the disparate treatment theory, a court would infer that the company had engaged in sex discrimination.

Taking the example one step further, if the evidence used by the employer supported only the exclusion of pregnant women but the employer fired all women from jobs involving exposure to the particular substance and reassigned men whose blood level exceeded that which is safe, then the employer would be guilty of discrimination on two counts. First, as to those women who are incapable of becoming pregnant, no grounds exist for excluding them from such jobs. Therefore, a strong discrimination case can be made in favor of the excluded class of women workers who are not susceptible to the effects of the hazardous substance. Second, pregnant women for whom exposure is unsafe as compared to men for whom exposure is unsafe have been discriminated against because they too have not been similarly reassigned to nonhazardous jobs.

The essence of the test is whether an employer can justify making distinctions which adversely affect one sex and whether an employer has treated similarly situated employees in a similar manner. The policy and its implementation are proper subjects for charges of illegal discrimination. Thus, in determining a policy's legality, employer justifications for the policy are considered on their own merits in terms of the known and unknown risks as well as in comparison to the company's overall employment practices.

A third question which must be asked is whether those who are assigned to high-risk jobs are being adequately protected. Today, some companies which refuse to place women in certain jobs based on so-called "health policies" are assigning men to work in other parts of the plants in jobs which expose them to substances in excess of the OSHA standard for safe exposure. The double-edged argument would tend to defeat a company's creditability in a private discrimination suit where the employer was asserting protectiveness as his only defense. Certainly in a governmental enforcement action, the employer would necessarily lose on at least the OSHAct or the discrimination count, if not on both.

Fourth, one must ask what is the employer's motive? Recent constitutional cases[38] which have been analogized to equal employment cases have held that effect alone may not be sufficient to sustain a discrimination charge. The Supreme Court has not given much guidance in determining the test for motivation, but certainly a specific exclusion of only one sex indicates a clear intention to exclude that sex from certain areas of employment. Within this context, the question becomes whether the employer has a discriminatory intent. The question cannot be answered without considering the facts of each case, but many companies will fight this issue by asserting the "necessity" for the exclusion of women. The success of their defense will depend on the feasibility of reducing the level of exposure and the alternatives available for reducing the degree of risk.

A fifth question is whether a union has aided or abetted in the adoption or implementation of the policy. Title VII and Executive Order 11246, as amended, allow suits against parties who have aided in an employer's discrimination against certain categories of workers. Through the collective bargaining process or other forms of approval, a union can be found liable for discrimination if the union was a participant in the formulation or effectuation of a discriminatory policy.

The possibility for union liability has prompted unions to recognize their obligation to represent women union members. An increasing number of unions are beginning to address the issues forthrightly. Although company health policies brought attention to women workers, union involvement has occasioned the disclosure of similar risks suffered by men. Many newly formed union health and safety committees have encouraged increased union activity in this area.

Finally, one must ask whether there has been an invasion of personal privacy. Women and men alike have been reluctant to submit to pregnancy and sperm tests on a regular basis. From a legal point of view, the privacy questions associated with compulsory testing are perhaps the most vague and difficult. Where does informed consent begin and liability end? How regularly or extensively can companies test employees? What tests are permissible? Can employment be conditioned upon employee testing?

The answers to the above questions lie in shades of gray. No legal conclusions have been established in the privacy field. However, in adopting a testing policy, privacy considerations cannot be ignored by any employer.

The legal significance of the exclusionary policies re arding women bear on discrimination allegations because an employer is, in effect, stating that only men are qualiied to work with particular substances. Sex is, thereby, made an occupational qualification for those jobs involving exposure to the identified chemicals. Employers who hire only men will seek to justify their actions by alleging that men's higher tolerance level constitutes a bona fide oocupational qualification (BFOQ). Section 703(e) of Title VII provides that: "... it shall not be an unlawful employment pracice ... to admit or employ any individual ... on the basis of ... sex ... in those certain instances where ... sex ... is a bona fide occupational qualification reasonably necessary to the normal operation of that particular enterprise."[39]

EEOC and the courts[40] have narrowly interpreted the applicability of the BFOQ defense in discrimination cases. The defense has been raised in other situations and has been upheld when sexual identification is an integral factor in the manufacturing or marketing of the business product. For example, a male model could be necessary to model male clothing.

Traditionally, BFOQ arguments have rarely prevailed. Like the business necessity defense, which is essentially a cost defense, the BFOQ defense does not usually come into play until there is a finding or an admission of discrimination.[41] The leading case articulating one view of the BFOQ defense recognized that the exception could be valid if the employer had "... a factual basis for believing that all or substantially all women would be unable to perform safely and efficiently the duties of the job involved."[42] The court in that case specifically rejected stereotypic chaacterizations[43] because it found that the required ability was not dependent on sexual identification and "... that using these class stereotypes denies desirable positions to a great many women perfectly capable of performing the duties involved."[44] In addition, other courts have rejected BFOQ defenses when the critical factor was "the physiological capabilities of individual employees"[45] or "the physical capabilities and endurance"[46] of employees rather than sex.

It would be hard to construct a winning BFOQ defense to the exclusion of all women because BFOQs have been recognized only when related to the employee's ability to perform a particular job and not the employee's personal safety on that job. In addition, most evidence indicates that men are also affected whenever toxins are identified as affecting women who have no childbearing capacity.

What about women who are capable of bearing children? This brings us to the question of whether pregnancy or childbearing capacity is a sex-based characteristic. Most people are surprised by the question because we all know that only women become pregnant.

However some lawyers and judges have a different view of pregnancy and sex characteristics. In the landmark U.S. Supreme Court case of *Gilbert* v. *General Electric*, Justice Rehnquist, writing for five justices, held that there are "... pregnant women and nonpregnant persons ...."[47] This distinction was perpetuated in the recent case of *City of Los Angeles, Department of Water and Power* v. *Manhart*.[48] In the area of employment, the Court has viewed pregnant women as having "a special physical disability"[49] which is not gender based. The Court has twice stated that pregnant women are different from nonpregnant persons in that "... the first group is exclusively female [and] the second includes members of both sexes."[50] The Court has never recognized that some "nonpregnant persons" may become "pregnant women", thereby losing some of the protections afforded the "nonpregnant persons" class. The Court has presumed pregnancy to be a "voluntary and desired condition."[51]

The Court's legalistic and theoretical base pretends that the distinction between the two groups is grounded on the identifiable and static characteristic of pregnancy, even though only women transverse the line of demarcation between the two categories. Consequently, the Court views all women's reproductive status and capability as having the characteristics of a few women.

The Court's opinions in *Gilbert* and *Manhart* obfuscate the Court's test in determining sex discrimination. Justice Blackmun's partial concurrence in *Manhart* best summarizes legal experts' confusion over the Court's rulings. He wrote: "The Court's distinction between the present case and *General Electric* — that the permitted classes there were 'pregnant women and nonpregnant persons,' both female and male, ante, p. 12 — seems to me to be just too easy. .... [F]or me, it does not serve to distinguish the case on any principled basis .... I feel, however, that we should meet the posture of the earlier cases head-on and not by thin rationalization that seeks to distinguish but fails in its quest."[52]

A general knowledge of the statutory and constitutional history of sex discrimination is critical to an understanding of the consequences of the 1976 and 1978 rulings. Title VII prohibits an employer, labor union, or employment agency from discriminating in employment on the basis of sex. Executive Order 11246, as amended, similarly prohibits federal contractors from adopting discriminatory policies and practices and requires Federal contractors to take affirmative action to ensure equal employment opportunity.[53]

By statute, equal employment laws are to be consistently construed.[54] Therefore, in general, the interpretations[55] and regulations[56] issued under both laws prohibit the same discriminatory policies and practices. Title VII and the Executive Order are applicable to the exclusion of pregnant women and women of childbearing capacity if the courts reach the threshold determination that any aspect of the particular exclusionary policy or its implementation is sex-based discrimination.

Many scholars once predicted that the Supreme Court would find the Title VII test for discrimination more stringent than the 14th Amendment tests under the Constitution. They began with the argument that Congress had specifically outlawed particular types of discrimination as compared to the Constitutional amendments which were designed to reach official action. They based their theory on a line of cases which held that Congress could legislate stricter requirements than those required by the constitutional standard.[57] Despite the fact that plaintiffs continue to include the argument in their briefs, the Supreme Court has repeatedly rejected that construction of Title VII in pregnancy cases. By analogy, the Court has applied the reasoning of the constitutional tests to Title VII cases. Therefore, a plaintiff alleging sex discrimination does not necessarily benefit by suing under Title VII as compared to a suit under the Constitution.

The first series of cases on pregnancy-related issues began about 8 years ago when courts were asked to consider the mandatory leave policies for pregnant teachers. The issues were finally resolved in the 1974 companion cases of *LaFleur* and *Cohen*.[58] There, the Supreme Court considered the question of whether a school board could constitutionally require every pregnant teacher to take maternity leave, without pay, at a specified time before and after her pregnancy, regardless of her ability to work.

The Court concluded that "... the arbitrary cut-off embodied in the mandatory leave rules ... [had] no rational relationship to the valid state interest of preserving continuity of instruction."[59] Finding a violation of the Due Process Clause of the 14th Amendment rather than a right to employment or an equal protection violation as pleaded, the Court invalidated the policies and held that "the rules contain no irrebuttable presumption of physical incompetency, and that the presumption applies even when medical evidence as to an individual woman's physical status might be wholly to the contrary."[60]

The Court based its opinion of the personal nature of pregnancy on the principle that "... the ability of any particular pregnant woman to continue to work past any fixed time in her pregnancy is very much an individual matter."[61] In a footnote, the Court recognized that the school board could require medical certification of fitness for duty as an alternative to the compulsory leave policy,[62] but the issue was not directly before the Court in *LaFleur* or *Cohen*.

In a second line of cases, women challenged the exclusion of pregnany and pregnancy-related disabilities from coverage under disability plans provided by a state and by an employer. The California plan was challenged as unconstitutional (*Geduldig* v. *Aeillo*),[63] and the later suit against General Electric was brought pursuant to Title VII (*Gilbert* v. *General Electric*).[64] The Supreme Court upheld the exclusion in both cases.

Relying on *Aeillo*, Justice Rehnquist's majority opinion in *Gilbert* stated without further explanation, that "pregnancy is of course confined to women, but it is in other ways different from the typical covered disease of disability."[65] He wrote that "an exclusion of pregnancy from a disability benefits plan providing general coverage is not a gender-based discrimination at all."[66] The essence of the ruling is that the plaintiffs never proved sex-based discrimination under any established standard. The Court reasoned that no discrimination was proven, because there was "no risk from which women are protected and men are not."[67] The core of the opinion is that as to those risks covered by the plan, both men and women are treated with complete equality.

In both *Aeillo* and *Gilbert,* the Court rejected the argument that because only women become pregnant, the exclusion of pregnancy has a disparate impact upon women. In *Gilbert,* the Court ignored the fact that women were not covered for other pregnancy-related disabilities during the period of their pregnancy or subsequent to childbirth. Thus, viewing the exclusion of pregnancy per se as a sex-neutral classification, the Court denied relief.

In a recent case,[68] the Supreme Court ruled that women employees could not be denied their accumulated seniority when they returned from pregnancy leave so long as men who were out on a disability leave did not suffer the same loss. The Court held the policy had a discriminatory impact because it deprived women of employment opportunities and adversely affected their status as employees.

In the same case, the Court rejected allegations of discrimination in the employers' denial of sick pay leave to pregnant employees, even though men are uniformly given such leave for male-related disabilities. Returning to the reasoning of the *Gilbert* case, the Court held that the policy was neutral on its face because women were not denied any benefits afforded to men. The Court again refused to link pregnancy with sex-based characteristics, and it imposed on women plaintiffs the burden of proving that the exclusion of pregnancy is a mere pretext "designed to effect an invidious discrimination against the members of one sex ...."[69]

Therefore, the apparent burden in pregnancy-related cases brought under the Constitution or Title VII is to demonstrate that, regardless of pregnancy, women are treated differently from similarly situated men. The difficulty in meeting this high burden arises from the Court's refusal to equate pregnancy or pregnancy-related disabilities with male disabilities for purposes of comparison. This seems to be particularly true when the issue involves money. The circuitry of their reasoning begins and ends with their adherence to the uniqueness of pregnancy and their refusal to link pregnancy and sex classifications.

Some believe that the Court has returned to a sex-plus theory whenever the sex-based question involves pregnancy. It may be that the only way to make sense out of the cases is to recognize the Court's reluctance to find discrimination when cost is introduced as a factor in pregnancy questions. The cost theory was recently supported by the ruling in the *Manhart* case.[70] There, the Court found discrimination in requiring women to contribute more to the pension fund than men, but denied retroactive relief to women workers because it could jeopardize "the insurer's solvency and, ultimately, the insureds' benefits."[71] Regardless of the Court's motives, these rulings will be applied in any litigation over the exclusion of women from certain jobs due to their childbearing potential.

Within this context, it is easy to foresee the development of several lines of cases which have different tests because of the variance in known risks, or each case may be one of first impression because prior case law will need to be continually reinterpreted as scientists and researchers introduce new evidence on known and unknown risks.

In any event, viewed in light of *Gilbert* and subsequent rulings, proving similarity of risks will be difficult because so few scientific studies have been adequately docu-

mented. The early cases may turn on the similarity of treatment among highly susceptible men and women with the increased susceptibility of women being defined as their
childbearing capacity, a class definition which will certainly be challenged by an affected class of women plaintiffs.

In October, 1978, Congress amended Title VII to require employers to treat pregnancy and related medical conditions the same as other disabilities. In doing so, the
holding of *Gilbert* was legislatively reversed. However, the reasoning of *Acillo* and
Gilbert still stands as precedent for pregnancy-related discrimination suits. Women
workers would be a step closer to enjoying equal employment opportunity.

In summary, the trend of future litigation in the health area will depend upon the
influence of the factors discussed above: the employee composition, the substance, the
extent of the harm, the policy — its support and implementation. No one can predict
how the issues will be finally resolved by the government or the courts. However, we
can be sure that the matter will not be resolved for several years.

IV. HOURS AND WAGES: THE FAIR LABOR STANDARDS ACT AND THE EQUAL PAY ACT

No discussion on women workers would be complete without mentioning the Fair
Labor Standards Act and the Equal Pay Act. Together, they add an important dimen-
sion to understanding the extent and nature of the governmental regulation of working
conditions.

The Fair Labor Standards Act (FLSA) establishes standards for minimum wage,
overtime pay, recordkeeping, and child labor. Although there is no provision for maximum or minimum hours, regulations of overtime pay has the effect of regulating
working hours.

Originally passed in 1938 when unemployment was widespread and business was
experiencing a depression, the Act has been amended a number of times over the years.
One significant amendment is the Equal Pay Act of 1963.

Unlike the state protective laws, the FLSA never made distinctions between male
and female workers. The Act has always been one of general application so long as
the employer met the coverage requirements.

The Equal Pay Act incorporates the coverage and enforcement provisions of the
FLSA. As a separate statute, the EPA prohibits wage differentials based solely on sex.
The EPA requires covered employers to pay equal wages to male and female employees
working in the same establishment and performing "equal work on jobs, the performance of which requires equal skill, effort, and responsibility, and which are performed
under similar working conditions."[73]

These Acts are good examples of the type of legislative formula which may be appropriate in regulating equal employment in light of chemical hazards. Certainly, the
OSHAct has the specific mandate to issue standards which ensure a safe and healthful
environment for every worker. Regardless of the course of events, a specific amendment requiring employers to practice equal employment opportunity by making the
workplace safe for everyone, including certain highly susceptible categories of workers,
might become necessary to ensure employment opportunity for women.

V. AGE AND RETIREMENT

A. Age Discrimination in Employment

The Age Discrimination in Employment Act (ADEA) prohibits discrimination in
employment based upon age with respect to employees between 40 and 70 years of

age. The same standards as those applied under Title VII have been judicially applied to suits brought under the ADEA. The full range of employment practices are covered including, *inter alia*, employment advertising, refusals to hire, decisions to fire or lay off, employment agency referrals, and other terms and conditions of employment.

Labor organizations and employment agencies as well as employers are subject to the prohibitions of the Act. The general test for finding discrimination is whether age was a factor in making the decision or taking the challenged action. Upon termination of a 60-day notice issued by the Equal Employment Opportunity Commission (EEOC), either the EEOC or the aggrieved party may sue to enforce the rights protected by the Act.

B. Pensions, Life Insurance, and Other Fringe Benefits

For decades, women have faced arbitrary distinctions in the receipt of fringe benefits when such distinctions could be supported by statistical evidence. Title VII and the Equal Pay Act declared such distinctions illegal when they were based solely on the employee's sex. However, not until the recent and landmark case of the *City of Los Angeles, Department of Water and Power et al. v. Manhart et al.*, which denied employers the right to require female employees to make larger contributions to pension funds than their male counterparts in order to receive equal benefits, were the subtle distinctions in fringe benefits identified by the courts as sex-based discriminatory practices.

Prior to *Manhart*, some "defined benefit" plans required women workers to make additional contributions because women on the average live longer than men on the average. This actuarial equivalency was based on the presumption that after retirement the average woman would receive the monthly benefits for several years longer than the average man. In many plans, no adjustment was made for joint and survivor options under which the female spouses of male employees are likely to have greater life expectancies than the male spouses of female employees.

The U.S. Supreme Court found these plans violative of Title VII and the Equal Pay Act because: (1) such plans "classify employees in terms of ... sex which tend to preserve traditional assumptions about groups rather than thoughtful scrutiny of individuals";[74] (2) the plan failed to allocate contribution differentials based on other types of risks, i.e., smokers and nonsmokers or married and unmarried persons, which are supported by similar life expectancy studies; (3) the Water Department had funded its death benefit plan, to the disadvantage of women as a class, by equal contributions from male and female employees in light of the same actuarial information they used in computing pension plan contributions; and (4) because the Equal Pay Act which requires employers to pay equal wages for equal work defines fringe benefits as a form of compensation.

The Court did not reach the question of whether "defined contribution" plans or "money purchase" plans which are based on equal contributions and which provide actuarially equivalent or lower monthly benefits are violative of equal employment statutes. Under such plans, upon retirement the employee receives the present value of the expected pensions which is equal for both sexes with identical work histories. When converted into a plan paying monthly benefits, a woman receives lower payments because she is actuarially expected to live longer. The Court stated that any differential in benefits paid to men and women will be based on "actual life span" and not on generalizations about the sexes. If applied, the reasoning would appear to require employers to offer plans which provide equal benefits.

The Court was careful to clarify that its ruling applied to employers or their agents and not to the insurance industry itself, but the impact on insurance carriers cannot be ignored. The decision indicates the Court's construction of the statutes. It will have the effect of revising all types of fringe benefits which involve distinctions based on sex.

No doubt there will be more litigation in this area. The passage of the Employment Retirement Income Security Act and the *Manhart* decision have revolutionized the pension and life insurance areas. Many issues regarding the permissible structure of pension plans are in a state of flux. Because women as a group live longer than men, women workers should participate to the greatest extent possible in the resolutions of these issues.

REFERENCES

1. The Occupational Safety and Health Act of 1970, 29 United States Code 651, 1970.
2. Title VII of the Civil Rights Act of 1964, as amended, 42 United States Code, 2000e.
3. Executive Order 11246, as amended, 42 United States Code 2000e.
4. The Fair Labor Standards Act, 29 United States Code 201 *et seq.*, regulations found at 29 Code of Federal Regulations Chapter V.
5. The Equal Pay Act of 1963, 29 United States Code 206(d). Interpretative Bulletins found at 29 Code of Federal Regulations *et seq.*
6. Age Discrimination in Employment Act, 29 United States Code 621 *et seq.*, 1967.
7. The Toxic Substances Cotrol Act, 15 United States Code 2601 *et seq.*, 1976.
8. Employee Retirement Income Security Act, 29 United States Code 1001 *et seq.*, 1974.
9. *Commonwealth* v. *Hamilton Manufacturing Company*, 120 Mass. 383, 1876.
10. *Muller* v. *Oregon*, 208 U.S. 412, 1908.
11. *Adkins* v. *Children's Hospital of the District of Columbia*, 261 U.S. 525, 1923.
12. *U.S.* v. *Darby*, 312 U.S. 100, 1941.
13. *Heidler* v. *Industrial Commission*, 482 P.2d 889, Ariz. 1971; see also *Puffer Mercantile Co.* v. *Arellano*, 546 P.2d 481, Colo. 1975, rev'g 528 P.2d 966, 1974; cf. *Fort* v. *Hood's Dairy Inc.*, 143 So. 2d 13, Fla. 1962.
14. Toxic Substance Control Act, 15 United States Code 2601.
15. *Intermountain Block and Pipe Corporation*, OSHRC Docket No. 298, 10 S.H.C. 3145, 1972.
16. *Arkansas-Best Freight System, Inc.*, OSHRC Docket No. 2375, 2 OSHC 1620, aff'd sub nom, *Arkansas-Best Freight System, Inc.* v. *OSHRC and Secretary of Labor*, 529 F. 2nd 649, 8th Cir., 1976.
17. *Mandell, Corsini, Inc.*, OSHRC Docket No. 2856, 1 OSHC 3310, 1944.
18. *The Joseph Bucheit and Sons Co.*, OSHRC Dockett No. 295, 1 OSHRC 3106, 1972.
19. *Reedy Tank Erectors, Inc.*, OSHRC Docket No. 5574, 2 OSHC 3310, 1975.
20. *American Petroleum Institute* v. *OSHA*, 581 F. 2d 493, 501—505 (5th Cir. 1978) *Cert. granted*, 47 U.S.L.W. 3541 (Febuary 21, 1979); see *RMI* v. *Secretary of Labor*, et. al., 594 F.2d 566 (6th Cir. 1979); cf. *AISI* v. *OSH®C*, 577 f. 2d 825 (3rd Cir. 1978); *The Society of Plastics Industry, Inc.* v. *OSHA*, 509, f. 2d 1301, 1309, 2nd Cir., 1975; see also *American Federation of Labor* v. *Brennan*,
21. *Gardner* v. *National Airlines*, 14 FEP 1806, May 17, 1977 (S.D. Fla.). The court had reserved its decision on two other questions until the Supreme Court rules on *Satty* v. *Nashville Gas Co.* 434 U.S. 136 (1977). *Harris* v. *Pan American World Airways*, Civil Action No. C74-1884 W.W.S. (N.D. Calif.). The case has been tried and a decision has been rendered in favor of the employer. The case is expected to be appealed. *Mauzy* v. *Delta Airlines*, Civil Action No. 75-H-619 (S.D. Tex.). This case was recently reassigned. A trial has not been held on the case. *Burwell* v. *Eastern Airlines*, Civil Action No. 74-0418-R. This case was tried in May, 1976, before Judge Mehridge in Richmond. The record was reopened this summer. No decision has been issued. *MacClennan et al.* v. *American Airlines*, Civil Action No. 76-2296 (E.D. Va.). Decision rendered October 21, 1977, BNA Daily Labor Report No. 270, E-1, October 26, 1977. *Condit* v. *United Airlines*, 558 F.2d 1176, 4th Cir. 1977, *cert. denied*, 46 U.S.L.W. 5381, March 21, 1978.
22. *Condit* v. *United Airlines*, supra, 558 F.2d, 1176.
23. *Martinez* v. *University of California*, Docket No. RA77-284 of the State District Court of New Mexico. Decision issued April 5, 1978.
24. The Office of Federal Contract Compliance Programs which enforces Executive Order 11246, as amended; the Equal Employment Opportunity Commission which enforces Title VII of the Civil Rights Act; and, The Department of Health, Education and Welfare's Office of Civil Rights which enforces Title IX of the Education Amendments of 1972.

25. 40 Federal Register 45934, October 3, 1975.

26. 29 United States Code 654 (a), Occuaptional Safety and Health Act.

27. 29 United States Code 651 (6), Occupational Safety and Health Act.

28. 29 United States Code 651 (6) and (7), Occupational Safety and Health Act.

29. 29 United States Code 655 (a), Occupational Safety and Health Act.

30. 29 United States Code 655(a), Occupational Safety and Health Act.

31. See 29 United States Code 655 (6) and (7).

32. 29 United States Code 655 (5) and (6).

33. *Industrial Union Department, AFL-CIO* v. *Hodgson*, 499 F.2d 467, D.C. Cir. 1974.

34. 29 United States Code 654.

35. 116 Cong. Rec. 3877, 1970; see also *National Realty and Construction Co., Inc.* v. *OSHRC*, 498, F.2d 1257, D.C. Cir. 1973, and *Brennan* v. *Vylactos Laboratories, Inc.*, 494 F.2d 460, 8th Cir. 1974.

36. *Robinson* v. *Lorillard Corp.*, 444 F.2d 791, 798, 4th Cir. 1971, *cert. denied*, 404 U.S. 1006, 1971.

37. Commission Decisions 75-072 and 75-055, CCH Employment Practices Decisions   6442 and   6413.

38. *Washington* v. *Davis*, 426 U.S. 229, 1976.

39. 42 U.S.C. 2000 2-e(3); see also 29 Code of Federal Regulations 1604.2(a) of the EEOC "Guidelines on Sex Discrimination" for its interpretation of the meaning of 703(e).

40. *Weeks* v. *Southern Bell Telephone and Telegraph Co.*, 408 F.2d 228, 5th Cir. 1969; *Rosenfeld* v. *Southern Pacific Co.*, 444 F.2d 1219, 9th Cir. 1971.

 4. *Weeks* v. *Southern Bell Telephone and Telegraph Co.*, 408 F.2d 228, 5th Cir. 1969; *Rosenfeld* v. *Southern Pacific Co.*, 444 F.2d 1219, 9th Cir. 1971.

42. *Weeks, supra*, 408 F.2d at 236.

43. See also Justice Marshall's concurring opinion in *Phillips* v. *Martin Marietta Corp.*, 400 U.S. 542, 1971.

44. *Weeks, supra*, 408 F.2d at 236.

45. *Bowe* v. *Colgate Palmolive Co.*, 416 F.2d 711, 718, 7th Cir. 1969.

46. *Rosenfeld, supra*, 444 F.2d at 1229.

47. *General Electric* v. *Gilbert*, 429 U.S. 125, 135, 1976, citing *Geduldig* v. *Aeillo*, 417 U.S. 484, 496-497, 1974.

48. *City of Los Ageles, Department of Water and Power et al.* v. *Manhart et al.*, 98 S. Ct. 1370 (1778) decision issued April 25, 1978, 12.

49. *Manhart, supra*, 98 S. Ct. at 1379.

50. *Manhart, supra*, 98 S. Ct. at 1379 citing *Gilbert*, 429 U.S. at 135.

51. *Gilbert, supra*, 429 U.S. at 135.

52. *City of Los Angeles, Department of Water and Power* v. *Manhart, supra*, concurring opinion of Justice Blackmun, 98 S. Ct. at 1384.

53. 42 United States Code 2000.

54. Section 715 of the Civil Rights Act of 1964, as amended, 42 United States Code 2000 14-e.

55. "Guidelines on Sex Discrimination," 29 Code of Federal Regulations 1604.

56. 41 Code of Federal Regulations Chapter 60.

57. *Washington* v. *Davis, supra*, 426 U.S. at 238-239.

58. *Cleveland Board of Education* v. *LaFleur*, 414 U.S. 632, 1974 and *Chesterfield Board of Education* v. *Cohen*, 414 U.S. 632, 1974.

59. *LaFleur* and *Cohen, supra*, 414 U.S. at 643.

60. *LaFleur* and *Cohen, supra*, 414 U.S. at 644.

61. *LaFleur* and *Cohen, supra*, 414 U.S. at 645.

62. *LaFleur* and *Cohen, supra*, 414 U.S. at 647.

63. *Geduldig* v. *Aeillo, supra*. 417 U.S. 484, 1974.

64. *General Electric* v. *Gilbert*, 429 U.S. 125, 1976.

65. *Gilbert*, 429 U.S. at 136.

66. *Gilbert*, 429 U.S. at 136.

67. *Gilbert*, 429 U.S. at 138, citing *Aeillo, supra*, 417, U.S. at 496-497.

68. *Nashville Gas Co.* v. *Satty*, Docket No. 75-536, 46 U.S.L.W. 4026, decision issued December 6, 1977.

69. *Satty, supra*, 46 U.S.L.W. 4028.

70. *Manhart, supra*, 98 S. Ct. at 1382.

71. *Manhart, supra*, 98 S. Ct. at 1382.

72. S. 995 and H.R. 6075 passed as P.L. 95—552 (October 31, 1978).

73. 29 United States Code 206(d).

74. *Manhart, supra*, 98 S. Ct. at 1376.

Chapter 8

THE HISTORICAL EXPERIENCE*

I. INTRODUCTION

Lead, benzene, beryllium, and ionizing radiation are examples of potentially dangerous health hazards for workers who are exposed to them. They are suitable examples for a discussion of the history of protective/restrictive regulations in the context of exclusion of women from work settings where exposure is possible.

There is irony to this choice — a natural choice because each one has been under scrutiny in relation to effects on the reproductive system of workers in the mid-1970s. The irony stems from the history of women workers who have always worked in industries where exposure to these physical and chemical agents has been severe. Their illnesses and deaths have contributed the primary information to epidemiologists and clinicians for our understanding of human tolerance of toxic exposures.

Three occupational hazards became part of the industrial development of Europe in the 19th century — lead and benzene by mid-century, ionizing radiation following on its discovery by Marie Curie, and others at the end of the century. Beryllium came into use in the 20th century.

II. LEAD

The history of the use of lead is well known and has been described through the centuries.[1-3] The ill effects were well enough known to be part of the social commentary in the 19th century writings of Dickens, Hardy, and Shaw.[4-6] In 1869, Dickens described the working conditions in an East London lead mill and the women who worked there, and it must be one of the best analyses we have of the relationship between working conditions, employer responsibilities, and worker risks.[6]

"...She was going back (to the lead mill) to get 'took on.' What could she do? Better be ulcerated and paralyzed for eighteen pence a day, while it lasted, than see the children starve," wrote Dickens. He was mystified by the conflicting information that he saw and heard from management and workers. He hoped that the Americans would soon develop a new method that would eliminate the dangers. That hope was somewhat misplaced. By the turn of the century, first Germany, then other European countries and England had found the toll of disability and death from lead poisoning to be too high. Rigorous controls to improve unsanitary and dangerous work conditions were imposed with the result that poisoning cases in Germany, for example, were reduced from 21.2% of workers in 1897 to 9.6% in 1889, and to 0.97% in 1912. In contrast, the U.S. by 1912 still had the same prevalence as Europe of 15 years before, and the "lead poisoning evil" was a phrase commonly used in the writing of the time. Alice Hamilton in her autobiography recounted her embarrassment at the 4th International Congress on Occupational Accidents and Diseases in Brussels in 1910, when she could not respond to questions from the participants concerning the rate of lead poisoning by industry, the regulations, and compensation system in the U.S.[7] Finally, the chairman dismissed the subject. "It is well known that there is no industrial hygiene in the U.S. Ça n'existe pas." Alice Hamilton's efforts to improve conditions in the

* This chapter includes material published in *Feminist Studies*, Volume 5, 1979. With permission.

lead industry, virtually single-handedly, are now part of our history of occupational health.[8]

Her concern for women workers was a very pragmatic one. Protective legislation, given the dangerous working conditions at the time for all workers, was a means to slightly improve the miserable lot of women in the trades.[9,10] The exclusion of women and children from many lead industries was the current practice in Europe where the long experience of centuries had shown that lead adversely affected reproduction. We can view the European prohibition on women and children working with lead as a direct effort to reduce the most obvious (and controllable) impact on the next generation, particularly in Germany where social concern for the integrity of race was fully developed at the end of the 19th century. "Race poison" was a term later used by Alice Hamilton and her contemporaries. Abortions among women lead workers were obvious under the deadly working conditions which prevailed in Europe until almost the end of the century and much later in the U.S. The acceptance of obvious work-associated illness was part of the worker's economic burden, with few, if any, alternatives for avoiding chronic debility and, all too often, death. Hamilton reported further on the international scene in 1919, noting that legislation in Great Britain barred women from some of the most dangerous lead work.

On the other hand, the Germans believe that the apparently greater susceptibility of women to lead poisoning is to be explained not by their sex, but by the fact that they are usually more poverty stricken than the men, are undernourished and obliged to do work for their families in addition to their factory work. Then also, a woman's skirt and hair collect the lead dust, so that she carries it home with her after work. Observations in the pottery industry in this country seemed to bear out the German theory, for while a much larger proportion of women than of men were found suffering from lead poisoning in the East Liverpool and Trenton districts (New Jersey), it was also found that in these districts the men are members of a strong union, are well paid, and have good living conditions, while the women are unorganized, underpaid, poorly housed, poorly fed, and subject to the worry and strain of supporting dependents on low wages. In the organized pottery fields, in the tile works, and in the art potteries of the Zanesville district (Ohio), the men and women were in the same economic class, all making low wages, with everything which that implies, and here the rate of lead poisoning was slightly greater among the men... But the most disasterous effect that lead has upon women is the effect on the generative organs. Women who suffer from lead poisoning are more likely to be sterile or to have miscarriages and stillbirths than are women not exposed to lead. If they bear living children, these are more likely to die during the first year of life th⁻ are children of women who have never been exposed to lead. This means that lead is a race poison, ε   that lead poisoning in women affects not only one generation, but two generations. Reports of British factory inspectors for the year 1897 showed . . . out of 77 married women, 15 never became pregnant. Of the 62 who became pregnant, 15 never bore a living child. Among all the 62 there were 212 pregnancies, but these resulted in only 61 living children; the stillbirths numbered 21, the miscarriages 90, and of the 101 children born alive, 40 died soon after birth. . . . Another British report shows:

	Miscarriages and stillbirths
100 mothers in housework	43.2
100 mothers in millwork, not lead	47.6
100 mothers in lead work before marriage	86.0
100 mothers in lead work after marriage	133.5

. . . A report to the French Government in 1905 . . . that 608 out of 1,000 pregnancies in lead workers resulted in premature birth. In certain Hungarian villages, where pottery glazing has been a home industry for generations, children born of lead-poisoned parents are not only subject to convulsions, but, if they live, often have abnormally large square heads, and this condition is associated with a lowered mentality.[11]

The changes that occurred in some of the worst industries from about 1895 to 1905 in Europe and England and considerably later in the U.S. cannot be overemphasized.

In Europe, the illness and death resulting from hazardous working conditions became unacceptable much earlier than was the case in the U.S., no doubt related to the stronger public health movement which was already dealing with other adverse results of the industrial revolution.[12] Improved industrial hygiene controls rapidly reduced acute illness and death, though the work environment was still far from safe from today's perspective.

Working women were seen to be more than doubly vulnerable to their unsanitary and hazardous home and work environment when they bore children. Alice Hamilton's approach (in the first quarter of the 20th century) was appropriate for the U.S. when we consider the extreme jeopardy in which women were placed socially and medically during a time when the social legislation affecting maternal and infant health was in its early stages.[13]

The Berne Conventions of 1906, upon which the League of Nations reported in the Washington International Labour Conference in 1919, described the pattern of exclusion of women from unhealthy trades due to regulation of their employment. Absolute exclusion of women was the practice in 18 countries, where there was contact with lead, mercury, phosphorous, and arsenic. Both New Jersey and Pennsylvania prohibited women from handling certain forms of lead.[14]

Alice Hamilton reported in "Hygiene of the Printing Trades" that at the meeting of the International Association of Labor Legislation in Lugano in 1910 and at the following meeting in Zurich in 1912, the Italians testified that

for the good of the race women must be forbidden to work in the printing trades, since the danger of lead poisoning is too great and not only are women more susceptible, but the results are transmitted to their offspring. The Austrians agreed and passed regulations in Austria to that effect, although the Italians could provide no proof of injury to women employed in Italy since their number was too small to warrant any conclusions. The British, on the other hand, maintained that it was entirely possible to do away with the danger of lead poisoning in the printing trade and that efforts should be directed toward that rather than toward the shutting out of women from an industry in which they had long been employed and which was in many ways suited to their powers. The French and the American delegates stood with the British.

The typographical industry is not the only one in which efforts have been made to prohibit work by women on the ground of danger to health, but whenever, as is certainly true in printing, the dangers are all avoidable, the only logical and fair thing to do is to abolish these dangers . . . Whatever process in printing is dangerous for women has dangers for men also, and, as we have repeatedly shown, all these dangers can and should be prevented.[15]

The transition over more than a hundred years of industrialization has been from the social tolerance of life-threatening levels of lead, through an abatement of the worst conditions, to the concern that we have today that the worker's health and well-being should not be jeopardized in any way by toxic substances. The final stage is far from universally recognized or accepted. Otherwise, we would be seeing regulations for total protection by means of zero or no-effect exposure to hazardous conditions. Instead, society is still confronted with choices. Is the economic cost of an exposure to a lead level low enough to show no biological effect less tolerable than excluding "susceptible" groups and/or accepting a risk of biological damage to some people? Discussion surrounding the proposed lead standard during 1978 would seem to indicate that there will be acceptance of a risk of biological damage to some people as well as efforts to exclude some "susceptible" groups and that economic considerations are more likely to prevail.

"Increased susceptibility" is a specious concept in the context of control of population exposure to toxic substances. Alice Hamilton's clear statements in 1919[11] are a sound base for this view. Lead is a toxic substance, which adversely affects biological systems. No human being is immune to its toxic effects, nor is it possible to predict any individual's dose response characteristics. George Bernard Shaw knew that well enough in 1894 when one of his characters said of her sister "She worked in a whitelead factory. She only expected to get her hands a little paralyzed; but she died."[6] Dickens was equally astute in 1869 when his informant told him " . . . and some of them gets lead-poisoned soon, and some of them gets lead-poisoned later, and some, but not many, niver."[4]

III. BENZENE

There are many comparable characteristics to the lead experience when we consider exposure of workers to benzene. In addition, there are some interesting contrasts in terms of the attitude toward the danger of benzene to reproduction.

The toxicity of benzene, most particularly its effect on the bone marrow, became evident in Sweden soon after its introduction into the rubber industry with the invention of the pneumatic tire in 1888. Workers in the rubber industry, boot and shoe industry, artificial leather manufacture, photogravure color printing, manufacturing of paints and varnishes, and dry cleaning were exposed to benzene used as a solvent and diluent.[16] Four fatal cases of benzene poisoning among nine young women in an Uppsala tire factory were reported at the 12th International Congress of Medicine in Moscow in 1897 by Santesson. His classic report described the purpuric skin spots, bleeding from the nose, gingiva, and vagina, symptoms which were considered to be quite unusual.[17] In the U.S., Selling in 1919 reported three cases, two of them fatal, of chronic benzene poisoning in a Baltimore tin can plant. The victims were 14-year-old girls working with 11 others sealing tin can ends with rubber dissolved in benzene.[18] Into the 1920s many of the cases reported were of young women, usually 16 or less. Vaginal bleeding was noted in some cases in all of these studies as well as hemorrhagic complications during pregnancy.[19,20] The general opinion, which Alice Hamilton shared, was that young girls were markedly susceptible to chronic benzene poisoning, with a more likely progression to severe and often fatal complications when vaginal bleeding was present. It is difficult for today's epidemiologist to guess the demographic characteristics of the work settings described, but the impression is that women and particularly very young women, 16 years or less, were more likely to be working on those jobs with persistent exposure to benzene in a great variety of rubber and paint operations. European studies also continued to report frequent and excessive menstruation and severe deterioration during pregnancy in chronic poisoning.[21-23] However, Greenburg of the U.S. Public Health Service was in accord with the European view that the susceptibility of young women particularly was due to their inherent ill health and was associated with tuberculosis, chlorosis (anemia), and pregnancy.[21] Obesity was also frequently noted as a possible predisposing characteristic. Many men during these same years died suddenly from acute poisoning when exposed to storage containers, stills, and other similar conditions, and they also suffered severely from chronic poisoning. As more men came to be poisoned in printing and other industries, the obvious wide variation in susceptibility from one person to another clearly overrode any presumed sex difference, because fatal blood changes were frequently unpredictable.

The important aspect of benzene exposure for women is that when poisoning occurs in the chronic form, which may be insidious in its progression to severe anemia and hemorrhagia purpura, there is bleeding from the nose, gingiva, and vagina.

Selling had shown that the life-threatening blood changes included extreme reduction of granular leucocytes.[18] The observation lead to a fortunately short-lived use of benzene as a therapeutic drug for the treatment of leukemia administered by mouth in gelatin capsules in 3- to 5-g doses. The drastic therapy, which generally resulted in death from chronic benzene poisoning before the final stages of leukemia, was clearly associated with menorrhagia.

The most reasonable explanation for the earlier view of increased susceptibility for women was the preponderance of women in poor health in the low-paying jobs where the benzene exposure had been persistent. The fact that bleeding from the vagina in association with bleeding from the nose and gingiva was a prominent presenting feature in severe chronic poisoning provided a female characteristic for the disease — a characteristic which all too frequently portended death.

Since the turn of the century there has been a gradual reduction of the severe and often sudden onset of fatal acute and chronic benzene poisoning due to high exposures. By the 1920s workers were experiencing a slower more insidious chronic poisoning even though improved ventilation was being attempted. However, a sudden deterioration was still probable wih a fatal result when there was protracted chronic exposure.

The International Labour Office in 1919 had reported restrictions in many countries on work involving contact with poisons additional to those of prime concern, i.e., lead, mercury, phosphorus, and arsenic. Most restrictions in both groups of toxic substances referred to employment of young persons under 18. Some countries excluded women altogether from certain lead processes, but benzene was not being specified other than as one of the constituents of varnish, rubber, etc.[14]

Despite the extensive medical reports concerning women, there were few examples of exclusion of women from working with benzene (Argentina, France, and pregnant women in Norway) early in the century, in marked contrast to the lead restrictions. In a few countries, exclusion was directed to young workers or women up to 18 or 21 years (Greece, Germany, Spain, and Italy.) By the 1920s, benzene poisoning was compensable and reportable in 15 of the U.S., though frequently, only if thee work was directly with benzene. Exposure in the same room was not necessarily recognized as occupational exposure for worker's compensation purposes even when poisoning occurred, if benzene was not being used by the worker.[20]

Alice Hamilton raised the danger flag for benzene in 1922 claiming that benzene poisoning was a growing menace in American industry.[24] In 1918, Britain had substituted whenever possible, a safer compound, xylene. Hamilton's extensive experience during World War I in the aircraft factories had shown her the dangers of solvent exposure and her efforts then had been crucial in maintaining some levels of control of the air environment in varnishing and spraying operations. Postwar, the rubber tire industry was expanding as were the dry cleaning industry and a vast, mechanized canning industry. An impetus to Alice Hamilton's campaign was the study by Adelaide Ross-Smith, Medical Investigator of the Bureau of Women in Industry of the New York Department of Labor. "Chronic Benzol Poisoning among Women Industrial Workers" was published in 1927 following a survey of six factories.[20] Chronic poisoning in the form of demonstrable blood changes was found in 33% of the 79 women who worked in the factories manufacturing tires and rubber goods, cameras, shoes, and sanitary tin cans. Another 33% reported general symptoms probably caused by benzene, but they were not considered to be clinically poisoned. Menstrual changes were reported in only 10% of the women and menstrual problems did not appear as a serious symptom. However, one death was associated with premature birth of a child due to postpartum hemorrhage. Ross-Smith found no marked differences in susceptibility between young and old workers. Alice Hamilton later described these cases a "mild" benzene poisoning.[25]

By 1928 she wrote that American conditions had improved.[26] She had worked through the U.S. National Safety Council to persuade industry that ventilation adequate to keep benzene concentrations below 100 ppm was necessary. At the beginning of her campaign, some chemists believed that 5% benzene vapor in factory air would not be poisonous, that is 50,000 ppm. It is interesting to note that the preliminary questionnaire for the study by the National Safety Council, sent to 324 U.S. industrial establishments known to be using benzene in 1923, included among the six questions: Have you considered benzol poisoning as a cause of illness, absenteeism, or labor turnover among your employees on account of any special type of sickness, for example: (a) anemia, purpura, hemorrhages, gastrointestinal or nervous disturbances, neurasthenia, disturbances of menstrual function in women workers or (b) sudden cases of collapse, shock, cyanosis, or heart failure.

Nearly 50 years later in 1971 the ILO adopted Convention 136 concerning "Protection Against Hazards of Poisoning Arising from Benzene," with 339 countries voting in favor, 0 against, with 6 abstentions.[27] Article 11 reads in part: "1) women medically certified as pregnant, and nursing mothers, shall not be employed in work processes involving exposure to benzene or products containing benzene."

In light of this long international experience, a reading of the recently proposed benzene standard presents some surprises. The emergency standard for benzene in the U.S. was 1 ppm averaged over an 8 hr period, with a 5 ppm ceiling limit, and stemmed from the recent studies of rubber workers showing a seven-fold increase in the risk of developing leukemia for those exposed to benzene.[28] This was not an unexpected finding in that leukemia was reported in people exposed to benzene in Italy in 1938, and similar findings have been reported since in most industrial countries. Alice Hamilton was saying in 1929 and others have repeated it since, that zero exposure was the only safe exposure and that less harmful substitutes should be used. The usual features of acute and chronic poisoning are presented under Signs and Symptoms in the *Appendix on Medical Surveillance Guidelines for Benzene,* including bleeding from the nose, gums, or mucous membranes and development of purpuric spots, but the menstrual taboo is apparent. There is no mention of abnormal menstruation as a symptom. Pregnancy is not mentioned.

There may be more than one explanation for these omissions. The OSHA lead standard is expected to set the precedent for the consideration of pregnancy in relation to toxic effects of a hazardous substance and is yet to be legally tested. Even so, ignoring the clinical evidence for benzene effects on the reproductive system when renal, liver, skin, and blood changes are noted as predisposing cautionary conditions seems shortsighted.

The effects of lead and benzene on the female reproductive system are of comparable severity, although there are clinical differences in the symptoms experienced. The real differences stem from the perceptions of lead and benzene in relation to women in the workplace. There are few examples of efforts to exclude women from working with benzene throughout the same 90 years that protective legislation and/or practices excluded women from working with lead. There is no strong explanation for this inconsistency, but it appears that the worker, man or woman, was expendable. The children of workers were not, and it was not the children of lead workers who were obviously affected.

The noticeable gap in the clinical literature is any mention of the pregnancy outcome of benzene workers. Other than the few reported cases of maternal deaths associated with postpartum hemorrhage there is no information on reproduction of men or women, which is so much a feature of the discussions concerning lead. There appear to be no marked demographic differences between workers who were exposed to lead and benzene and yet there is no commentary at all in the literature on fertility, miscarriages and abortions or congenital malformations in the case of benzene. We could assume that no pathological problems occurred in relation to children born of benzene workers or that they were not observed. Alice Hamilton published a complete review of the European and American experience up to 1930 and did not mention reproductive effects, other than six reported maternal deaths in association with pregnancy of the 36 autopsies published up to that time. Hemorrhage in the ovaries was noted in three other cases at autopsy. Alice Hamilton was particularly interested in what she called "race poisons", a term used by her and others to particularly denote those toxic substances which also affected the next generation, so that she must not have recognized evidence of the effects of benzene on the conceptus or live-born children.[25]

IV. BERYLLIUM

The possibility that no adverse effects were observable in the fetus and the live-born child leads one to a reconsideration of the proposed beryllium standard,[29] where again the particular hazard for pregnant women is not mentioned. There is no evidence that beryllium affects the fetus or the live-born child, although the placenta does not provide a complete barrier. However, it is difficult to ignore Harriet Hardy's frequently reported observation that the Beryllium Registry formerly at the Massachusetts General Hospital shows that of the 96 women who died, 64 of them died from exacerbation of beryllium poisoning symptoms in association with pregnancy.[30] Although that experience in the 1950s was under conditions of exposure far more severe than are likely to occur today, the fact remains that a judgment was made that the effect of beryllium poisoning on the pregnant woman could be ignored, just as the benzene hazard to the pregnant woman has been forgotten, at least in the U.S. There is no mention of the clinical relationship in any obstetrics or toxicology textbook.

Is the hazard to the future generations the key consideration that makes the concern for lead exposure different? Is there a concern for the health of the pregnant worker herself?

These questions are pertinent from a historical perspective because it is evident from the review of a century's writing on lead and benzene and only 25 years on beryllium that the immediate issue of today's equal employment opportunity legislation is not a controlling factor in the long development of these attitudes. A review of policies developed for the control of ionizing radiation may throw some additional light on the idea.

V. IONIZING RADIATION

An evaluation of radiation exposure and protection in the occupational health setting provides a marked contrast with the lead and benzene experience. Indeed, it is difficult to identify an example comparable to ionizing radiation where the work practices and protective constraints have been so extensively analyzed and described. The contrast also strongly suggests that the philosophy of protection of workers from the vast range of industrial hazards is far from being a unitary concept.

A short summary of the history of the human experience with ionizing radiation is useful because in our generation the level of conscious concern has been higher and more sophisticated than for any other environmental hazard. (Tobacco smoking may be comparable.)

Marie Curie and her husband, Pierre discovered polonium and radium in 1898, for which they were awarded the Nobel Prize. X-rays had also been discovered and similarly recognized. There was an immediate development of new medical, scientific, and industrial uses with a proliferation of inventions using X-rays and radioisotopes in many parts of the world. Almost immediately adverse effects of X-rays on the health of physicists, chemists, and radiologists were recognized. For example, within 3 months of Roentgen's discovery of X-rays, Thomas Edison in the U.S. experienced conjunctivitis from X-ray exposure. More serious skin burns and ulceration became evident within a year and malignancies were being documented by 1911. The victims were research workers, radiologists, laboratory assistants, technicians, and nurses. By the time radiography was coming into industrial use, the need for protection by shielding and controlled exposure had been recognized. However, the protection itself was slow in coming and not universally used, even though the efficacy of lead shielding was known from before 1903. The disfigurement, chronic illness, severe anemias, and terminal cancers of health professionals and scientists were in marked contrast to the expectant public view that X-rays provided remarkable diagnoses and miraculous cures.[16]

The accumulated experience came into focus in the mid-1920s with the identification of necrosis of the jaw among workers using luminous paint in New Jersey. The dental profession, which had played an important role in controlling other occupational diseases with severe oral pathology through prophylactic and preventive dentistry, now found that more extensive medical care and hospitalization was necessary for "radium necrosis" as it came to be called. Dentists in New Jersey refused to extract teeth from radium dial painters because of the severe and possibly fatal sequelae. Several men who died had been chemists formulating the luminous paint, and they suffered from symptoms similar to chronic benzene poisoning, acute leukemia, and other acute blood dyscrasias. Bone cancer and leukemia appeared as later terminal illnesses among many of the young women who had been radium dial painters in their youth, licking the paint brushes to a fine point and ingesting radium.[31]

The Consumer's League of the Oranges aided the young women in bringing suits against the U.S. Radium Corporation when they had exhausted their families' financial resources for medical costs. The long litigation which ensued, in part related to the inadequacy of worker's compensation in New Jersey, made world-wide headlines.

There was a sudden revival of interest in the experience of the radium dial painters and chemists in the 1940s and early 1950s because of the development and use of nuclear weapons. Workers were being exposed to radioactive elements in a greater variety of occupations — uranium mining and milling, metal fabrication, laboratory extraction, etc. Although the diagnostic and therapeutic experience with external radiation in the form of X-rays was extensive, the only documented information on internally deposited radioactive substances concerned the radium dial painters and chemists. The relationship between the dose of radioactivity deposited in the body for a period of years and the biological effect were unknown.[32] The administrator of the Manhattan Project had a responsibility to ensure that there would not be an unacceptable level of adverse health effects on workers exposed to ionizing radiation so that estimates of "safe" radiation exposure levels had to be rapidly obtained. An initial review of the radium dial painters experience 25 years before provided the first evaluation, but it was obvious that more exact and detailed information would be needed as the nuclear industry moved beyond the immediate military demands. By 1955, radioactive fallout contaminated the whole world with the deposition of strontium-90 in the skeletons of every living person and there were demands for a more detailed understanding of the biological effects of internally deposited radioactive material. The deceased (by means of exhumed remains) and living radium dial painters have been and are still being intensively studied to establish the level of radioactivity associated with cancer and other changes in the skeleton and soft tissues.[33,34] These data have been, in part, used to establish maximum permissible standards for all workers exposed to radiation. However, it is difficult to understand why virtually no useful information has been reported on their reproductive experience. Belated attempts are now being made with the result that detailed accurate information on menstrual changes, fetal deaths, miscarriages, and congenital abnormalities is now virtually impossible to obtain. Similarly there is no reproductive information available for those working with external radiation — X-ray technicians, for example.

It is still difficult to explain the low level of concern for the reproductive experience of those in the health professions, other than in terms of consistent disregard for the health and safety of hospital employees in all areas, for example, infectious disease control and exposure to anesthetic gases. Diagnostic and therapeutic radiation procedures involving technicians, nurses, and radiologists have provided a probable risk for adverse pregnancy outcome at least comparable with that for lead exposure over the past 20 years. Survey programs of radiation monitoring, extended by extrapolation to the total population, have resulted in estimates of genetic dose to the U.S. population from medical X-rays, natural background radiation, and radioactive fallout to date. There is then a quantitative sense of the total radiation impact on the genetic pool, but no detailed epidemiologic studies of high risk groups, such as hospital workers, to provide detailed information.

Evaluation of reproductive effects relies heavily on laboratory animal experiments, the Hiroshima-Nagasaki victims, and clinical reports of patients undergoing therapeutic X-irradiation.[35]

VI. CONCLUSION

Lead has not been found to cause cancer in the human population. Fatalities from kidney failure and other lead-related causes are just as inevitable, but do not engender the same fear and public response that is seen when cancer is recognized. Cancer is the overriding health concern evident in our society today. Those chemical hazards which are associated with cancer produce a quality of fear which generates a consistent demand that workers should experience no exposure. Under such conditions the effects on the reproductive system are also controlled. Benzene falls in this category. However, there is the problem of dealing with accidental and unrecognized exposures. Symptoms of those excessively exposed will continue to lead us to identification of poor working conditions, for as long as industrial pollution is inadequately regulated. It is important then to prevent reproductive information from being ignored.

Our perception of the dose effect relationships differs in the examples I have discussed. For benzene and ionizing radiation, a high dose may be associated with a high probability of cancer and lower doses are assumed (on the basis of epidemiologic information) to only lower the probability of cancer and not necessarily eliminate the risk. This is a conservative view, which means that standards based on this philosophy assure maximum worker protection, i.e., minimum worker risk. In contrast, lower doses of lead reduce the severity of the poisoning without altering as markedly the probability of being affected. The reduction of severe effects is the aim of the proposed lead standard issued OSHA. The concept of "race poison" affecting all future generations has long been associated with lead, and yet historically we see a consistent view toward protecting the unborn by protecting the mother from exposure, but not the father. It appears today that this view has been more focused on the individual fetus but, its protection still demands, on the basis of a very conservative viewpoint, "control" of all women, which may mean nonemployment of women where they would be exposed to lead. The wider generalization to the good of future generations no longer appears to hold so strongly for lead, in contrast to the danger that was perceived in the 19th century potteries and white lead mills.

In the case of ionizing radiation the concern for future generations developed more recently in the context of war. Public attitudes were moulded by the use of atomic weapons, the politics of the cold war, and concern for the future of the human race on our planet. In addition, many radiation workers had considerable sophistication and understanding of the potential biological effects of radiation, both in terms of cancer and reproduction. The pressure for continued reevaluation of safe conditions for radiation exposure has therefore been stronger and a more complex view of risk benefit relationships has developed. In addition, more reliance was placed on theoretical extrapolations of the possible effects of low levels of ionizing radiation, a more straightforward procedure for most physical phenomena than is the case for chemical agents where assumptions concerning physiological and biochemical pathways are complex.

In conclusion, the philosophy of radiation protection (despite the deficiencies in details of implementation) can be viewed as a development of our modern history, with public scrutiny becoming more and more influential over the past 30 years.

Can we attribute the slow progress toward worker protection in industries with chemical exposures to attitudes and working practices developed in the industrial revolution? Is the more holistic view apparent for radiation exposure and, of recent origin, likely to lead to a more rational approach to the setting of standards for chemical contaminants and ensure the protection of all workers and their children?

Zero exposure conditions have been seriously proposed for carcinogenic substances. Reproductive hazards are then also eliminated. The central issue of hazard to the reproductive system remains, with its associated social complexity, when the worker is expected to tolerate subclinical changes in other body systems with little likelihood of fatal outcome. We know that each physical, chemical, or biological agent, if it affects the reproductive system, is likely to be unique in its action. The male or female reproductive system may be affected, or both. The effect on a subsequent pregnancy cannot be attributed solely to the woman's work experience. If the fetus itself is affected, it is unlikely to be affected by a level that has no biological effect at all on others in the workplace.

It is evident that no single pathway to the damaged child exists, although our industrial society has emphasized one only — the working pregnant woman. Her protection, historically, has been of concern only to a few. In contrast, the fetus has been considered in terms of the integrity of the country's race, so that protection from "race poisons" was necessary, in terms of the future of the world population and most recently as an individual adventitiously present in the workplace. The concept of the right to procreate healthy children has now been proposed by the Occupational Safety and Health Administration.

There is one striking example of international resolution of a severe chemical hazard. White (yellow) phosphorus is no longer a toxic substance of concern in the workplace. Its biological effect on workers in the match industry earlier in the century was so severe, with excruciating agony, deformity, and death, that international legislation and vigorous control measures were introduced. Despite intensive regulatory efforts, cases of phosphorus necrosis ("phossy jaw") continued to appear so that prohibition was seen as the only solution. The international treaty of Berne in 1906 prohibited the manufacture, importation, and sale of matches containing white (yellow) phosphorus, and by 1925 the International Labour Office could report that most nations of the world were signatories of the Berne convention. The U.S. Bureau of Labor had published a study "Phosphorus Poisoning in the Match Industry in the United States" in 1910 reporting on 15 of the 16 match factories in the U.S.[36] There were 3591 persons employed — 2024 men, 1253 women, and 314 children under 16 years of age (121 boys and 193 girls), with 65% of them working with direct exposure to phosphorus. However, 95% of the women and 83% of the children worked in phosphorus processes, i.e., most of the women and children were at high risk. Phosphorus necrosis which involved loss of large amounts of the bones of the jaw and face under conditions of extreme suffering, including intolerable smell to those around them, occurred in 150, 4 of whom died. The U.S., which did not belong to the ILO, passed the Esch-Hughes Act in 1912 imposing a tax of 2 cents per hundred on all white phosphorus matches manufactured after July, 1913 and also prohibiting the importation of such matches after that date and exportation after July 1, 1914. The Diamond Match Company, which held the patent for nonpoisonous (sesquisulphide of phosphorus) matches, allowed the use of the patent to the other match manufacturers. The generation of such vast international effort to control a toxic substance has not been matched since.

In the U.S. white phosphorus continued to be used in fireworks until 1926, when the Bureau of Labor Statistics reported further cases of phosphorus necrosis including six deaths. However, since that time the dangers seem to have been controlled.

It could be conjectured that the severity of the appearance of the victims in the case of the phosphorus workers and the radium dial painters was a factor in the control of the hazard. Historians of the period could no doubt offer other suggestions.

REFERENCES

1. Ramazzini, B., *Diseases of Workers*, (trans. from the Latin text by Wilmer Cave Wright, De Morbis Artificum of 1713), Hafner, New York, 1964.
2. Agricola, G., *De Re Metallica, 1556*,(trans. Hoover, H. C. and Hoover, L. H.), 1912.
3. Paracelsus, T., *Von der Bergsucht*, Bilingen, 1567.
4. Dickens, C., *The Uncommercial Traveller — All the Year Round*, New Series 1:13, 25, 1869.
5. Hardy, T., *Desperate Remedies*, 1871.
6. Shaw, G. B., *Mrs. Warren's Profession*, 1894.
7. Hamilton, A., *Exploring the Dangerous Trades*, Little, Brown, Boston, 1943.
8. Hamilton, A., Lead Poisoning in the Manufacture of Storage Batteries, Bull. No. 165, Bureau of Labor Statistics, U.S. Department of Labor, Washington, D.C., 1914.
9. Corn, J. K., Alice Hamilton, M.D., and women's welfare, *New Engl. J. Med.*, 294, 316, 1976.
10. Butler, E. B., *Women and the Trades, Pittsburgh 1907—8*, Russell Sage Foundation, 1911.
11. Hamilton, A., Women in the Lead Industries, Bull. No. 253, Bureau of Labor Statistics, U.S. Department of Labor, Washington, D.C., 1919.
12. Rozen, G., What is social medicine, in *From Medical Police to Social Medicine, Essays on the History of Health Care*, Science History Publication, New York, 1974, 60.
13. Lemmons, J. S., The Sheppard-Towner Act: progressiveness in the 1920's, *J. Am. Hist.*, 55, 776, 1969.
14. League of Nations, *Report on the Employment of Women and Children and the Berne Conventions of 1906*, Harrison and Sons, London, 1919.
15. Hamilton, A., Hygiene of the Printing Trades, Bulletin No. 209, Bureau of Labor Statistics, U.S. Department of Labor, Washington, D.C., 1917.
16. Hunter, D., *Diseases of Occupations*, 4th ed., Little, Brown, Boston, 1969.
17. Santesson, C. G., Ueber chronische Vergiftungen mit, Steinkolen-theerbenzin, Vier Todesfalle, *Arch. Hyg.*, 31, 336, 1897.
18. Selling, L., A preliminary report of some cases of purpura hemorrhagia due to benzol poisoning, *Johns Hopkins Hosp. Bull.*, 21, 33, 1910.
19. Hogan, J. F. and Schrader, J. H., Benzol poisoning, *Am. J. Public Health*, 13, 279, 1923.
20. Ross-Smith, A., Chronic Benzol Poisoning Among Women Industrial Workers, Special Bull. No. 150, New York State Department of Labor, 1927.
21. U.S. Public Health Service, Benzol poisoning as an industrial hazard, *Public Health Rep.*, 41, 1410, 1926.

22. **Meda, G.,** Il benzolismo professionale, Il Lavoro, 13, 264.

23. **Brücken,** Ueber Chronische Benzolvergiftung, *Dsch. Med. Wochenschr.,* 49, 1120, 1923.

24. **Hamilton, A.,** The growing menace of benzene (benzol) poisoning in American industry, JAMA, 78, 627, 1922.

25. **Hamilton, A.,** Benzene (benzol) poisoning, *Arch. Pathol.,* 11, 434, 1931.

26. **Hamilton, A.,** Lessening menace of benzol poisoning in American industry, *J. Ind. Hyg.,* 10, 227, 1928.

27. International Labour Office, Protection Against Hazards of Poisoning Arising from Benzene, 54, 246, 1971.

28. Fed. Reg., May 3, 1977.

29. U.S. Department of Labor, Occupational Safety and Health Administration, Proposed standard for occupational exposure to beryllium, *Occup. Safety Health Rep.,* 5, 811, 1975.

30. **Hardy, H.,** Beryllium poisoning — lessons in control of man-made disease, *New Engl. J. Med.,* 273, 119, 1965.

31. U.S. Department of Labor, Radium poisoning. Industrial poisoning from radioactive substances, *Monthly Labor Review,* 28, 1200, 1929.

32. **Evans, R.,** Protection of radium dial workers and radiologists from injury by radium, *J. Ind. Hyg. Toxicol.,* 25, 253, 1943.

33. **Maletskos, C. J., Braun, A. G., Shanahan, M. M., and Evans, R. D.,** Quantitative Evaluation of Dose-Response Relationships in Human Beings with Skeletal Burdens of Radium 226 and Radium 228, in *Assessment of Radioactivity in Man,* Vol. 2, International Atomic Energy Agency, Vienna, 1964.

34. **Polednak, A. P.,** Long term effects of radium exposure in female dial workers, *Environ. Res., 13* (237), 396, 1977.

35. Ionizing Radiation: Levels and Effects. A Report of the United Nations Scientific Committee on the Effects of Atomic Radiation (UNSCEAR Report), Vol. 2, United Nations, 1972.

36. Phosphorus Poisoning, Bull. No. 86, Bureau of Labor Statistics, U.S. Department of Labor, Washington, D.C., 1910.

37. Phosphorus Necrosis in the Manufacture of Fireworks and in the Preparation of Phosphorus, Bull. No. 405, Bureau of Labor Statistics, U.S. Department of Labor, Washington, D.C., 1926.

Chapter 9

THE FUTURE

I. PSYCHOGENIC ILLNESS

The information in foregoing chapters makes only passing reference to those conditions which are associated with behavioral, psychological, and emotional stress. As research in behavorial toxicology and industrial psychology expands into a more direct application to women and their working conditions, the linkage between physiological and biochemical effects and the currently subjective measures of job dissatisfaction and stress should become clearer. Smith et al. have recently reported three incidents of industrial mass psychogenic illness in which the majority of workers affected were women.[1] The locations were an electronics assembly plant, an aluminum furniture assembly plant, and a frozen fish packing plant. Symptoms included headaches, dizziness, light-headedness, weakness, sleepiness, nausea, bad taste and dry mouths, and breathing difficulties — all symptoms which may be associated with exposure to toxic substances. The analyses of data from biomedical examinations and sociodemographic and behavioral interviews lead to a conclusion that all three episodes had similarities which appeared to indicate mass psychogenic illness for each. The male workers in a predominantly female work force were also experiencing physical and psychological job stress and concomitant physical strain. Colligan and Smith in commenting on the methodological approach needed for evaluating outbreaks of mass psychogenic illness in industry stated that such outbreaks have rarely been reported in the scientific literature in the U.S. although their occurrence is not uncommon.[2] The responsibility of state and federal health agencies is to ensure that a toxic environment is not causing the symptoms but following that "the whole episode thus ends as abruptly and mysteriously as it began and the final report is unceremoniously buried in the agency files." The fact that men have also been affected in these episodes, although they have been the minority employees in the episodes examined, indicates that they are not immune. We can also conjecture that comparable episodes of severe stress do occur in male intensive occupations, e.g., military service and upper management. Psychogenic illness with symptoms more compatible with the social expectations for male behavior occurs. The stresses may act more intensely on susceptible workers who then respond in their own particular way. The higher suicide and accident rates observed in many occupational cohort studies of male workers could in part be explained by such responses. Outbreaks of violence and aggression have always been part of the male work environment and viewed as a traditional social pattern of behavior in response to stress.

The National Institute for Occupational Safety and Health now has a Behavioral and Motivational Factors Branch so that there will possibly be more frequent recognition of the effects of stressful conditions and toxic contaminants on the work tolerance of women and men. It may also be observed that there is a sex difference in the responses to unsatisfactory work environments.

II. EFFECT OF CIGARETTE SMOKING

The impact of increased cigarette smoking among young women is an additional factor that must be taken into account in our belated attempts to describe the occupational health of women workers. The National Center for Health Statistics has exam-

TABLE 1

25 Detailed Occupation Categories for White Females with Lowest Percent Smoking Only Cigarettes —
1970

	Percent current smokers	Percent smoking a pack or more	Percent started younger than 20
Accountants and auditors	30.83	67.57	45.95
Bus drivers	29.03	66.67	44.44
Charwomen and cleaners	28.57	58.33	41.67
Janitors and sextons	28.57	50.00	57.14
Private household workers (not elsewhere classified)	28.50	52.73	43.64
Stenographers	28.36	63.16	63.16
Housewives, retired and unemployed	28.30	54.71	53.33
Nongroup social, welfare workers	27.27	83.33	61.11
File clerks	27.16	36.36	77.27
Service workers public (not elsewhere classified)	26.67	25.00	12.50
Teachers (not elsewhere classified)	26.19	50.00	50.00
Counter/fountain workers	25.51	36.00	52.00
Sewers, stitching, manufacturing	25.61	50.43	48.70
Payroll and timekeeping clerks	24.44	63.64	36.36
Teachers secondary school	24.02	36.07	54.10
Technicians, medical and dental	23.58	36.00	44.00
Attendants, assistants, library	23.26	20.00	40.00
Attendants professional/personal service	22.41	46.15	53.85
Musicians, music teachers	21.33	31.25	18.75
Babysitters, private household	21.33	55.56	51.11
Dressmakers, seamstress not factories	20.25	56.25	56.25
Therapists, healers (not elsewhere classified)	20.00	66.67	66.67
Farmers (owners and tenant)	20.00	50.00	33.33
Teachers elementary school	19.38	36.13	46.22
Librarians	16.39	40.00	40.00

ined smoking habits in a probability sample of 75,827 American white women and men from the 1970 Household Interview Survey.[3] The prevalence of smoking among employed white women was approaching that for males in many occupations and was lowest among professionals, managers, and proprietors (Tables 1 and 2). Overall the prevalence of cigarette smoking among women in 1970 had remained relatively constant since the estimates of the mid-fifties when 67.5% of women were nonsmokers. However, a detailed analysis by occupation showed a marked variability for the 25 detailed occupations with the highest percentage of cigarette smoking and the 25 occupations with the lowest percentage of cigarette smoking. For 42 out of the total 70 occupations (60%) the smoking prevalence was 30% or greater, which was similar to the prevalence seen among men in similar occupations. However, the number of cigarettes smoked was less among women. The effects of the remarkable increase in smoking among adolescent girls during the mid-seventies along with the extensive cigarette advertising in women's magazines and support of women's sports events by the tobacco industry will become slowly apparent over the next 10 to 15 years. High-risk occupations[4] which in 1970 showed high smoking prevalence were hairdressers and cosmetologists (44.6%), assemblers (43.6%), nurses (38.4%), laundry and dry cleaning operatives (38.3%), and packers and wrappers (37.4%), whereas some low-risk occupations such as elementary schoolteachers and librarians had smoking prevalences of 19.4 and 16.4%, respectively. Most epidemiologic studies of women workers have not yet been able to take smoking into account.

TABLE 2

25 Detailed Occupation Categories for White Females with Highest Percent Smoking Only Cigarettes —
1970

	Percent current smokers	Percent smoking a pack or more	Percent started younger than 20
Waiters and waitresses	49.65	62.63	62.99
Buyers, department heads, store	46.48	48.48	42.42
Shipping and receiving clerks	48.48	75.00	68.75
Real estate agents, brokers	44.83	73.08	38.46
Hairdressers/cosmetologists	44.57	55.65	61.74
Professional, technical, kindred workers	43.97	58.82	66.67
Foremen (not elsewhere classified)	43.75	64.29	39.29
Assemblers	43.62	62.26	52.83
Managers, officials, props (not elsewhere classified)	41.76	61.27	43.66
Hucksters and peddlers	40.40	62.50	55.00
Technical, other engineers, physical sciences	40.00	66.67	66.67
Agents (not elsewhere classified)	41.86	72.22	61.11
Editors and reporters	41.94	53.85	61.54
Bookkeepers	38.63	63.55	56.19
Nurses, professional	38.42	50.68	43.84
Laundry, drycleaning, operatives	38.32	56.10	60.98
Operatives, kindred (not elsewhere classified)	38.51	52.27	53.69
Secretaries	37.79	55.83	57.09
Packers, wrappers (not elsewhere classified)	37.44	55.70	56.96
Telephone operators	37.43	47.76	53.73
Checkers, examiners, inspectors, manufacturing	37.34	55.93	55.93
Office machine operators	36.49	55.56	65.43
Attendants, hospital, other institutions	36.45	54.55	57.02
Cashiers	36.08	55.56	58.17
Personnel, labor-related workers	35.71	40.00	53.33

The additional confounding factor for women is the use of oral contraceptives. Interactive effects between smoking and oral contraceptive use are now being detected epidemiologically so that it seems unlikely that all other toxic contaminants would act independently of altered endocrine conditions.[5]

Epidemiologically the complications of a gradual increase in smoking, the introduction of oral contraceptives, the choice not to bear children, and entry into new occupations before the long experience in the old has been fully evaluated place on today's investigator an awesome task, whether the outcome under examination is restricted to women workers or to their reproductive experience.

III. MORTALITY SEX RATIO

Andjelkovich et al. have raised a series of critical issues in the analysis of cohorts of female working populations.[6] A study similar to that of Monson and Nakano of female rubber workers confirmed the excess of lung, uterus, bladder, and lymphatic cancer and myeloma and a significant deficit for breast cancer.[7] Although Andjelkovich's sample was smaller, 1649 women, it was not diluted by salaried and hourly employees with no industrial exposure. The central problem in the study of occupational health experience of women workers is the "virtual nonexistence of mortality data for females in other industries," a general problem also identified for the study of reproductive effects. Andjelkovich et al. and Waldron have all conjectured on the potential influence of hazardous occupations on women workers.[6,8] The former concluded that the advantageous sex difference in mortality for women may be moderated by the change to more hazardous occupations. Waldron examined the factors contributing to the 60% higher mortality of U.S. men when compared with women and identified them as higher rates of suicide, fatal motor vehicle and other accidents, cirrhosis of the liver, respiratory cancers, and emphysema, all of which are related to behaviors which are encouraged or accepted more in males. If as she suggests cigarette smoking contributes more than one third of the sex differential in adult mortality, increased smoking by women in addition to any other behavior components that could affect female accident rates would make the death rate in women more comparable to that in men. There is as yet little firm data to indicate any marked change in the advantageous mortality sex ratio for women and discussion of the possibilities for the future and causes for the past can become convoluted.

The central question is whether some segments of the working population are more or less susceptible to the variety of stresses which are characteristic for most occupations. So far there are no epidemiologic data which provide any indication that women are more prone than men to the adverse effects of any working conditions. Epidemiological studies (should they be done in the future) may show a heterogeneous response from one occupation to another, but in the meantime the marked differential in the death rates of men and women should be evidence enough that the vulnerable half of the country's population is not now being adequately protected from fatal influences.

IV. REPRODUCTION

Women tend to marry men older than themselves despite all the obvious long-term social disadvantages. There is evidence that older paternal age is a factor in sporadic fresh mutational cases of autosomal dominant and X-linked recessive disorders.[9] Jones et al. state, "The precise reason for the older paternal age factor in fresh gene mutation is unknown." Estimates of the likelihood of mutation leading to sporadic cases of achondroplasia, fibrodysplasia ossificans progressiva, the Apert syndrome, and hemophilia A are tenfold from the third to the sixth decade of life. However, older maternal age is associated with gross chromosomal aneuploidy, a more frequent cause of congenital abnormalities of known genetic origin. At least 60% of congenital abnormalities are of unknown origin. The larger and more intensive occupational exposure of men has not yet been examined in relation to adverse reproductive outcome of unknown etiology.

The more sensitive approach developed by Stein et al. is the examination of spontaneous abortions for anomalies.[10] Strobino et al. have suggested the use of their method for systematic epidemiologic study extending across maternal and paternal occupational exposures and across pregnancy outcomes.[11] They note that although the nonsystematic, empirical approach to environmental hazards has been useful in the past, reliable observations have resulted only where there are large populations available, enormous odds ratios, or extraordinary effects. In contrast, monitoring for mutagenic and teratogenic substances by routine investigation of the incidence of defects among spontaneous abortions is far more practical and efficient. It seems possible with the development of routine use of occupational history questionnaires which include questions appropriate for reproductive studies that the three categories of parental exposure, maternal exposure during pregnancy, maternal and paternal exposure before conception could be more adequately examined. When the full range of reproductive outcomes is considered (infertility, spontaneous abortions, low birthweight, late fetal deaths and neonatal deaths, morphologic abnormalities and chromosome anomalies, developmental disabilities including physical and mental abnormalities) it is evident that more sensitive, short-term statistically rigorous approaches are needed. Stein et al. have shown that chromosome studies of aborted fetuses provide such economy because of the high concentration of anomalies among spontaneous abortions.[10] They have also established a set of relationships between incidence of anomalies, fetal loss, and birth defects among recognized pregnancies, which should markedly improve the evaluation of associations between occupational exposures and adverse pregnancy outcome.

The most critical gap in our understanding of human reproduction is the influence of adverse work conditions. The evidence of the adverse effects of lead, pesticides, ionizing radiation, and microwaves on the reproductive experience of men and women should be enough to direct epidemiologic curiosity in some new directions. Yet there are in all probability many work conditions where reproductive hazards are very low. At present, it is difficult to assess risk for reproductive effect at all.

V. PREGNANCY AND WORK

British interest in the social factors affecting pregnancy outcome has lead to a more extensive literature concerned with working women over a long period of time than we have seen in the U.S.[12-17] Illsley concluded from the experience in Britain that, "The hypothesis that excessive maternal activity — particularly heavy and prolonged manual work — may adversely affect the course of pregnancy has had a long and persistent history. Although no systematic evidence is available in relation to pre-eclampsia and perinatal death, the association between work and low birth weight undoubtedly exists."[18]

Douglas had corrected the earlier calculation error in the Committee Report of the Royal College of Obstetricians and Gynecologists and showed virtually no relationship between prematurity and work and Drillien had found no relationship in Glasgow.[12,13,16] Stewart found that babies born to women gainfully employed outside their home had lower birth weights than babies born to full-time housewives.[17] However, there were inconsistencies in the matched populations of housewives and her conclusion could not be considered to be strongly based. Illsley noted that negative findings in developed countries did not necessarily indicate that work is irrelevant to pregnancy outcome in other cultures.[18] In those countries where a labor intensive economy still holds it may be more difficult to evaluate the effect of physical activity even though the adverse conditions may provide a more extreme effect on reproduction. The transfer of hazardous factories from those countries with strong regulatory control of occupational hazards and the introduction of women of childbearing age into employment to reduce population growth are two external economic forces which are having a direct effect on the physical and chemical environment of women in developing countries today.

Kavoussi in his analysis of workers in the textile industry in Iran particularly points to the problems of data collection and analysis in reproductive studies, even in a country with low worker turnover, long employment from adolescence, and very few induced abortions.[19] A comparison was made between 272 working women and 217 nonworking wives. A rate of assumed spontaneous abortion was found to be 12% of pregnancies for workers over 40 vs. only 8% of the pregnancies of nonworking wives over 40, a statistically significant difference. The more comparable experience for those under 40 may be in part a reflection of the improved living conditions and medical care in Iran for the younger mothers. There is also a problem of differential recall by age for questions concerned with previous pregnancies, particularly where the average number of pregnancies was high — over seven per woman in this study. Indeed, a firm conclusion cannot be reached from the data provided.

In the U.S. the relationship between occupational exposure to an adverse physical, chemical, or biological environment and reproductive outcome has only recently been acknowledged. The available data for examining the relationship are sparse. The National Survey of Family Growth found that in a 12 month period (1972 to 1973) about 1,260,000 women worked during pregnancy, about 9% of the female labor force of reproductive age.[20] The work participation of the pregnant population was comparable to that of other women, about 42%. In addition, the percentage working in the last trimester of pregnancy (48%) was comparable to that 10 years earlier.[21] The latest report of the Bureau of Labor Statistics shows that 46.4 million women aged 16 and over were employed at some time during the year 1977, a number that is in excess of the total population of many countries where studies of women workers has been considered to be practicable.[22] Well over a million American women workers became pregnant, about 2%. However, about 4% of working men fathered children that year, based on a work force made up of 81% of the men of working age in the country, 61 million workers.

VI. CHILD LABOR

The underlying assumption in discussions concerning workers in the U.S. is that they are at least 16 years of age. However, for employment in agriculture the Fair Labor Standards Act, Section 12 allows workers to be 14 and 15 years of age outside school hours except in occupations found and declared by the Secretary of Labor to be particularly hazardous for the employment of minors under 16 years of age, workers of 12 and 13 years of age in nonhazardous occupations outside school hours, and workers 10 and 11 years of age in nonhazardous occupations outside of school hours employed to hand-harvest short season crops for 8 hr a day, 40 hr a week. Department of Labor proposed rules governing the procedures for obtaining permission to use 10- and 11-year-old workers were published in the Federal Register on April 4, 1978 and included a description of supporting data needed for such an application, e.g., that the level and type of pesticides and other chemicals used would not have an adverse effect on the health and well-being of minors.[23] It is impossible to make such an evaluation on the basis of current biological information of the effects of toxic substances on prepubescent children. The period of rapid growth for the ovaries and uterus occurs from 9 to 13 years, with a doubling of the weight of the ovaries and more than trebling of the uterus weight.[24,25] Widholm et al. have shown that a girl's sexual and endocrine development begins before she reaches a bone age of 8 years.[26] They measured urinary excretion of estrogen, follicle stimulating hormone (FSH), luteinizing hormone (LH), and serum levels of progesterone in 148 school girls and student nurses ranging in age from 7 to 20 years. There were 80 premenarcheal and 68 menstruating girls and women. The very detailed study of growth and development in adolescent girls showed that puberty is not a sudden event in physiological and biochemical terms. Instead, sexual maturity takes place as a moderate, almost linear increase of both gonadotropins and steroids starting before the age of 8 years with steady hormone levels remaining constant for 1 or 2 years following menarche. Endocrine changes leading to sexual maturity and cyclic interaction between the central nervous system and the ovaries are virtually unknown, but it can be assumed that introduction of toxic contaminants into the prepubertal and adolescent environment is undesirable if there is any chance that they may interfere with the endocrine system. For male development at comparable ages there is progressive maturation of the testes under the influence of gradually rising levels of pituitary gonadotropin.[25] The normal low levels of FSH and LH begin to rise slowly at about 6 years of age as the rate of testes growth begins to increase. Seminiferous tubules develop and gonocytes begin to proliferate. Enlargement of the genitalia begins between 9.5 and 13.5 years of age and is complete in 95% of males between 13 and 17 years of age.

The adequacy of pesticide control measures for protection of young farm workers can be questioned when reentry standards have been set only with adult males in mind. In the U.S., migrant families harvest many crops and tenant farm families grow and harvest cotton and tobacco with inadequate education and surveillance for safe working practices. Exposure of young workers at a critical period of reproductive development in developing countries without child labor laws must be given more serious attention.

VII. CAUSE AND EFFECT

Kasl has devised a scheme which very well applies to both the residential and occupational world most people inhabit throughout their lives.[27] Epidemiologists are frequently confronted with the statement "there is no evidence" to support or refute a suspected relationship between an occupational hazard and an adverse health effect. Kasl uses a series of descriptors which could well be applied to many of the examples used in the foregoing chapters:

The matter has not yet been adequately studied.
Only poor studies have examined the matter and the results cannot be trusted.
The results of various studies are all over the place and in effect cancel each other out.
The association can be trusted, but a causal interpretation is unclear.
A causal relation exists but it is powerfully mediated or influenced by social, psychological or individual difference variables.
Good studies agree that no association exists.

There are good studies of women workers on the way which will show "no evidence". Unfortunately, many others of them will.

REFERENCES

1. Smith, M. J., Colligan, M. J., and Hurrell, J. J., Three incidents of industrial mass psychogenic illness, *J. Occup. Med.*, 20, 399, 1978.
2. Colligan, M. J. and Smith, M. J., A methodological approach for evaluating outbreaks of mass psychogenic illness in industry, *J. Occup. Med.*, 20, 401, 1978.
3. Sterling, T. D. and Weinkam, J. J., Smoking characteristics by type of employment, *J. Occup. Med.*, 18, 743, 1976.
4. De Coufle, P., Stanislawczyk, K., Houten, L., Bross, I. D. J., and Viadana, E., A Retrospective Survey of Cancer in Relation to Occupation, No. 77—178, National Institute for Occupational Health and Safety, U.S. Department of Health, Education and Welfare, Washington, D.C., 1977.
5. Mann, J. I., Doll, R., Thorogood, M., Vessey, M. P., and Waters, W. E., Risk factors for myocardial infarction in young women, *Br. J. Prev. Soc. Med.*, 30, 94, 1976.
6. Andjelkovich, D., Taulbee, J., and Blum, S., Mortality of female workers in a rubber manufacturing plant, *J. Occup. Med.*, 20, 409, 1978.
7. Monson, R. R. and Nakanno, K. K., Mortality among rubber workers. II. Other employees, *Am. J. Epidemiol.*, 103, 297, 1976.
8. Waldron, I., Why do women live longer than men?, *Soc. Sci. Med.*, 10, 349, 1976.
9. Jones, K. L., Smith, D. W., Harvey, M. A. S., Hall, B. D., and Quan, L., Older paternal age and fresh gene mutation. Data on additional disorders, *J. Pediatr.*, 86, 84, 1975.

10. **Stein, Z., Susser, M., Warburton, D., Wittes, J., and Kline, J.,** Spontaneous abortion as a screening device, *Am. J. Epidemiol.,* 102, 275, 1975.
11. **Strobino, B. R., Kline, J., and Stein, Z.,** Chemical and physical exposures of parents: effects on human reproduction and offspring, *Early Hum. Dev.,* 1, 371, 1978.
12. Royal College of Obstetricians and Gynecologists and Population Investigation Committee, *Maternity in Great Britain,* Oxford University Press, London, 1948.
13. **Douglas, J. W. B.,** Some factors associated with prematurity, *J. Obstet. Gynaecol. Br. Emp.,* 57, 143, 1950.
14. **Ferguson, T. and Logan, J. C.,** Mothers employed out of home, *Glasgow Med. J.,* 34, 221, 1953.
15. **Illsley, R., Billewicz, W. Z., and Thomson, A. M.,** Prematurity and paid work during pregnancy, *Br. J. Prev. Soc. Med.,* 8, 153, 1954.
16. **Drillian, C. M.,** The social and economic factors affecting the incidence of premature birth, *J. Obstet. Gynaecol. Br. Emp.,* 64, 161, 1957.
17. **Stewart, A. M.,** A note on the obstetric effects of work during pregnancy, *Br. J. Prev. Soc. Med.,* 9, 159, 1955.
18. **Illsley, R.,** The sociological study of reproduction and its outcome, in *Childbearing — Its Social and Psychological Aspects,* Richardson, S. A. and Guttmacher, A. F., Eds., Williams & Wilkins, Baltimore, 1973, 75.
19. **Kavoussi, N.,** The effect of industrialization on spontaneous abortion in Iran, *J. Occup. Med.,* 19, 419, 1977.
20. **Hendershot, G. E.,** Pregnant Workers in the United States, Advance Data from Bureau of Vital and Health Statistics, No. 11, National Center for Health Statistics, U.S. Department of Health, Education and Welfare, Washington, D.C., 1978.
21. Employment During Pregnancy, Ser. 22, No. 7, National Center for Health Statistics, U.S. Department of Health, Education and Welfare, Washington, D.C., 1968.
22. Patterns of Employment before and after Childbirth, Vital and Health Statistics Series 23, National Center for Health Statistics, U.S. Department of Health, Education and Welfare, Washington, D.C., 1978.
23. U.S. Department of Labor, Wage and Hourly Division, Waiver of child labor provisions for agricultural employment of 10 and 11 year old minors in hand-harvesting of short season crops, *Fed. Reg.,* 43, 14068, 1978.
24. **Ross, G. T. and Vande Wiele, R. L.,** The ovaries, in *Textbook of Endocrinology,* 5th ed., Williams, R. H., Ed., W. B. Saunders, Philadelphia, 1974, 372.
25. **Paulsen, G. A.,** The testes, in *Textbook of Endocrinology,* 5th ed., Williams, R. H., Ed., W. B. Saunders, Philadelphia, 1974, 323.
26. **Widholm, O., Kantero, R. L., Axelson, E., Johansson, E. D. B., and Wide, L.,** Endocrine changes before and after the menarche, *Acta Obstet. Gynec. Scand.,* 53, 197, 1974.
27. **Kasl, V.,** The effects of the residential environment on health and behavior, a review, in The Effect of the Man-made Environment on Health and Behavior, No. 77—8318, Hinkle, L. E. and Loring, W. C., Eds., Center for Disease Control, U.S. Department of Health, Education and Welfare, Washington, D.C., 1977.

INDEX

A

D

N

O